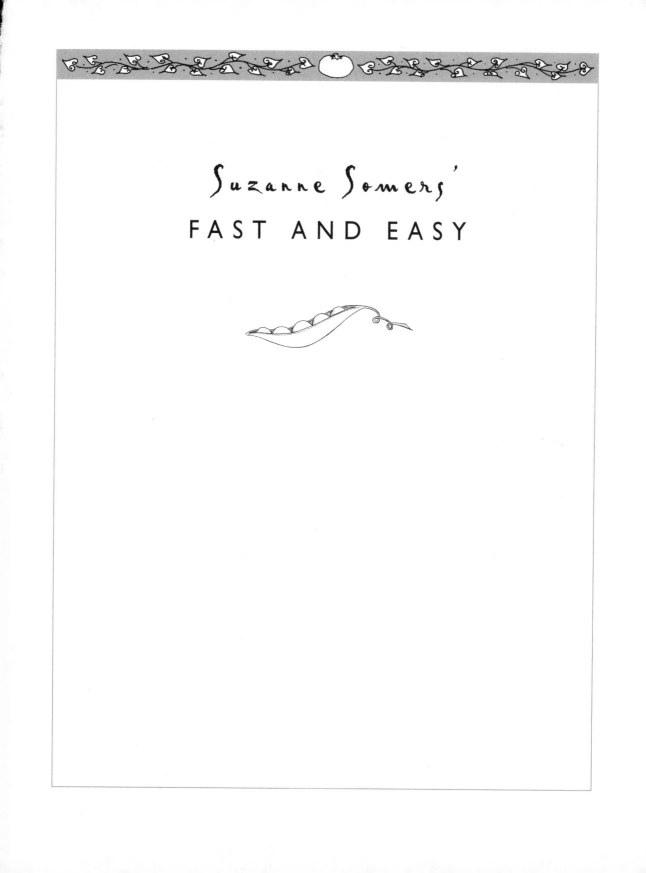

Suzanne Somers'
FAST AND EASY

Suzanne Somers'
FAST AND EASY

Lose Weight the Somersize Way with Quick,

Delicious Meals for the Entire Family!

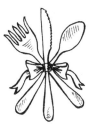

BY SUZANNE SOMERS

Illustrations by Leslie Hamel

Foreword by Michael Galitzer, M.D.

CROWN PUBLISHERS • NEW YORK

Author's Note: This book proposes dietary recommendations for the reader to follow. However, before starting this or any other diet regimen, you should consult your physician.

Published by Crown Publishers, New York, New York.

Member of the Crown Publishing Group, a division of Random House, Inc.

www.randomhouse.com

CROWN is a trademark and the Crown colophon is a registered trademark of Random House, Inc.

Printed in the United States of America

Design by Debbie Glasserman and Lauren Dong

Library of Congress Cataloging-in-Publication Data
Somers, Suzanne
Suzanne Somers' fast and easy : lose weight the Somersize way with quick, delicious meals for the entire family! / by Suzanne Somers ; illustrations by Leslie Hamel ; foreword by Michael Galitzer
p. cm.
Includes bibliographical references and index.
1. Reducing diets. 2. Food combining. 3. Quick and easy cookery.
4. Carbohydrates, Refined—Physiological effect. I. Title.
RM222.2.S6556 2002
613.2'5—dc21 2002006887

ISBN: 1-4000-4643-2

10 9 8 7 6 5 4 3 2 1

First Edition

To all those who suffered as a result of September 11, 2001.

My thoughts and prayers are with you.

Acknowledgments

Once again it is my pleasure to thank all those who helped me put this book together.

My agent, Al Lowman, is the backbone of this entire series of books. He is like no other agent I have ever worked with. The "deal" is only part of what he brings to the table. He is there on every page with every photograph, with every cover suggestion. He is also part of the marketing and advertising strategy. In other words, Al is full-service, and he brings to every aspect his wit, wisdom, and brilliance. Thank you, Al.

Caroline Somers is my "ace." She is my daughter, my daughter-in-law, the mother of my grandchildren, and my son's wife. She is also smart, savvy, and incredibly talented. She brings so much to this series of books and the entire division of Somersize foods. I really couldn't do this project without her. She cares deeply about this program and is involved in every aspect. I depend upon her to concur with me that the recipes we are bringing to you are the best-tasting and most incredible foods we are able to concoct. It is a rich and rewarding experience to work so closely with her. I love you, Caroline.

My other "daughter," my stepdaughter, Leslie Hamel, has illustrated all of the books in the Somersize series. She is incredibly talented, and her drawings always make me crack up. She has a funny take on things that is evident in her illustrations. They clearly establish the guidelines of Somersizing through her humor and talent. I love working with her and love her dearly, as if she were my own daughter.

Dr. Michael Galitzer is a fresh face in the Somersize program. Denise Vivaldo, who runs my test kitchen, is one of his patients, and he has been so impressed with her progress, with the Somersize program, and with Somer-Sweet as a means to get people off of refined sugar that he was eager to write the foreword. He is now passing our SomerSweet to many of his patients, which is the greatest testament of all. Dr. Galitzer is one of the new cutting-edge doctors who uses the best of Western, Eastern, and holistic medicines, and I thank him for his informative foreword and his enthusiasm for this way of eating.

Paul Schulick, master herbalist, has been a dear friend for many years. He is one of the first people in my life who helped me to understand the importance of supplements in today's polluted environment. Sadly, our food supply has been so badly damaged that it is now necessary to get our vital nutrients and minerals through supplements, because the food we eat can no longer meet our nutritional requirements. Paul is a purist and cares deeply about healing, not harming. The supplements he is packaging under the Somersize name are of the highest quality in integrity and ingredients. Do not miss the chapter that he wrote for this book. It is extremely enlightening. Thank, you, Paul.

My editor, Kristin Kiser, has been with me now for my last five books. Kristin is great to work with. She never interferes with my "voice," but is right there whenever I need her to pick up the slack. It was Kristin who organized the jumble of "Frequently Asked Questions," which is a sizeable amount of this book.

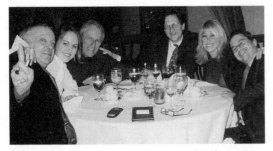

My "Crown" team: my agent Al Lowman, my editor Kristin Kiser, Alan, Andy Martin, me, and Chip Gibson.

Over the years I have been asked these questions over and over by so many of you that we realized a portion of the book should be dedicated to answering them. Frankly, I never would have had the patience to organize all those questions, and that is where Kristin comes through for me. She has an excellent eye, great literary taste, and every suggestion she gives me comes from intelligence and experience. I wouldn't want to do a book without her. Thank you so much, Kristin.

My husband, Alan Hamel, is always a big part of everything I do. While I sit at my computer, writing, he is on the phone mapping out strategy for the selling and marketing of the product. He lays out the advertising, and he thinks up the marketing approach with his clever and savvy intelligence. Alan and I are a team. We are partners in life and in business. We get along like two happy puppies, spending 365 days a year together, twenty-four hours a day, and we never tire of being with one another. It is a lucky and miraculous thing to find a "life mate," "soul mate." I love you dearly, Alan

Sandi Mendelson and Judy Hilsinger are publicists extraordinaire. We start on the "Today Show," and blitz the entire country after that. Thanks for a stellar job, girls.

My dream team at Crown: Chip Gibson, my former publisher, who spearheaded the Somersize series, has been an absolute joy to work with. He has moved onward and upward, but I will always give him credit for initially seeing the potential in this idea.

Jenny Frost, my new publisher, Andy Martin, the funniest guy around, Steve Ross, Tina Constable, and Wendy Schuman. This is the most enjoyable group of extraordinarily talented people in all of publishing. I feel so blessed.

Once again, my lawyer, who "gets it," Marc Chamlin. This is our sixth book together. I look forward to many more. Thanks for all the good advice.

And then there is Jeff Katz, who is the only photographer I choose to work with. He puts his heart and soul into these photographs. There are countless meetings beforehand and he comes with enthusiasm and creativity. Jeff will do anything to get the perfect shot. If it means climbing mountains or hundreds of stairs (as is the case in my house), then that's what he does. He makes the food jump off the plate, and makes me look so great that I wish I could walk around in life with his beautiful lighting surrounding me. Thank you once again, sweet friend, for giving me these beautiful and quality photographs.

And thank you to Jeff's stellar team, Victor Boghossian, Jack Coyier, Michael Negrete, Gabriel Hutchison—you are all the greatest.

Brian Toffoli, my incredible food stylist, and his assistant Steven Lichtscheidl, bring such restraint and loveliness to every setup. Brian does it simply and beautifully, never allowing his ego to get in the way while we all pull and fuss with the shot. He knows that sometimes a simple daisy is all that is needed to finish the effect. Thank you for your great work once again.

Denise Vivaldo, Andy Sheen-Turner, Cindie Flannigan, and Blake Machamer run my test kitchen. Denise heads up the kitchen, and without her and her team there would be no Somersize food. She takes my recipes, which are always "a handful of this and a handful of that," and breaks them down to bring you exact measurements. She is also excellent at such assignments as: "Denise, see if you can make up a Pavlova recipe using SomerSweet." Two days later, she'll present me with a perfect meringue cake. Denise and her team are invaluable to both myself and Caroline. While I am writing and Caroline is researching, Denise and her team are testing recipe after recipe to ensure that you are able to make these delicious foods with ease. It was Denise and Andy who came up with the spinach "bread," which will rock your world. Thank you to all of you.

Samantha Degen is my stylist of choice again and again. I just let her loose in my closet and she finds things I forgot that I have. She makes sure I am looking nice for these photographs, because I am so involved with all the other aspects of the shoot that I forget about how I look. Thanks for another great job, Sam.

Shannon Frost is a talented and caring makeup artist. Again, when I am involved with these Somersize shoots I am too impatient to sit in front of the mirror and fix myself. So I leave that to Shannon. I rarely look in the mirror because I know she will make me look right. Thanks, Shannon.

Mary Schuck designs my beautiful covers and I love the style of them. The "look" of this book is classic Mary, and I appreciate the time and patience you put in to please me. Thank you also to Amy Boorstein, Jane Searle, Jean Lynch, and Lauren Dong, my fabulous production team, who make sure my books get published without a hitch, and to Claudia Gabel, who assists Kristin so capably.

A big "thank you" to all the girls in my office, especially Marsha Yanchuck, my assistant of twenty-five years, who corrects all the grammar and spelling and organizes the testimonials from all of you who send in your beautiful letters and your "before" and "after" photos. Thank you, Marsha, you know I love you. A big thanks also to Anka Brazzell, who runs our office, Liz Kozakowski, and Julie Turkel. I love you all.

Special thanks to Sarah D'Agostino, our coordinator on the photo shoot, who did just about everything, and for what she wasn't able to do, a big "thank you" to Trish Gardner and Christy Blaser, who picked up the slack.

And thank you to my darling grandchildren, who were background for so many of these beautiful photographs. They made the days fun. Laughing, giggling, skipping, sneaking food off the display table, becoming the darlings of everyone. Thank you to my yummy, irresistible, adorable grandchildren. I love you so-oooo much!

And thank you to Bruce, my darling son, who cheerfully leaves his successful business, Sincbox Productions, to help us with the kids for the several days it takes to produce these photos, and never complains when I grab him to sit in for the occasional picture. Bruce is never without a smile and a good attitude. You were full of goodness from the moment of your birth, and I've always been honored to be your mother. I love you.

And certainly, my friend Dr. Diana Schwarzbein continues to constantly instruct and inform me about the latest breakthroughs in science and physiology. She has been my mentor and teacher over the years and is the person who helped me to understand the "insulin connection" that is the crux of this program. Her input has been invaluable. She is one of the leading endocrinologists in this country and is one of the "cutting edge" doc-

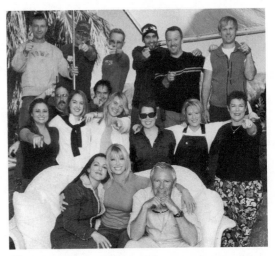

The photo team. From left to right, front row: Caroline Somers, Suzanne Somers, Alan Hamel. Second row: Sarah D'Agostino, Kristin Kiser, Shannon Frost, Samantha Degen, Cindie Flannigan, Denise Vivaldo. Third row: Blake Machamer, Andy Sheen-Turner. Fourth row: Jack Coyier, Jeff Katz, Michael Negrete, Gabriel Hutchison, Brian Toffoli, Steven Lichtscheidl.

tors that I seek out, who uses the best of Western medicine in conjunction with Eastern and holistic. Diana has a keen understanding of the necessity to supplement our damaged food supply with vitamins, herbs, and essential amino acids. Thank you, Diana, for all the information you have so generously shared.

And to you, my fabulous readers, and all my friends on HSN: You inspire and amaze me. You teach me and force me to grow and move forward. What great friends you have all become. I listen to you and take your suggestions, use and incorporate the recipes you send, and am continually impressed by your creativity. Thanks so much. I love you all.

Contents

Part Two—Everything You Need to Know About Somersizing • 75

Part Three—The Somersize Recipes • 177

Foreword

My medical career began in Los Angeles, where I was a board-certified emergency room physician from 1974 through 1988. During that time I participated in the response to many "code blues" (cardiac arrests). By the time the patient got to the ER, it was often too late. We continued CPR, but after twenty minutes, we ended the resuscitation.

Then, in 1991, at a self-improvement seminar on the Big Island of Hawaii, my beliefs about life and death were radically changed. I had just climbed to the top of a fifty-foot pole (attached by ropes), and I leaped to catch a trapeze and missed. I was extremely dismayed as I was slowly lowered down from the pole. I began to walk away from my group of sixty people, and as I did I noticed that one of the people in my group was crying because he had also missed the trapeze. Realizing that my emotional state was far better than his, I decided to rejoin my group and cheer for my fellow teammates.

One of my teammates, Howard, had just missed the trapeze. He was smiling as he was lowered to the ground, but as his feet gently landed, fifteen feet directly in front of me, he went into cardiac arrest. I immediately began CPR, had two teammates massage the inner aspect of the little fingers (the heart meridian in acupuncture), and called for the paramedics. It took thirty minutes for the paramedics to arrive. We started the IV, put a tube in his trachea, gave him all the cardiac drugs, defibrillated him with the paddles, but to no avail. He was flat-lined. I continued to work on him as we transferred him to the ambulance. As I moved to board the ambulance, the paramedics thanked me for my help and informed me that my services were no longer needed (it was now their turf). I looked them straight in the eye and said, "No way, I'm not leaving now."

We took a thirty-minute ride to the hospital (it turned out to be an urgent care center), during which time the defibrillator stopped working. We had done an hour of CPR and I was exhausted, Howard was purple and gray, and it didn't look good.

We were five minutes from the hospital when the paramedic smacked the defibrillator, like you would do to an old TV set to get it to work. Suddenly a heart rhythm magically appeared on the monitor. Five minutes later, as we pulled up to the hospital, Howard had a blood pressure of 100/60, and five minutes later, he woke up. Howard went on to make a complete recovery, after being without a heartbeat for an hour. For the next seven years I received the most beautiful cards from Howard, thanking me for saving his life. We were taught in medical school that the brain can only go five minutes without oxygen before irreversible changes occur, but Howard didn't agree with that theory. My lesson was "Never say never," and don't fall into the trap of using old beliefs to guide present actions and behaviors.

Yes, miracles do happen. Everything is possible. You can do anything and everything that you want. You can lose weight. You can regain your health. All you need to do is alter your beliefs about what you want to change. A belief is nothing more than a feeling of certainty about something. We all had beliefs about the world when we were younger that no longer serve us. I remember being a kid and thinking that thirty was old!

We also keep looking back to the past to define possibilities for the future. This is what people do about losing weight. They go back to the past when they were unable to lose weight for a sustained period of time, and get frustrated when attempting to lose weight in the present. The key is to change the beliefs that no longer serve you. How do you change those beliefs? The best way is to start developing new attitudes and experiences that cause you to question your old beliefs.

Suzanne Somers, in her new book, *Suzanne Somers' Fast and Easy*, gives you an incredible amount of information that is both scientifically based and medically correct. She wonderfully debunks the old thinking that fats are bad for you and carbs are good for you. Suzanne understands that people want to feel better and have more energy, but don't want to deprive themselves. She knows that the key is to focus on what people can have. As soon as we start to think about what we can't have and how 0we have to limit ourselves, we don't feel well. When we have great choices and tastes, we become more enthusiastic about life. Somersizing offers great ways to both feel and look better.

I have been practicing anti-aging medicine since 1986. I use many different modalities, including nutrition, homeopathy, herbs, acupuncture, heavy metal detoxification, sensory resonance, and natural hormone replacement therapy. In 1986 I was a burnt-out ER doc. When I added all the hours of all the shifts that I worked in the ER, I had spent the equivalent of three full years living in a hospital! For most of my ER years, there were no trauma centers in LA. The trauma cases went to the nearest ER. They used to call me Dr. Trauma, for I seemed to attract those cases, whenever I worked.

In 1986 I came across an opportunity in Los Angeles. A holistic clinic was looking for a medical doctor to do general practice and nutrition. I knew general practice from being an ER doc, but didn't have a clue about nutrition. I went about learning nutrition, reading everything I could get my hands on. I took countless seminars, listened to numerous audiotapes, and hired a nutritionist to help me. I figured the best way to start was to get blood tests that showed the foods that people were allergic to. I thought that if you identified the allergenic foods and had people avoid those foods, they had to get better. Wrong. Nobody felt better, nobody lost weight, and the GI symptoms of gas, bloating, and constipation persisted. In those days, I never asked why people were allergic to those foods. Could it be that they were allergic to those foods because of poor food-combining choices? Were they eating those foods every day, even two to three times a day, because they were addicted to how they reacted to those foods? Were they tired because they ate far too many carbs? Did they gain weight because they ate too many carbs, and not enough healthy fats? What I needed in those days were Suzanne's wonderful books about Somersizing.

I have since come to understand that health is our natural state of being—disease and illness are an aberration. Regaining your health is not always fast, but it can be easy. The first thing that someone who wants to get healthier must do is to improve his or her nutrition. How should you eat? One of the key tenets in medicine is that obesity is a risk factor for many diseases, including heart dis-

ease, cancer, hypertension, and stroke. So the next question is: how does one eat in order to prevent obesity? Should you avoid fats and eat lots of carbohydrates, or as Somersizing says, should you eat fats and avoid most carbohydrates, and thereby lower blood insulin levels, which prevent storage of excess calories as fat? The evidence overwhelmingly points to Somersizing as the most effective approach. Let's look at history for proof.

In *The Physiology of Taste,* written in 1825 and considered to be one of the most famous books ever printed about food, the French gastronome Jean Anthelme Brillat-Savarin says that he could easily identify the causes of obesity after thirty years of listening to "one stout party" after another proclaiming the joys of bread, rice, and potatoes. But more than one hundred years later medical professionals decided that bread, rice, and potatoes weren't causing obesity; that eating fat was making us sick. Ancel Keys, a University of Minnesota physician, introduced the low-fat-is-good-health dogma in the 1950s with his theory that dietary fat raises cholesterol levels and gives you heart disease. This started an anti-fat trend that gripped the country in the twentieth century. In January 1977 a Senate committee led by George McGovern published its "Dietary Goals for the United States," advising that Americans significantly curb their fat intake to abate an epidemic of "killer diseases" supposedly sweeping the country. In 1984 the National Institutes of Health officially recommended that all Americans over the age of two eat less fat. By now the model American breakfast of eggs and bacon had given way to a bowl of Special K with low-fat milk, a glass of orange juice, and toast (hold the butter, please). Over the past twenty years most Americans have followed this low-fat, high-carbohydrate approach, resulting in skyrocketing levels of obesity in both adults and children!

Enter twenty-first-century science. Walter Willet, chairman of the department of nutrition at the Harvard School of Public Health, is the spokesperson of the longest-running, most comprehensive diet and health study ever performed, costing upward of $100 million and including data on nearly 300,000 individuals. His conclusion is that the "data clearly contradict the low-fat-is-good-health message."

Americans not only eat way too many carbohydrates, but they eat the wrong kind of carbohydrates. Here is a list of the top twenty sources of carbohydrate in the American diet.

1. potatoes
2. white bread
3. cold breakfast cereal
4. dark bread
5. orange juice
6. bananas
7. white rice
8. pizza
9. pasta
10. muffins
11. fruit punch
12. carbonated soft drinks
13. apples
14. skim milk
15. pancakes
16. table sugar
17. jam
18. cranberry juice
19. french fries
20. candy

When eaten regularly, most of these foods are guaranteed to produce the following symptoms:

1. weight gain
2. fatigue
3. irritability
4. mood swings
5. poor sleep
6. gas and bloating

Suzanne is being very kind when she refers to most of these foods as "Funky Foods." She doesn't feel that all carbohydrates are bad; the carbs in whole-grain form, such as whole wheat pasta and whole wheat bread, are actually beneficial for you, since they contain large amounts of fiber, which causes blood sugar to rise more slowly after eating, resulting in less insulin release. She makes a further distinction in that she does not want you to combine these healthy carbs with foods in the Proteins/Fats group, so that digestion is optimized, with no gas or bloating.

Suzanne wants all of us to be the best that we can be, to radiate health, to have passion, to have boundless energy, and to be emotionally balanced. You can't get to these physical and emotional states by eating the funky carbohydrates. Additionally, by regularly eating most of these Funky Foods, you will not only throw your body out of balance but gain a whole lot of weight, since excess insulin release causes your body to store calories as fat.

Another area Suzanne skillfully addresses in *Fast and Easy* is bone loss, or osteoporosis. The United States has the highest level of calcium consumption in the world, yet also has one of the highest incidences of osteoporosis. How can that be? The major reason is increased cellular acidity. The major causes of cellular acidity are stress, poor nutrition, and lack of exercise.

Cellular acidity (or cellular toxicity) can occur at any age. As a rule, the older we are, the more toxic we are, because our elimination systems become more sluggish. Toxins accumulate in and around cells. The cellular environment thus becomes more acidic. The easiest way for the body to neutralize cellular acidity is to mobilize alkaline minerals such as calcium and magnesium. The greatest reservoir of these alkaline minerals is in the bone. Consequently, calcium and magnesium leave the bone in order to neutralize cellular acidity, resulting in osteoporosis. Just taking calcium is not enough. We need to follow Suzanne's advice to improve our nutrition, exercise more, and find more effective ways to deal with stress. One good way to deal with stress is to see stress as a challenge instead of a threat. By giving more desirable meaning to those circumstances or events in our lives that we might label as stressors, we elicit healthier emotional responses.

There are three main causes of chronic stress:

1. Long-term unhealthy beliefs that cause us to perceive life events as "dangers," and thus trigger an alarm response;

2. Long-term or persistent deprivation of our emotional need for "bonding" or closeness;

3. Not getting enough of our psychological needs met in our daily environments that are unique to our specific personality type. Some of us need to have fun and excitement; others need acknowledgement of our values; others need acknowledgment of our ability to think clearly and logically; other people need solitude; and some of us need our senses to be richly stimulated.

Suzanne Somers speaks to all of us in the important work that she is doing in nutrition and health. She's like a friend we can trust and believe, and also have fun with as we reshape our thoughts and beliefs along with reshaping our bodies!

I am very impressed that *Fast and Easy* addresses the role of supplements in optimizing health. It is a fact that most Americans eat a diet that contains foods that are processed and full of preservatives and colorings. Therefore, we are unable to obtain the necessary amount of nutrients—the vitamins, minerals, and enzymes that are needed to drive chemical reactions in the body that create energy and detoxify the body from the toxins that we are exposed to on a daily basis. Some of the major toxins in our environment are:

1. The city water that we drink, bathe in, and shower with;

2. The insecticides and pesticides that contaminate our fruits and vegetables;

3. The hormones and antibiotics that are given to animals to fatten them up and accelerate their growth, and to prevent infection that might result from their less-than-optimal living conditions;
4. Exhaust pollution from automobiles and industry;
5. Substances such as cigarette smoke and alcohol.

These toxins must be eliminated from the body by our liver, lymph, and kidney systems. If they are not eliminated efficiently, they begin to be stored in the body. Over time they will interfere with organ function and hormone production, resulting in clinical symptoms such as fatigue, insomnia, and irritability.

With this in mind, there is a great need for all of us to supplement our daily food intake with vitamins, minerals, and enzymes, and to also use herbs to help our organs (especially the liver) excrete toxins out of the body. Suzanne is to be commended for addressing the subject in an elegant and very understandable way, and for creating products that improve our health.

One day, a patient of mine, who is an associate of Suzanne's, returned for her second visit. She was feeling much better, and gave me a gift of SomerSweet Chocolate Truffles, which my assistant and I thought were quite delicious. She also gave me a can of the sweetener, SomerSweet, to try. Among other things, I practice German Biological Medicine, which allows me to test all sorts of products, from herbs and homeopathics, to vitamins and other supplements, to make sure that the product is both effective and tolerated by the body. Some products are quite effective but are very poorly tolerated—an example is cancer chemotherapy. I want my patients to have products that both work and have no side effects. I began testing Somer-Sweet with all my patients and found it to be both effective and tolerated by everyone. It appears to be a far superior product than stevia, the sweetener derived from an herb from the Amazon. To my amazement, Somer-Sweet also appears to normalize insulin levels in patients that have varying degrees of insulin resistance. While much more definitive research needs to be done, this product is clearly a winner, and is extremely safe. My congratulations to Suzanne for developing such a wonderful product.

Health is much, much more than the absence of disease. Health is energy, vitality, passion. Healthy people have physical energy, emotional balance, and spiritual awareness. We now have the tools to slow the aging process and accelerate the regeneration of the cells and tissues of the body. *Suzanne Somers' Fast and Easy* gives all of us the information we need to take our health to the next level. It is fun and factual reading. I heartily recommend this book to everyone who is interested in using nutrition to slow the aging process. Suzanne Somers is clearly a health hero, for she is determined to improve the health of Americans, by creating a way of eating that reduces obesity, increases vitality, and thus promotes happiness.

As Suzanne says,

To Your Health!

MICHAEL GALITZER, M.D.

Suzanne Somers'
FAST AND EASY

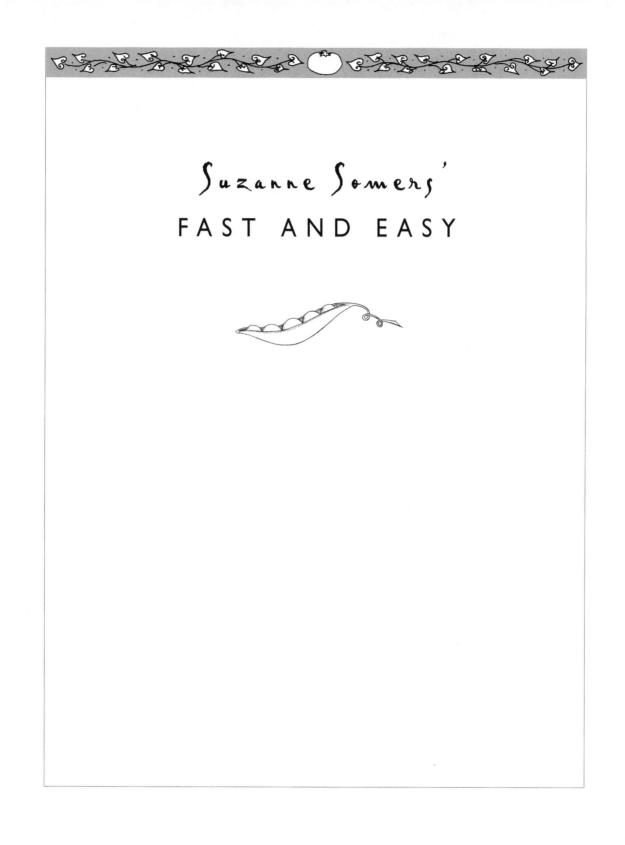

Introduction

You've bought the book. You've opened it. You've started reading. You are on your way to learning about the most effective, satisfying way to lose weight that you'll ever experience. It's called Somersizing, and it's not a diet at all, but a way of eating that has transformed figures, improved health, and increased energy for millions of Somersizers across the globe. Congratulations, you're about to become part of the club.

Here's your test for Somersize Club Membership:

Do you like to eat rich and delicious foods?

Do you enjoy eating meals without weighing and measuring portions?

Do you prefer eating without counting calories?

Do you believe in a healthy variety of foods from every food group?

Do you like to eat until you are completely satisfied?

Do you like the option of cooking for yourself or eating in restaurants?

Do you like to have at least three meals a day, plus snacks in between?

Do you like to eat guilt-free sweets?

If you answered "Yes" to these questions, you've passed. Welcome to the world of Somersizing. Your life is about to change. Your body is on its way to its ideal weight. Your taste buds will dance with glee. Your health will improve. And you are going to have a great time doing it.

Somersize is celebrating its tenth anniversary in 2002. It was in 1992 that I took the famed trip to France where I was introduced to this way of eating. The French, even with all their butter and cream sauces, are so dang skinny. They eat the richest food, and yet they boast the second-lowest risk of heart disease in the world. It was here that the seeds of Somersizing began to grow.

It sounds too good to be true, but you've no doubt learned about the amazing results from your friends and coworkers who have tried the program. Maybe you've seen me on television and heard Somersizers call in to share their success stories. Perhaps you've been on SuzanneSomers.com and chatted with people on the program. Or you've thumbed through the Somersize books and seen the numerous before and after photos. You've heard about the incredible food in magazine articles. You've read that people are including fats in their diets and watching their cholesterol levels improve. This is the real deal.

For those of you who have already read my earlier books and started to lose weight on the program, you already know what a treat you are in for reading *Fast and Easy*. Each Somersize book has evolved from the previous one. I thank you for your input. Your suggestions are very important to me. So what about this book is different from my first three Somersize books, *Eat Great, Lose Weight; Get Skinny on Fabulous Foods;* and *Eat, Cheat, and Melt the Fat Away*? It is *Fast and Easy*. I keep hearing how much you love the program, but that you want it to be faster and easier. As always, I listened to your comments, and I wrote a fourth Somersize book that addresses your concerns.

Our lives are crazy. We're running from here to there with no time to cook. We're all juggling busy schedules, but we want to stay healthy and fit. Now we can. In *Fast and Easy*, I take my tried-and-true program

and adapt it for people with no time to cook. Many single people do not like to spend a lot of time in the kitchen cooking for one. Even couples feel that it's a lot of work for only two people. And families don't have time to make a dinner for the kids and then a separate Somersize meal for the adults. I'm here to help.

In this book I have created over 100 simple and delicious recipes that take very little preparation time, like Somersize Shake It and Bake It Chicken, Turkey Taco Wraps, and Somersize Double Double Cheese-burgers with Somersize Fast and Easy Onion Rings. All of these recipes are made with ingredients that are readily available at mainstream grocery stores, so you don't have to go searching for unusual and expensive ingredients at specialty shops. The preparation time for most of the recipes is no more than fifteen minutes, and the cooking time is no more than thirty minutes. Even if you have no time to cook, you can find time for these quick, easy, and delicious meals.

Not only do I give you recipes that you can make in half an hour or less, but I also show you how you can make Somersizing appealing for the whole family, especially children. I am so worried about our kids. There is a growing epidemic in our country of children who are becoming overweight and obese. I will share with you later in the book staggering statistics about the decrease of activity in kids' lives and the increase of their sugar consumption. It's a recipe for disaster in terms of their health and well-being. But who wants to put a kid on a diet? Who wants to deny a kid dessert? We love spoiling our children and with my program you can. Somersizing can be a family way of life, and your children will thank you. They will love the food! And there's no portion control, so if they're still hungry for more, you may always give them as much food as it takes to fill them up. We have all sorts of family favorites, like Somersize Macaroni and Cheese, Somersize Chicken Nuggets, and Mini–Pepperoni Pizzas! You don't have to feel like you are depriving your children when you all Somersize together. I guarantee you won't hear any complaints from the kids.

To get you and your family jump-started on the road to good health, I have provided a fast and easy explanation of the program up front. There's a special section that cuts through the extended scientific backup and gets you started on the program immediately. This will be a great refresher course if you are already familiar with the program. That being said, if you are new to the program, I highly recommend you read the sections on why sugar is the body's greatest enemy and why fat is truly your friend. You must undo the notion that a low-fat diet is the key to weight loss. Understanding how our bodies work and why they respond to this program helps keep you motivated and on track. You'll learn why cutting calories is only a short-term fix that will keep you on the endless diet roller coaster. It's fascinating information about our physiology. Once everyone starts asking how you lost the weight, you'll want to explain exactly how and why this amazing program works.

The real culprit is the hormone insulin that is released by the pancreas when we eat sugar or foods that turn to sugar upon digestion, like white flour, potatoes, and pasta. The whole key to the Somersize program is controlling our insulin levels. Insulin must be present for foods to be stored as fat. Therefore, the most important part of Somersizing is to minimize the foods that cause the release of insulin. You will soon understand just how important it is to eliminate sugar (and hidden sugars) from your diet. Then we learn to eat real foods in combinations that aid in digestion, like Chicken Kiev, Warm Steak and Arugula Salad with Parmesan Shavings, and Lemony Artichokes with Artichoke and Onion Dip. Without the presence of insulin, none of these foods can be stored as fat. Isn't that just peachy? You can eat like a queen and end up with the waistline of a princess.

Once you learn the basic tenets of the program, it's so easy! The pounds will literally melt away as your body learns to use its stored fuel (your fat reserves) as an energy source. This constant source of energy keeps you feeling great while you melt down to your goal weight. Just read the testimonial letters included in the book. Almost everyone speaks of the amazing energy they have while Somersizing. That's because you are no longer overloading your body with empty carbohydrates that are not being burned off. Carbohydrates are used for energy. If you consume too much "energy," your body will store the extra in your fat reserves. Once you give up sugar and empty carbohydrates, your body will convert your fat reserves and use them as an energy source. That's when you start to melt down to your ideal weight.

It all sounds great, but are you still adjusting to the fact that you're going to have to give up sugar and white bread? Are you running to the fridge for your last can of sugary soda pop? Are you thinking that maybe you can't do this program if you have to give up the dreaded sweet stuff? Not to worry. We have SomerSweet . . . the most exciting product I have ever developed. I am truly off sugar and no longer crave the poison. SomerSweet fills all my sweet needs. It tastes like sugar, with no nasty aftertaste. It bakes like sugar. In fact, it even caramelizes. And it's blended with natural, sweet fiber, so you can feel good about using it. With SomerSweet you will not miss the sugar! Somersize desserts are a gift, whether you're trying to lose weight or not. Could you go for Somersize Coffee Toffee Ice Cream, Chocolate Dipped Strawberries, or Chocolate Cupcakes with Whipped Cream Filling? What more could you ask for?

Fast and Easy also contains a new section devoted to our health. I receive numerous letters and e-mails at SuzanneSomers.com asking me what type of supplements I take, and why, so I have included a detailed section about the importance of vitamins and supplements. I have learned so much about this field from Paul Schulick, a revered expert, a friend, and a man of true integrity. After many discussions with Paul about the needs of Somersizers, we have developed an entire line of Somersize Supplements that help you maximize your results. And you'll just love hearing about Somersize Crave Control to help curb those little cravings for sugar.

In the health section I have also included vital information about how Somersizing will help keep your serotonin levels healthy and balanced, so your moods will be even and you won't crave carbohydrates; I also include important information about why we need to keep our bones healthy to ward off osteoporosis. Men, women, and children of all ages will be surprised to learn that the foods you eat from the time you are young can have a dramatic effect on your risk of bone loss as an adult. Don't wait until it's too late to build your bone density. Somersizing not only helps you lose weight, it helps build bone density so you can maintain an active, healthy life.

I take new Somersizers and veteran Somersizers—if they want a refresher—through Level One, the weight-loss portion of the program, explaining step by step how to get started and stay on track. Almost Level One is for folks who are already losing steadily and can handle a few minor imbalances without disrupting their progress. Level Two is the maintenance portion of the program where we learn to Somersize for life. I have new information in this section about keeping our bodies in perfect balance. In Level Two, you'll learn the importance of adding a little carbohydrate back into our protein meals to keep our metabolism at optimum speed.

I can't tell you how many e-mails and questions I get about bringing food to work. I'll give you a whole week's worth of lunchbox ideas that are perfect for work and school. Brown bagging it has never been so easy! You'll get tips on how to order Somer-

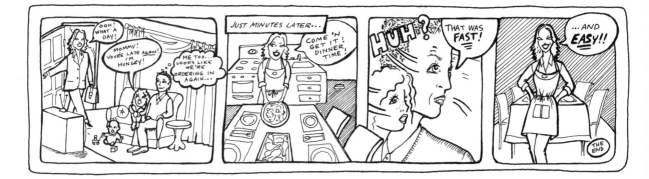

size meals, even in fast-food restaurants. I've created menus you can use for a week if you are really pressed for time and need some help coming up with delicious Somersized meals. And I'll give you great snack ideas to keep the whole family away from the bags of chips. There is no deprivation on this program, just a shift in thinking that can literally transform your family from the inside out.

Even if you are a longtime member of the Somersize Club, you are going to find so many great tips in this new book on how to incorporate Somersizing into your busy life, particularly if you have a family. I have really tried to anticipate all the questions you could have. To make answering your questions extra convenient, I have cataloged hundreds of the most frequently asked Somersize questions. This easy-to-use format will allow you to look up questions in any category. I have been building this list for close to a decade, and all the answers are printed right here.

For the first time in my Somersize books I can fill you in on some exciting developments coming out of the Somersize test kitchen, great new pre-packaged foods, protein bars and shakes, and appliances that will make Somersizing a breeze. Check out Chapter 14 to learn more about these products.

But let's not forget about the most important section of the book—the food! With over 100 new recipes, you'll learn to make meals in minutes. Twenty-Minute Turkey Chili with sour cream and cheddar cheese, Fried Shrimp with Spicy Cocktail Sauce, Baby-Back Barbecue Ribs with Somersize Barbecue Sauce. These are meals you and your family will devour; meals with ingredients that won't break the bank; meals that won't keep you in the kitchen all day; meals that taste too good to be true. And don't forget dessert. We have SomerSweet desserts that will rock your world! Somersize Jiggly Fruit Gels with Perfectly Whipped Cream, Boston Cream Pie Cake, and even Chocolate Cream Pie. Imagine all this incredible food, while you slip into those jeans that haven't fit you in years. Ah, this is good.

Hey, you . . . new club member . . . are you ready? I thought so. Let's Somersize.

Part One

THE FAST AND EASY WAY

TO START SOMERSIZING—AND

WHY YOU NEED TO

GET STARTED *RIGHT NOW*

THE

SOMERSIZE WAY OF LIFE

How to Somersize: The Fast and Easy Explanation

If you're ready to start this program right now, then this is the section for you. I'll take you right to the basics and show you the fast track to find the slim new you. You won't believe how easy this program is. All it takes is a shift in your thinking about how to eat right. Once you learn the Seven Easy Steps to Somersizing, you will be able to eat sinfully rich food, in abundant portions, in a way that reprograms your metabolism to burn fat and give you a constant source of energy.

Level One is the weight-loss portion of the program. You want to lose weight, gain energy, and eat delicious food? Here we go. The most important aspect of Somersizing is controlling our insulin levels. You will learn all about the hormone insulin and its effects on our bodies in later chapters. All you need to know right now is that when you Somersize, the first step is to eliminate a small list of foods that raise our insulin levels, like sugar, white flour, potatoes, white rice, and alcohol. These foods are called Funky Foods. You will find a complete list of Funky Foods in the Reference Guide in the back of the book. Say good-bye to them for now, and get ready to say hello to the skinny person that is about to emerge from your cocoon.

After we eliminate the Funky Foods, we separate normal, everyday foods into groups. Then we combine these foods in a way that aids in digestion and weight control. Here are the four Somersize Food Groups:

Pro/Fats: Includes proteins like meat, poultry, fish, eggs, and fats in their natural state like oil, butter, cream, and cheese.

Veggies: Includes a whole host of low-starch, fresh vegetables, from artichokes to peppers to zucchini and more.

Carbos: Includes whole-grain pastas, cereals, breads, beans, and nonfat dairy products.

Fruit: Includes a huge variety of fresh fruits, from apples to peaches to tangerines and more.

Again, you will find complete lists of these food groups in the back of the book in the Reference Guide. Now that you have the four Somersize Food Groups, you just follow the Seven Easy Steps to Somersizing.

1. Eliminate all Funky Foods.
2. Eat Fruit alone, on an empty stomach: twenty minutes before a Carbos meal, one hour before a Pro/Fats meal, two hours after your last meal.
3. Eat Pro/Fats with Veggies.
4. Eat Carbos with Veggies.
5. Keep Pro/Fats separate from Carbos.
6. Wait three hours between meals if switching from a Pro/Fats meal to a Carbos meal, or vice versa.
7. Do not skip meals. Eat at least three meals a day, and eat until you feel satisfied and comfortably full.

That's it. You may eat whenever you are hungry. You should eat until you feel comfortably full and you should not skip meals. Start now! Go to the refrigerator and get a slice of salami (a Pro/Fat) and a slice of cheese (a Pro/Fat) and spread a little mayo (a Pro/Fat) on it. Roll it up with a piece of lettuce (a Veggie) and you have a nice little Pro/Fats and Veggies snack. There are endless, wonderful combinations of food that you may eat while you are losing weight.

Let's start with the top of the day. First, you pick the food group you would like for your meal: Fruit, Pro/Fats, Veggies, or Carbos. If you want a Fruit meal for breakfast, you may have anything in the Somersize Fruit group. You could have a bowl of freshly cut fruit salad, or you could have a fruit smoothie. We eat fruit on an empty stomach (twenty minutes before a Carbos meal, one hour before a Pro/Fats meal, or two hours after your last meal). Fruit can upset the digestive process when combined with other foods. You'll read more about that later. Remember, this is the fast and easy explanation! Or, instead of Fruit, you could choose a Pro/Fats and Veggies breakfast by combining any of the foods from the Pro/Fats group with any of the foods from the Veggies group. In this breakfast you could have eggs with bacon or sausage. Fry them in butter or oil and serve them with a side of asparagus or spinach. Anything on the Pro/Fats and Veggies lists is fair game. As a third choice you could have a Carbo breakfast and enjoy a whole array of whole-grain cereals and breads with nonfat dairy products. All of these foods appear in the Carbos group, so you may eat any of them together. Have Shredded Wheat with nonfat milk or oatmeal with nonfat milk. Have whole-grain toast with nonfat cottage cheese and a touch of cinnamon. And feel free to sprinkle SomerSweet, my amazing answer to sugar, on top to sweeten things up a bit.

As for portions, you do not have to weigh or measure anything. Isn't that a miracle! All I ask is that you eat until you are comfortably full. Listen to your body. Satisfy your hunger

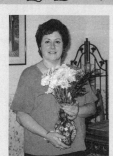

before

Dear Suzanne,

The words "thank you" just do not seem to be enough. All of my life, I have been struggling with losing the same 20 pounds. A few years ago, I decided to join a local diet center, and after weighing and measuring my high-carbohydrate, fat-free food, I finally lost the weight. But every day I felt hungry and deprived.

It didn't take long to gain it all back again, with a few added extra pounds. I was feeling depressed, desperate, and totally disgusted with myself, and that is when I had a light-bulb moment. I remembered my Aunt Nancy had lost all of her weight on your program, and she did so by eating wonderful, delicious food. I knew I just had to try this way of eating. In March of 2001, I started to Somersize, and in six months, I had lost 22 pounds. I have maintained my weight for five months now, and it was and still is so easy. I went for my annual physical a few weeks ago and was so pleased with my cholesterol results, and so was my doctor.

This October, my daughter will be getting married. It was such a thrill to shop for the gown I will wear on her wedding day. For the first time in my adult life I am happy when I look in the mirror. Sugar can never taste as good as thin feels.

Fondly,
Christine Doran

after

and know when you have eaten enough to satiate your appetite. Unlike restrictive diets, you will always have enough to eat on this program. Do not skip meals. You must eat three meals a day, and you may have as many snacks as you want. In order to increase your metabolism, you must eat! That being said, you also do not want to overstuff yourself with food, just because there are no restrictions on portion sizes.

Let's continue with our day. For lunch or dinner you may choose to have a Pro/Fats and Veggies meal, or a Carbos and Veggies meal. For a Pro/Fats and Veggies meal, you could have a big salad filled with lots of fresh leafy greens, chopped fresh vegetables, chicken, ham, cheese, eggs, and bacon. You may top it with salad dressing of your choice, like blue cheese, Italian, or Caesar. Just make sure the dressing you choose does not contain any sugar or other Funky Foods. Many bottles of salad dressings have added sugars or starches. Thousand Island dressing usually has sugar in it. Ranch has buttermilk, which is a Funky Food. I have included several salad dressing recipes in my series of Somersize books. I also have Somersize Salad Dressing Mixes that make it really fast and easy. All you add are the fresh ingredients like olive oil, vinegar, mayonnaise, or sour cream.

That's right, when you Somersize, you may have the fat; in fact, you *should* have the fat! Fat is essential to health and to life—it's sugar that is the enemy. (Extensive explanations on this to come.) Beware of the bottled "fat-free" dressings because they are often loaded with starches and sugars to make up for the missing fat.

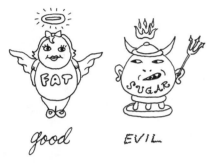

good   EVIL

There are many, many options for lunch and dinner with the Pro/Fats and Veggies meal. Look at the list for Pro/Fats: meat, poultry, seafood, cheese, cream, oil, and butter. And the Veggies list includes all your favorite low-starch vegetables, so anything on the list is okay to combine with anything on the Pro/Fats list. That means you can have a big steak with a mushroom cream sauce and a side of broccoli. If you like butter or a sprinkling of cheese on your broccoli, go for it. What you need to stay away from in this meal are the potatoes, rice, pasta, or bread. Have a hearty salad to start. Eat extra vegetables. You will not miss the starch with your protein and vegetables because you still get to have the flavor! You may have the sauce, the dressing . . . all the good stuff. You may even have dessert!

Somersize Cheesecake, Somersize Ice Cream, Somersize Crème Brûlée. You may have the sweets as long as they are made only with foods from the Pro/Fats group and without any sugar. SomerSweet, which is five times sweeter than sugar, makes it easy to have your sweets while you're losing weight.

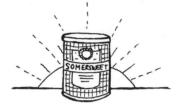

Fat is your friend. It's my Somersize mantra and the one thing I hope you take away from this book. Dietary fats are essential to good health and can be eaten freely when you Somersize. Eat roasted chicken . . . with the skin! Eat eggs . . . as many as you like! Eat seafood . . . it's like a free food! Look at your Pro/Fats and Veggies meal: meat, seafood, poultry, eggs, cheese, cream, salad dressings, vegetables, even dessert! The reason you can eat all of these delicious, flavorful foods is that you are not combining them with carbohydrates. If you were to add a significant amount of carbohydrates to this meal, then you would be spoiling a perfectly combined Somersize meal and you would reverse your results.

Here is a fast and easy explanation of how your body receives carbohydrates and sugars. Carbohydrates and sugars are used by the body as an energy source. When your body needs energy, it first looks to the dietary sugars and carbs that you eat. If you are not giving your body a significant source of "quick energy" in the form of sugar and carbs, your body will say, "Hey, where is my energy source? I guess I better find some other form of fuel to keep this machine running." And do you know where your body looks for fuel? In your fat reserves! Without a significant amount of dietary carbohydrates, your body will convert your stored fat to fuel and burn it as energy. So you convert your body from a carbo-burning machine to a fat-burning machine. You eat rich, divine food and your body begins melting away your stored fat, supplying you with a constant, even source of energy while you slim down to your goal weight. Fabulous! That's the Somersize secret.

So does that mean that you have to eliminate all carbohydrates when you Somersize? No. That is what separates my program from other high-protein programs. When you Somersize, you may eat any of the carbohydrates in the Carbos group as long as you do not combine them with any Pro/Fats. These foods have been carefully selected because they are in their whole-grain form. For example, you'll find brown rice, but not white rice. You'll find whole-wheat pasta, but not white pasta. You'll find whole-grain bread, but not white bread. Carbohydrates in their whole-grain form are filled with fiber and do not cause your insulin to spike as much as their refined counterparts. Also, fruits and vegetables both contain carbohydrates, and I do not ask you to eliminate these foods, as many other programs do.

If you are not having a Pro/Fats and Veggies lunch or dinner, you may occasionally choose the Carbos and Veggies meal. In this meal, you may have things like whole-grain pasta with marinara sauce, or brown rice with steamed vegetables, or vegetarian lasagna or lentil soup. Any of these foods in the Carbos group may be eaten with any of the foods from the Veggies group. What you won't find in either group are any added fats. Hold the Parmesan cheese on your pasta and make sure your sauce is made without oil. You can top your brown rice and vegetables with soy sauce, but not butter, and you must make your vegetarian lasagna with nonfat ricotta cheese. You could also try my line of whole-grain Somersize Pastas with my fat-free Somersize Sauces—then you know you are following all the guidelines.

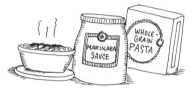

When switching from a Pro/Fats meal to a Carbos meal, you must wait three hours between meals. The same rules apply for snacks. That way your system is cleared of one combination before you add a different combination. I have included a Sample Somersize Week (p. 98) so you can get an idea of what a whole week's worth of menus looks like. As for when to choose Pro/Fats meals and when to choose Carbos meals, I recommend you eat mostly Pro/Fats meals when you are first beginning the program. This is the most effective way to jump-start your weight loss. The best time to eat your Carbos is in the morning; that way, your body has the whole day to burn off the energy supplied from that meal.

When you're first starting, I usually recommend that you have Carbos for breakfast three to four times a week, and make the rest of your breakfasts, lunches, and dinners Pro/Fats and Veggies meals. (Remember, when you have Carbos for breakfast, you may begin with Fruit, wait twenty minutes, then have your Carbos meal. You may also incorporate fruit as a snack as long as it is two hours after your last meal.)

For lunches and dinners, I would stick to Pro/Fats and Veggies as a rule with Carbos and Veggies as the exception. Just make sure you are balancing your Pro/Fats with plenty of fresh vegetables. You do not want to live on meat and cheese alone! You need vegetables because they supply your body with necessary roughage, and they also give you a small amount of carbohydrates to keep your system balanced.

Somersizing is not a diet. It's a way of eating that is healthy, delicious, and effective. Overall, look at the balance of foods—we eat plenty of fresh fruits and vegetables to provide fiber, vitamins, and minerals; we get whole-grain carbohydrates for energy and additional fiber; and we supply our body with the protein and fat from meat and dairy products that are so essential to our good health. By eating *real* foods instead of processed and refined foods, we are supplying our bodies with the building materials it needs to keep us healthy—not just on the outside, but on the inside as well. What a revelation! All you need to do is follow the simple guidelines, and you can enjoy a slim new body and a healthy new outlook on life.

When Somersizing, you are eating delicious foods in combinations that make your digestive system run like clockwork. Food is digested smoothly and efficiently. Your body extracts what it needs and discards the remainder while you melt away pounds and have more energy than ever before. And because it's so easy to eat this way, you can easily dine in just about any restaurant, prepare meals for yourself by using any of my Somersize recipes, or make meals in minutes with my Somersize food products. And you can create Somersize favorites of your own. Simple. Effective. Incredible!

You probably still have many questions, but this is the fast and easy overview of the program to help get you started. Later in the book I will describe Level One, the weight-loss portion of the program, in detail. Once you have started losing weight, I will describe how to incorporate little cheats in a new category called Almost Level One. Plus, I will outline Level Two for those of you who are ready for maintenance. This program is for life. This is the last weight-loss book you will ever have to read.

If you have not read the previous Somersize books, make sure to read the next sections of *Fast and Easy*. They will supply you with the extended information about the importance of fats, the dangers of sugar, and the truth about insulin, the fat-storing hormone. With cutting-edge research from Dr. Diana Schwarzbein, we'll uncover the scam of the last two decades in regard to the whole fat-free movement and how new medical studies have convinced the greatest skeptics. You'll also learn how deprivation diets will keep you strapped into the diet roller coaster forever. No more! Your ticket off the ride is right here.

The Princess and the Pooch:
A Weight-Loss Fairy Tale

This is a great way to explain Somersizing to your kids. It is a story that may sound like a fairy tale at first but is unfortunately all too real. At least this story can have a happy ending!

Once upon a time, in a faraway land, there was a lovely princess named Penelope. Penelope had everything a young princess could ask for . . . beautiful clothes, a stunning palace, sparkling gems, and suitors from across the land. She loved boat rides on the lake, strolling through the countryside, and riding her horse around the palace grounds. But of all her favorite activities, her very favorite was eating. She'd been seen on the boat gnawing on a baguette. Her walks through the countryside included baskets filled with salami sandwiches and blueberry pie. She was often holding the reins of her horse with one hand and shoveling chocolate cake into her mouth with the other. Indeed,

Penelope loved her food. She was accustomed to royal feasts, and ate to her heart's content at each and every meal. In fact, the kitchen staff had a hard time keeping up with her voracious appetite.

As the years passed, Penelope really started putting on the pounds; she was getting downright poochy for the first time in her life. At first the royal tailors let out all the seams in her gowns, but she kept growing. Soon she had grown out of her clothes completely and the tailors were busy at work making her larger gowns. The townspeople started whispering and nicknamed the Princess "Penelope and the Pooch."

One day Penelope looked at herself in the glass and said, "The people are right. I've got to lose the pooch." Penelope went to her parents for help. The King and the Queen vowed to do whatever they could to help their beautiful young daughter. The King issued an edict across the land to find a diet that could help Penelope lose weight. The King was barraged with doctors, nutritionists, and weight-loss gurus who came with one diet after the other, all with the promise that Penelope could lose weight with ease. Poor poochy Penelope was willing to try whatever it took.

The first diet required Penelope to count calories and fat grams. The staff weighed and measured her food, and when they presented Penelope with her meals, she couldn't believe how minuscule the portions were. She was determined to stick with it and lose the weight, but how she despised the plain food with no flavor. She suffered—she was hungry, cranky, and listless—but the weight started coming off. All the townspeople commented on how slim and lovely Penelope looked. "By golly, Penelope's lost her pooch!"

The Princess was proud of her new slim figure, but this was no way to live! *After weeks of deprivation, she couldn't take it anymore. She burst into the kitchen in the middle of the night and tore into the refrigerator. She devoured whole chickens, mashed potatoes, and an entire platter of chocolate-filled éclairs. Within a short amount of time, she gained back all of the*

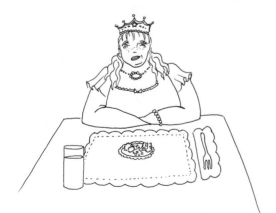

weight, plus a few extra pounds. Penelope's pooch was back.

The Princess was depressed; all that hard work and now she was worse off than when she had started. She was not going to lose this battle of the bulge. She went back to her father, who once again summoned the experts for a new diet for the Princess. This time, Penelope was given a powdered shake for breakfast, a powdered shake for lunch, and a small serving of food for dinner. Steadfast, she stuck with it and choked down the nasty drinks. Oh, how she missed eating real food! By and by the weight came off, and once again the townspeople applauded her efforts while she found herself tired and hungry. The staff commented on how quick she was to anger. She was downright bratty!

The Princess was proud of her new slim figure, but this was no way to live! *Once again, deprivation got the best of her and she slipped into the kitchen and feasted through the night. She ate roasted meats with gravy, bowls of pasta, and an entire cheesecake. Once she was back to her normal eating habits, the weight came back quickly. How she hated being in the spotlight as she rode up and down the scale! Just like the time before, she gained back even more than she had lost.*

Penelope tried to get comfortable in her larger body. Perhaps she was destined to be overweight. She just loved food too much to give it up. If only she

could take away her desire to eat. Once again, she went to her father with this request, and her father summoned the weight-loss experts. *"What Princess Penelope needs is a magic pill to take away her desire for food,"* said the King. The next morning the Princess was given bottles of pills . . . magic pills that would take away her appetite. She took one every day to curb her cravings for food and sweets. It worked! She lost her appetite and soon the weight came off.

The Princess was proud of her new slim figure, but this was no way to live! *Her mother started noticing that Penelope was running in circles, speaking rapid-fire, and shaking uncontrollably. The Queen demanded that the royal doctor examine Penelope. Yes, she was slim, but these "magic" pills were dangerous to her health! The doctor took her off them immediately and warned all the people in the kingdom to stay away from these pills.*

The Princess's pooch returned with force. This time Penelope's weight hit an all-time high, and poor Princess Penelope hit an all-time low. Up and down the diet roller coaster she rode with no end in sight. If only she could find a way to eat the food she loved and still lose weight. It seemed impossible. Even the King felt he had run out of options.

Then one day, a little old lady approached the palace. (Okay, she wasn't that *old.) She introduced herself as Suzanne and asked to speak to the King, claiming that she had the solution for the Princess and the Pooch. The King was not interested because all the experts had led his daughter astray. He wanted to know her credentials. Suzanne explained, "I'm not a doctor. I'm not a nutritionist, but I have found a way to eat incredible food in abundant portions while the pounds melt away. It's called Somersize and it's a revolutionary way of eating that reprograms your metabolism to burn off your stored fat reserves."*

The King was cautious, but intrigued. The woman asked if she could prepare a Somersize meal for the Princess and her family. The King

agreed. Suzanne went to work in the kitchen, searing steaks and roasting chickens. She grilled fish and boiled lobsters. She made cream sauces and butter sauces. She made huge salads and tossed them with real cheese and dressings made from the finest olive oil. She chopped, steamed, and sautéed vegetables, then tossed them in butter and sprinkled them with Parmesan cheese. And then she went to town on desserts. She made rich and creamy cheesecakes, homemade ice cream with hot fudge sauce, and fluffy chocolate mousse. It was a feast fit for a king!

When Princess Penelope sat at the table and saw the spectacular spread, she sighed and said, "Thank goodness I'm no longer on a diet. This food looks incredible. All of my favorite things!" Her father watched her eat with delight. At the end of her meal, the King introduced the Princess to Suzanne and explained that indeed, she had just begun her new diet. Suzanne interrupted, "Forgive me, your Highness, but Somersize is not a diet, it's way of eating that helps you lose weight and gain energy."

The Princess couldn't believe it. Could it really be true? Could she really eat all this amaz-

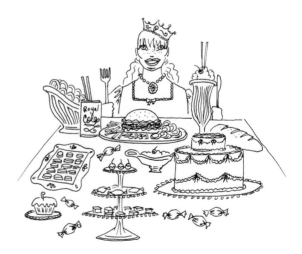

ing food and still lose weight? Suzanne assured her that eating incredible food and losing weight is the premise of Somersizing. The Princess was thrilled! She ate the greatest food of her life, and just as Suzanne had promised, soon the pounds started melting away. Penelope couldn't believe it! The pooch was gone for good. The Princess was so proud of her new slim figure and she said to all the townspeople, "Now this is the way to live . . . the Somersize way!"

And she did . . . slim, healthy, and happily ever after.

COUNTING CALORIES: THE REAL TRUTH BEHIND THE FAIRY TALE

I think many of us see a bit of ourselves in Penelope. We've all tried diets, lost the weight, and then watched the pounds creep back on. All my life I had been thin. Then I hit my forties and my metabolism betrayed me. I put on twenty pounds and could not seem to shake it. I tried one diet after the

next. They all worked . . . but not for long. Dieting was a destructive cycle that always made me feel like a failure. Now I realize I could not have been more wrong. *I was not to blame. And neither are you.* Ninety-five percent of us who go on diets gain back all the weight and often more. Why? Are we all just lazy slobs with no willpower? Conventional dieting in the past few decades has presumed that cutting calories and fat and increasing activity level are the keys to weight loss. We've all tried it and succeeded

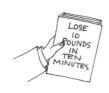

for limited periods of time, but *cutting calories is only a temporary weight-loss solution.* It is also a potentially dangerous weight-loss solution.

SENDING YOUR BODY INTO SURVIVAL INSTINCT

Here's what happens physiologically when you reduce your calorie intake. Let's say your body is used to 1,500 calories a day and you reduce your intake to 1,000 a day. Since your body is used to running on 1,500 calories a day, it must make up for the missing fuel source first by burning off your glycogen and protein stores. (Glycogen is stored with water and, therefore, weighs more than fat. The scale may reflect a substantial weight loss due mostly to the loss of water, not fat. That's what the term "water weight" means.) After your glycogen and protein stores have been depleted, then your body will begin to burn off your fat reserves to provide you with enough energy to get you through the day. This initial burning of fuel is why you will lose weight when you cut your calories.

After this initial weight loss, many of us reach that frustrating plateau. We're still counting every calorie, yet we've stopped losing weight. Why won't our damn bodies cooperate? *It's survival instinct.* As our glycogen and protein stores are being depleted, our metabolism will actually slow down to keep us from starving to death. Your body adapts to

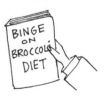

survive on, say 1,000 calories a day, even less fuel than it needed before. Plus, your new lower metabolism means you have a slower-running machine—quite simply, less energy to get through the day, leaving you tired and listless!

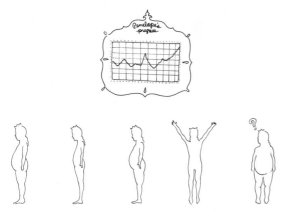

Sound familiar? Tired, deprived, and a halt in weight loss. These are all the trappings of a low-calorie diet. But it gets even worse. Your body recognizes that it's not getting enough food, so it starts to store away a portion of the food. It may use, say, 800 calories for fuel and store 200 as fat for later use. So even though you're still living on poached chicken, rice cakes, and celery sticks, you may actually start to gain a couple of pounds. That's when the deprivation outweighs the results and Penelope bursts into the pantry to binge on any and every morsel of food. It gets worse still. By cutting our calories in the first place, we have forced our bodies to slow down our metabolism, so our bodies actually need fewer calories to survive than they did before the diet. When we go back to eating our previously "normal" 1,500 calories a day, our bodies will have an *excess* of fuel, because they have adapted to

survive on 800 calories a day. That leaves 700 calories that will be stored as fat for later use! That's why we gain all the weight back and then a little extra—it's our new lower metabolism, all thanks to cutting back on those calories.

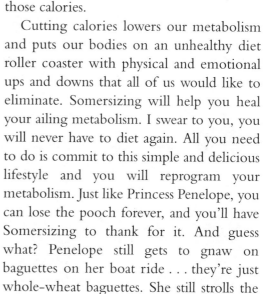

Cutting calories lowers our metabolism and puts our bodies on an unhealthy diet roller coaster with physical and emotional ups and downs that all of us would like to eliminate. Somersizing will help you heal your ailing metabolism. I swear to you, you will never have to diet again. All you need to do is commit to this simple and delicious lifestyle and you will reprogram your metabolism. Just like Princess Penelope, you can lose the pooch forever, and you'll have Somersizing to thank for it. And guess what? Penelope still gets to gnaw on baguettes on her boat ride . . . they're just whole-wheat baguettes. She still strolls the countryside munching on salami (she just eats it without the bread). And she still enjoys chocolate cake; she just makes it with SomerSweet instead of sugar. Hardly a sacrifice at all to lose all the weight you want and feel infused with energy along the way. With Somersizing, you really can live happily ever after.

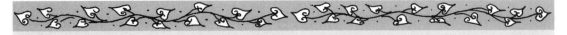

Dear Suzanne,

Little did I know the day I bought your first book that my life was about to change. Being overweight for so many years, and one failed dieting attempt after another, I sighed and thought, "Well, I may as well read *this* book." As you can imagine, I wasn't expecting much when I cracked the cover, thinking I had heard it, read it, and tried it all before. However, the more I read, the more excited I became, and before I finished the book, I thought I could probably eat this way without much trouble. I figured I should at least give it a try.

Soon after I began your program, the weight started dropping off. Encouraged and happy with my results, I bought your other books and started collecting Somersized recipes. That was eleven months and four big ring binders ago! I've lost 75 pounds so far and I'll move on to Level Two when I lose 20 to 30 more. My husband has joined in, and he's lost 36 pounds with just a few more to go. That's over 100 pounds lost between us!

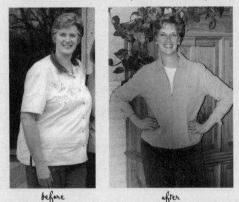

before   after

We sit down to a meal and look at this delicious food, look at each other and start laughing. Who would dream that we could eat like we do and lose weight? So I'd like to offer you my sincerest thanks, Suzanne. You've simply handed me the key I was searching so long for and almost gave up hope of ever finding, the key to not only getting the weight off, but just as important—keeping it off.

With much gratitude,
Debbie Bruce

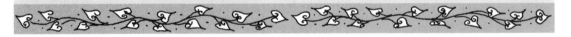

THREE

❖

Sugar: The Evil Villain

No fairy tale would be complete without an evil villain. Enter the most evil one of all . . . *sugar*. It may look like a white knight, all dressed up in "fat-free" rhetoric, but don't be deceived. Sugar is the body's greatest enemy and the most important element to eliminate from our diet.

I know it's not easy. We are addicted to sugar in this country. Do you know that the average American eats over 150 pounds of sugar and sweeteners (like corn syrup) every year? That's up 28 pounds since the early 1970s! We start our mornings off with sugary cereals, Pop-Tarts, or danish. Or we look for low-fat, supposedly healthy alternatives like NutriGrain bars, granola, and bagels made from white flour. These products are still loaded with sugar, starches, and often plenty of chemicals and preservatives.

I have always loved sugar and sweets. I started baking at a very early age with my mother. It was one of the wonderful ways we connected in my otherwise crazy household. I still remember the smells, the tastes, and the thrill of taking a perfectly baked cake out the oven. Baking is still one of my favorite pastimes. When my grandchildren come over, I pull up chairs to the kitchen counter, and they take turns adding the ingredients and stirring the batter. They butter the pans for me, and then we pour the batter, carefully scraping the bowl. Is there anything as cute as a child with flour all over her face as she bites into a piece of freshly baked cake?

Cake . . . baked from scratch. This is how my sugar addiction began. For the rest of my life I would crave the sweet stuff. When I was younger I didn't have a problem eating sugar. I could basically eat whatever I wanted and still stay thin. My body had no trouble metabolizing sugar or any other foods. Then I hit forty and suddenly the party was over. I started noticing a thickness in my midsection. My hips were rounder than ever and I had a hard time holding my stomach in. I would eat a meal and then feel bloated and uncomfortable.

In the eighties everyone started talking about fats, so I tried cutting back. I would carry those little containers of instant noodles so I always had a fat-free snack on hand. The problem got worse, not better. Little did I know those noodles may have been fat-free, but because they were made with white flour, it was the same as eating sugar. They may as well call it "Cup of Sugar"! Like most of us, I was convinced that fat was the problem. I never linked my dips in energy to my sugar intake. I never knew my sugar intake was responsible for my irritability. I never knew my sugar intake was responsible for my rolling hips. And I never knew that eating sugar made me crave even more and more sugar. Then I finally learned that *sugar is the body's greatest enemy!* Surprisingly, sugar is more fattening than fat.

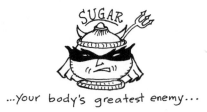

...your body's greatest enemy...

Sugars and starches are carbohydrates, and your body metabolizes them both the same way. Carbohydrates are one of the body's main sources of fuel. The other is fat. In order to understand why some carbohydrates can cause weight problems, let's look at what happens when you eat carbos. When you eat carbos, they break down into glucose, which causes your blood sugar to rise. When the blood sugar is elevated, it is the job of the pancreas to secrete a hormone called insulin. Insulin balances the blood sugar by carrying the glucose to the cells where it will be burned off for energy. By storing the sugar away in the cells, your blood sugar level becomes balanced. If your cells are filled with sugar and will not accept any more, then the insulin will send the sugar to be stored as fat reserves for later use.

INSULIN—THE SWORD OF TRUTH

Insulin is called the "fat-storing hormone" because insulin is responsible for determining whether food will be burned off as energy or stored as fat. *Insulin must be present for food to be stored as fat.* That is why it is vitally important to identify the foods that cause our bodies to secrete insulin. If we can control our insulin levels, we can control our weight.

As I said, when we eat sugar or carbohydrates, our blood sugar is elevated. If your metabolism is working at optimum, first your pancreas secretes insulin; then along with the sugar, the insulin travels to the liver where the sugar will be converted to fat. The fat will be burned off immediately as fuel, or it will be stored as fat. Here's the hitch. We say people are "insulin resistant" when their cells will not accept any additional sugar. When the cells are filled with excess energy and do not need any more sugar or fats for energy this initiates a further release of insulin from the pancreas.

This leads to even higher insulin levels. If the blood sugar and fats are not burned as fuel, they will be stored for later use. *Therefore, even fat-free carbohydrates, like sugar and white flour, can be converted to fat if we do not need the energy at the time we eat.* With this information, one can see how the elevation of our blood sugar can lead to weight gain if we eat too many carbohydrates at one time.

Most of us will experience some degree of insulin resistance because it occurs naturally as we get older (explaining why many of us gain weight as we age). Quite simply, as we get older, our metabolic processes slow down and we do not need as many carbohydrates as we did when we were young. But if we don't change our eating habits, those carbohydrates we used to burn off get stored as fat and we get thick around the middle as the decades stack up.

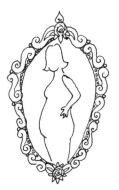

MIRROR, MIRROR ON THE WALL . . . WHO'S GOT THE THICKEST MIDSECTION OF ALL?

Here's the true test, taught to me by Dr. Schwarzbein. Take off your clothes and stand naked in front of the mirror. If you are thick through the middle, then at some point you have had a raised insulin level. If you are a man with love handles and a pot belly, then you have had raised insulin levels. If you are a woman with a thickness around the reproductive areas, such as stomach, hips, thighs, and buttocks, then you have had raised insulin levels. If you have raised insulin levels, that means your cells are filled with sugar and will not accept any more! When your insulin levels are raised and your cells are filled, sugar in any form (a piece of candy, a bowl of pasta, or a potato) will be converted into fat and stored for later use.

Remember—insulin is a hormone, and when we have too much insulin, we throw off our body's entire hormonal balance. Hormonal imbalance leads to weight gain, increased cholesterol, and disease. *Stop listening to those who blame fat . . . I believe that raised insulin is the medical culprit for all of these ills.* The fat-free movement has been a hoax and has finally been revealed to the medical community by two new studies that prove high-protein programs are more effective for losing weight and improving cholesterol than low-fat/high-carb programs.

Many of us have varying degrees of high insulin levels leading to weight gain and disease. Even some children have a genetic predisposition to insulin resistance. Why is it that some kids can eat as much sugar and junk food as they want and they stay thin as rails, and others eat the sugar and junk and end up overweight? Some of it is genetics, but the majority of it is due to the fact that our kids are living on sugar and processed foods. Many kids do not eat enough real food and they think that ketchup and french fries count as vegetables. Their little cells also become overloaded with energy (sugar), and suddenly you have a child with the beginnings of a weight problem . . . a problem that can last a lifetime.

This is not a guilt trip, but if you are a parent of an overweight child, it is time to stop blaming genetics and time to change your family's eating habits. Bad habits can be changed with great food. Your kids will love the food on this program, and they'll never feel like they are on a diet. In the coming chapters I will take you step by step through the program and show you how to Somersize for your kids and turn your home and health around.

Whether you're an adult or a child, a few pounds overweight or obese, it's never too late to improve your health and appearance from the inside out. Now that the true evil villain is exposed, I will show you how to destroy it! That's why the crux of this program is to teach you how to keep your pancreas from oversecreting insulin, which will keep your blood sugar and your hormones balanced. With balance comes weight loss. With balance comes improved cholesterol levels. With balance and weight loss comes decreased risk of heart disease and cancer. When you heal your insulin resistance, your body will unload the stored-up sugar in your cells. That's when "The Melt" begins. Your body will release all that stored sugar, then it will turn to your fat reserves and break them down to use as an energy source. The result? You get thinner and thinner while your body is being fed a constant source of energy.

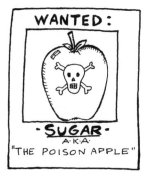

SUGAR—ALSO KNOWN AS "THE POISON APPLE"

Now that we understand the importance of controlling insulin, let's look at the foods that cause our bodies to secrete insulin. The amount your blood sugar is elevated depends upon the amount and the *type* of sugars you are eating. We must learn what sugars are. Sugar is not only the granulated white stuff you use to sweeten your coffee. Potatoes are sugar. White pasta is sugar. Rice is sugar. Bread is sugar. Alcohol is sugar. Cereal is sugar. Milk is sugar. Fruit is sugar.

However, some sugars cause more of an insulin release than others. Carbohydrates in their refined form are much harder on our systems than those in their natural form. In the last century we have refined most of the nutrients out of our foods. White rice is simply brown rice without the nutty exterior. Brown rice has a wonderful flavor and is loaded with fiber you won't find in white rice. Fiber is essential when we are eating carbohydrates because fiber helps lower insulin levels. And how about white flour? Breads and pastas used to be made with natural whole grains, and as the grains became more refined, we as a society gained more and more weight. We can all improve our health by replacing these processed foods with their whole-grain counterparts.

Some studies show that 75 percent of the average American diet is made up of refined carbohydrates like sugar, white flour, white pasta, and instant potatoes. It's no wonder that obesity is epidemic in our country! And being thin is not just a vanity issue. It is a cause for great concern regarding our health. Obesity is the second leading cause of premature death after cigarette smoking. The statistics are staggering. As a country we are becoming more and more obese, especially since we have adopted the "fat-free" mania that has swept the country over the last two decades. These products replace real fats with refined carbohydrates, like sugar, starchy thickeners, and white flour. Here's why the consumption of so many refined carbohydrates is hard on our systems.

Complex carbohydrates (like whole grains and vegetables low in starch) cause only moderate to minimal increases in your

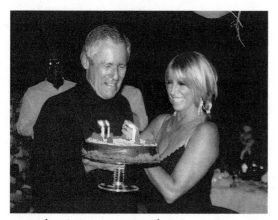

My birthday, my husband, and a Somersized cake.

blood sugar, meaning less insulin is needed to balance the blood sugar. But simple carbohydrates (like sugar, white flour, and potatoes) cause a sharp increase in blood sugar. This surge of blood sugar gives us a "sugar rush" or a "sugar high." I see it with the grandkids. They come over to the house happy, happy, happy. We have a great lunch and then they run around and play. They come back asking for treats, and as the grandmother, I love to spoil them. I give them some form of sugar, and guess what? They go into a major hyper mode while they are experiencing their sugar high and then they crash. The whining and complaining begin. The temper tantrums follow. Yes, I *spoil* them all right. After they come down from the sugar, they are ruined. They go from being happy wonderful little people to irritable kids who need time-outs. Now I have learned my lesson. No more sugar.

Let's recap: Here's what happens to us physiologically when we eat the sugar. As we now know, when we eat sugar, our blood sugar spikes. When the blood sugar is elevated to such a high level, insulin is released; the sugar is carried to the liver, where it is converted to fat. If the insulin is successful, the fat will be burned off as fuel; however, if your cells are filled with sugar, they will not accept any more. When your cells are filled, it's like the doors are closed and the insulin has nowhere to store the blood sugar. Then the pancreas secretes even more insulin to attempt to balance the blood sugar. This results in an excess amount of insulin in the bloodstream, which causes a condition called "hyperinsulinemia." The insulin must find a place to store the blood sugar. If the cells are filled with sugar and won't accept any more, the insulin will then go to the fat cells and store the blood sugar there.

Insulin must be present for food to be stored as fat. This very powerful hormone is the most important decision maker as to whether sugar gets burned as fuel or stored as fat for later use. You may be one of those people who can eat a ton of sugar and just keep burning it off. You're lucky now, but eventually it will probably catch up with you. With a perfect metabolism, sugar will be converted to fat, then sent to the muscle cells, where it will be burned off as energy. Over time, if you consume too much sugar and you become insulin resistant, your muscle cells will become filled with energy and will not accept any more. At this point, the converted sugar is stored in the fat cells, particularly around the midsection. It is at this point that we start to gain weight. The next progression of insulin resistance is Type II diabetes. If the muscle cells are filled, and the fat cells are filled, the liver cannot convert the sugar to fat, so it remains in the bloodstream. This disease is becoming more and more prevalent in our society, even among children. Sugar is poison, and we are slowly killing ourselves with it.

It makes me crazy when I see companies promoting fat-free items loaded with sugar and carbohydrates that will make your insulin levels go through the roof. I see kids eating bags of Jelly Bellies because they are fat free! We have been fooled, and parents . . . we need to wake up. We have been led to believe that fat is the only danger. Fat-free cookies are not going to help us lose weight! Fat-free frozen yogurt is not going to help us lose weight. Fat-free chips are not a free treat. The fat is not the problem. In fact, it is the sugar, the white flour, and the potato that cause the weight gain! And the chemicals that accompany many fat-free products are harmful to your health. Olestra, the fake fat recently approved by the FDA, must carry a warning label because some vitamins and nutrients adhere to it so they cannot be absorbed by your body. We are also warned that eating Olestra may cause abdominal cramping and loose stool syndrome. Is this anything you want to put into your body, or your child's body? If the warning "may cause anal leakage" doesn't turn you off, what will?

If fat-free cookies, cakes, and potato chips sound too good to be true, it's because they are. Fat has been made the fall guy, but sugar is the body's greatest enemy. Effective marketing has duped our society into thinking if we are eating low fat, we are safely eating food that is healthier for us and will not make us fat. But they don't tell us that *sugar turns right to fat and can be harmful to your health!*

After this extra insulin has sent the sugar to the fat cells, eventually our blood sugar is lowered to even below its starting point. That's when we feel the letdown or the "sugar low." This sugar low leaves us feeling tired, listless, and artificially hungry. This is when my grandkids have their tizzy fits. During this time we often feel like taking a nap, or we reach for something sweet or caffeinated to give us more energy—then the vicious cycle repeats. Sugar goes in, blood sugar goes up, pancreas secretes insulin, then blood sugar drops and we feel tired and hungry again, causing us to eat more and more without ever satisfying our nutritional needs.

Now you are beginning to see the importance of insulin in determining whether the broken-down sugar will be burned as fuel or stored as fat. As I mentioned, some complex carbos cause smaller insulin responses (whole grains, green vegetables) and will usually be burned off from the sugar cells as readily available fuel. Other carbos cause larger insulin responses (sugar, white flour, potatoes) and will often be stored as fat because they contain way more energy than our bodies need for immediate use. A single potato is so high in starch, it provides us with more energy than most people need in an entire day. Think about how many excess carbohydrates you eat in a normal day and imagine how much your body actually needs for fuel and how much gets stored as fat. Unless you're a marathon runner, you're probably storing an ample supply of fat reserves from overindulging in the wrong kind of carbohydrates.

You may know people who seem to contradict what I just told you. They live on bad carbs and junk food, wolfing down fries and chips and candy bars and never gaining weight. Keep in mind that each of us is created differently with a unique and ever-changing metabolism. Some people have a perfect metabolism that will always burn the food they eat as fuel—even if it's bad food like refined carbs—rather than storing it as fat. Other people start out with a perfect metabolism, and as they get older their metabolism changes and suddenly they find themselves with a weight problem. But nothing is free. Even if your friends don't

gain weight, they still can be damaged by eating junk food—they are prone to heart attacks, decreased energy, mood swings, and possible early death from poor nutrition.

Whether you have an imperfect metabolism and want to lose weight or your weight is fine and you want to achieve maximum health, Somersizing can help you and your family. By eliminating foods that cause large fluctuations in our blood sugar and by properly combining nutritious, delicious foods, we are able to lose weight and gain energy while achieving our maximum health. Most of us do not have a perfect metabolism, but Somersizing can show you how to *get control* over your metabolism. This program can actually heal your ailing metabolism. It's never too late to change and it's never too late to start better eating habits for you and your whole family.

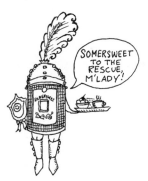

SOMERSWEET—YOUR WHITE KNIGHT IN SHINING ARMOR

Now that we have SomerSweet, saying good-bye to sugar is a piece of cake! Somer-Sweet is the most exciting product I have ever developed. It's five times sweeter than sugar, and because it's blended with natural, sweet fiber, it's something you can feel good about using. It tastes like sugar, it bakes like sugar, it even caramelizes like sugar. With SomerSweet, Somersizing is easier than ever before! Using this remarkable product makes this program no sacrifice at all. You do not have to give up sweets; you just have to give up sugar. I sprinkle SomerSweet on my cereal and oatmeal. I sweeten my decaf coffee and tea. I treat myself with Somer-Sweet Cheesecake, Crème Brûlée, and Ice Cream. It sure doesn't feel like I gave up sugar, except I feel a whole lot better, I look a whole lot slimmer, and my moods are a heck of a lot more even. This is a revolution in taste sensation and weight management.

THE SOMERSIZE SOLUTION: YOUR HAPPILY EVER AFTER

I hope you have a clear picture of how Somersizing works. When your body needs energy, it will first go to the carbohydrates you eat to burn as fuel. If there are fewer carbohydrate sources available, your body will break down your fat reserves when you need energy. By cutting back on sugar and highly starchy foods, you force your body to melt away your fat reserves as an energy source.

That's the key to Somersizing. We convert our bodies from carbo-burning machines into fat-burning machines. By limiting our sugars and starches, we force our bodies to break down our fat reserves to use as a constant source of energy. No sugar highs and lows—just an even source of energy to get through the day as we watch our fat melt away.

The good news is that you don't have to say good-bye to sugar and starches forever. While you are on the weight-loss portion of the program, Level One, the built-up sugar is being emptied from your cells. When you reach your goal weight, you will advance to Level Two, the maintenance portion of Somersizing. On Level Two you may incorporate some sugar and starches back into your eating plans (in moderation). Because your cells are no longer filled with sugar, they can handle moderate amounts without becoming overloaded. That is why on Level Two some previously forbidden sugars and starches are permitted, because they will be burned off rather than stored as fat.

It's time for you to live happily ever after in the world of Somersize, but first, read on about your new best friend, fat!

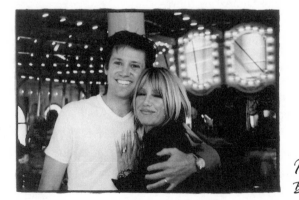

I adore my son Bruce.

FOUR

Fat: Your Friend for Life

In every good story there's a protagonist who is accompanied by a friendly sidekick. This friend is often good-natured, sensible, supportive, and a little chubby. That's right, I'm talking about the "lovable fat friend." Our Somersize story is no different. When you Somersize, fat is your lovable friend. Eating fats is sensible. Fats support healthy cellular function and healthy cellular reproduction. Fats can help you lose weight . . . and they taste incredible! It's true; when you Somersize, you may eat fats and still lose weight. Fats are your friend for life.

I've spent a great deal of time defending my position on fats. The mainstream medical establishment certainly does not share my opinions about fat! They believe that dietary fats are the primary cause of weight gain, obesity, and poor health. I just don't agree. How can I make a statement as bold as that? I've done my homework; countless hours of research reading medical journals

and having long discussions with my greatest teacher, Dr. Schwarzbein. We've been led to believe that eating fats will make us gain weight, increase our cholesterol, and eventually make us die from heart disease. If you accept that as the truth, then how do you explain the following facts? In the last two decades Americans have cut their fat intake from 38 percent to 34 percent of their daily calories, and yet in that same time period the average weight per person has increased by eight pounds! How can that be? Isn't a reduced-fat diet supposed to help us lose weight? Doesn't less fat in our diets mean less fat on our bodies? Not necessarily. We keep hearing, "Eat less fat. Eat less fat," and we have obeyed. When I wrote the first Somersize book in 1996 I quoted the following statistic:

"The percentage of adults who are overweight has *increased* by 10% since 1980. Over 37% of females and 34% of males are now overweight. Obesity is rampant in our country, and everyone thinks fat is to blame."

I was shocked when I looked at my research and learned that today, 54.9 percent of Americans are overweight! In eight years we've gone from 37 percent to over half the nation. Yes, we have a problem, but fat is not to blame.

When you Somersize, you may eat steak with melted herb butter. You may eat eggs fried in bacon fat. You may eat chicken with mushroom cream sauce. You may pour full-fat dressings on your salads. You may freely snack on cheese. "Impossible," you say. Hark back to the previous chapter and remember what we learned about insulin. Insulin is the fat-storing hormone. Insulin is solely responsible for deciding whether food will be burned as fuel or stored as fat. *Insulin must be present for food to be stored as fat.* Eating dietary fat causes virtually no secretion of insulin. Without the presence of insulin, food cannot be stored as fat. Regardless of how much fat you eat, the pancreas will not secrete insulin, *which is the only way fat can be stored as body fat.* As long as you are eating in Somersize combinations, you may eat fat and still lose weight.

On the contrary, you can gain weight if you eat proteins or fats *with* sugars or carbohydrates. Here's why. If you eat a Pro/Fat alone, like a piece of meat, your body will break it down easily. Pro/Fats will not cause weight gain when eaten alone because they trigger virtually no increase in your blood sugar levels, so there is not a significant insulin response. Pro/Fats can also be eaten in combination with vegetables low in

starch (which are also foods that cause little to no insulin production). Therefore, eating Pro/Fats, like eggs, meat, cheese, and butter, will not make you fat when eaten in the suggested Somersize combinations.

Let's say you eat Pro/Fats *with* a carbohydrate, like meat with potatoes. The body

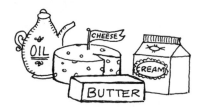

should use the carbohydrates in the potato for energy, extract the protein and healthy fats from the meat, and discard the remainder. But the carbohydrates in the potato will trigger an insulin response that can lead to both the potato *and* the meat being sent to the fat cells. So say good-bye to meat and potatoes, white bread with cheese, or turkey with yams. I know this may sound difficult, but there are so many other things you can eat in the right combinations you won't even miss these foods. Once your body is back in balance you may enjoy this combination in moderation.

Believe it or not, fat is not fattening when eaten alone. You can eat fat with other fats, with proteins, or with vegetables in Somersize combinations and still lose weight. This is a sinfully indulgent way to lose weight! No more poached fish served only with lemon . . . bring on the lemon-caper butter sauce. No more plain steamed vegetables . . . bring on the hollandaise sauce. No more dry chicken breasts . . . leave the skin on and serve it with pan drippings! No more sugary, starchy, fat-free desserts . . . bring on the SomerSweet Crème Brûlée made with real cream!

Okay, so now you know you can eat fat. Does that mean you should chug down a gallon of duck fat, or live on a diet of meat and cheese? Of course not. There is no need to gorge on fats or any of the Somersize foods. Somersize promotes balanced eating filled with essential nutrients from several food groups. Besides, your body will tell you when you've had enough fat and signal you to stop. What a thrill it is to know that I can enjoy a piece of Brie without guilt. How wonderful not to feel deprived when you're trying to lose weight! I think that's the main reason Somersizing has been so successful with everyone who has tried it. You can incorporate rich, flavorful foods into your diet and still lose all the weight you want; that helps people stick to the program.

FAT—EAT TO YOUR HEART'S CONTENT

I hope at this point I have convinced you that you may eat fat in Somersize combinations and still lose weight. If you have embraced that lovely thought, you are probably still concerned about increasing your cholesterol levels, increased risk of heart disease, and certain types of cancer. We've been told that a diet low in fat will help improve our risk of these health problems. I'm going to change your thinking about this as well. When you Somersize, you may eat fat to your heart's content . . . and I mean that literally.

The preliminary medical research I found on cholesterol, heart disease, and cancer from the 1970s to the present all placed significant blame for these illnesses on dietary fat. However, the deeper I dug, the more information I found that led me to different conclusions. Actually, insulin resistance is one of the main ingredients in your recipe for high cholesterol and heart disease. (Later in this book you can read about the numerous studies that back up these claims.) Eating in proper Somersize combinations helps control your insulin levels, which subsequently helps improve your cholesterol. I've heard it time and time again from all of you who have seen the results for yourself. I cannot count the hundreds and hundreds of testimonial letters from people who tell me how their cholesterol profile is improving while they are eating the richest foods of their lives. Their doctors are stunned!

Fortunately, I have begun to see the medical community sit up and take notice. On the news the other night, I saw a segment about a medical study that proved high insulin levels were responsible for increased cholesterol. The newscasters warned people that perhaps fat isn't the problem . . . maybe we should watch our sugar and carbohydrate intake. The anchors seemed a little miffed: "Hmm, what do you know?" This is hardly new information! This is not even controversial in the medical community. Over twenty years of studies link high insulin levels to raised cholesterol levels and heart disease. This information is undisputed. Fat just took center stage because one lone study about dietary fat in the early eighties changed everyone's thinking about

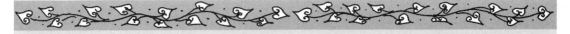

Dear Suzanne,

Somersizing has changed my life. Before starting your plan almost two years ago, I was nearly 100 pounds heavier. I didn't believe in diets so I did nothing about my weight problem. I wanted to find something I could stick with for the rest of my life, a total eating-habit change. When my friend Kathy told me about your plan, I was totally resistant. What, give up my peanut butter toast? A month later while surfing the Web, I ran into some testimonials for your plan. Then I decided to buy your book.

I couldn't believe how much yummy food I could eat and still lose weight. I eat more veggies than I did before, and even though I eat all the stuff doctors tell you to avoid when trying to lower your cholesterol, mine has gone down 60 points since starting your program. It has been surprisingly easy

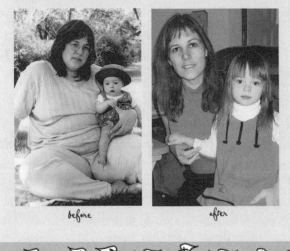

before   after

to stick with Somersizing because I am so satisfied with what I can eat. When I do have that rare craving or temptation, I tell myself that if I eat that funky thing, then I won't be able to eat all the "fattening" stuff I have been enjoying to lose weight.

I feel I have finally found the miracle diet that I have been waiting for all these years. Thank you, Suzanne, for the difference you've made in my life.

Sincerely,
Nancy Ward

the role of fat in heart disease. Since then, our country has been on a fat-free frenzy that's hotter than Britney Spears.

When I wrote the very first Somersize book, *Eat Great, Lose Weight,* I had enough knowledge to know that you could eat fats and still lose weight. I learned about the insulin connection and how this hormone is responsible for weight gain. Still, I was worried about overall fat consumption because of the apparent connection to cholesterol, so I advised that we consume fats in moder-

ation. It was not until I was writing my second Somersize book, *Get Skinny on Fabulous Food,* that I gained a wealth of knowledge about the real reason for raised cholesterol. Once again, the culprit is raised insulin levels! This information came to me from a doctor who would become one of the most influential people in my life, Dr. Diana Schwarzbein.

I felt like I had met my soul sister in defending fat. Her clinical findings prove not only that fat is not dangerous to our health, but also that it is essential to our health! Now, with more conviction than ever, I proudly preach my Somersize mantra that *fat is your friend!* I will also share here all the up-to-date findings that show how important fat is to our diet. Dr. Schwarzbein explains in her book, *The Schwarzbein Principle,* the important role of fat in creating healthy cells. If we do not eat enough dietary fat, we are damaging our cells and our bodies' ability to reproduce new cells. When cell abnormalities develop, disease can set in.

MEET YOUR FATS—POLY, MONO, UNSATURATED, SATURATED, AND TRANS

A balanced diet, including fat, is essential to life. When I say fat, I don't mean the fat you give your body in the form of cake, or fat from a candy bar, or fat from french fries. There are several different types of fat. Some are good, in fact essential to your health and well-being. Other fats should be eliminated from your diet. There are two main types of fats: saturated and unsaturated. Saturated fats include butter, lard, coconut oil, and palm oil. These types of fats are usually solid at room temperature. Unsaturated fats are generally liquid at room temperature. These liquid types of fat are categorized as monounsaturated—such as olive oil, canola oil, and nut oil—or polyunsaturated—such as corn oil or safflower oil. All of these fats are included in the Somersize program.

Trans fats are the fats that come from polyunsaturated fat, like partially hydro-genated oil. These trans fats are the most unhealthy kind because they are completely unnatural. Margarine is an excellent example. We've been led to believe that margarine is a healthier choice than real butter, because butter is saturated and margarine is unsaturated. But margarine is made by taking a vegetable oil and stripping it of its essential fatty acids. The remainder is processed by forcing hydrogen atoms into it. When complete, margarine, which comes in a solid state, is actually more saturated than its original liquid form. Trans fats also occur when we heat polyunsaturated fats (like vegetable oil) to high temperatures for frying. I know it sounds ironic, but you are actually better off frying food in saturated fat—like butter, lard, or palm kernel oil—or in monounsaturated fat—like peanut oil—than you are frying it in polyunsaturated oil like corn, safflower, or vegetable oil. We've been led to believe these polyunsaturated oils are a healthier choice, but beware of frying foods with them because when heated too high, they become the most unhealthy types of fats—trans fats.

In response to the fat scare, many restaurants and food chains boast that they fry only in "cholesterol free" oils, like vegetable, corn, or safflower oil. These "healthy" oils in their natural state become dangerous trans fats when heated to high temperatures for frying! Don't be duped by fat-free propaganda. Eating foods filled with these trans fats is bad for our health. Trans fats are rampant in the processed foods we eat. It's not just the fries at restaurants. They appear in almost every snack food that comes in a bag or a box at the grocery store—cakes, cookies, crackers, breads, chips, margarine, bottled salad dressings, and more. Many of the low-fat varieties of these foods are filled with trans fats.

And why are trans fats so bad for us? They raise your bad cholesterol (LDL) and lower your good cholesterol (HDL). Plus, they muck up your cells with these fake fats and actually block your body from accepting the good fats it needs to produce healthy cells. Sadly, people are eliminating saturated fats, like eggs, cheese, butter, and red meat, thinking they are the culprits for raised cholesterol and heart disease, when in actuality raised insulin levels and trans fats are the problems. Since the introduction of fake foods into our society, we have been on a fast road to weight gain and disease. When I was a child, my mother baked me cookies made with real butter. That was considered a treat. Now cookies are prepackaged in the grocery store, depleted of any real fats and filled with unhealthful trans fats.

Get back to eating real fats like butter, cream, cheese, sour cream, and eggs! Most doctors will tell you that eating foods high in saturated fats is a recipe for weight gain and a heart attack. They will tell you these are the types of "fatty" foods that will raise our cholesterol. They advise us to stick to unsaturated fats in minimal amounts. So how can I share with you my program with a clear conscience when Somersizing supports eating saturated fats to your heart's content? Because I have done the research and have seen that the majority of the medical community is wrong! Finally, in 2002, we have the mainstream medical establishment sitting up and taking notice of the health benefits of low-carbohydrate programs. Saturated fats are good fats and essential to life. They must be included in our daily meals.

There has been an ongoing study in Framingham, Massachusetts, that has followed the diets and health of a large test group of citizens of this city. For many years this study supported the notion that saturated fats increase our risk of cholesterol. However, Dr. William Castelli, who was the director of the study, has changed his tune. In 1992 he was quoted:

> In Framingham, Massachusetts, the more saturated fats one ate, the more cholesterol one ate, the more calories one ate, the lower people's serum cholesterol. . . . We found that the people who ate the most cholesterol, the most saturated fat, ate the most calories, weighed the least, and were the most physically active.

Most of the women who had better health reports got their fats from eating creamy salad dressings two to three times per week. The moral of the story is: Bring on the blue cheese, creamy Italian, and Caesar dressings and stay away from the tasteless fat-free dressings with ingredient lists that no one can pronounce.

After I read all the dramatic Somersize testimonial letters, it makes more sense to me than ever. People are bringing cheese, cream, and bacon back into their lives, and they have healthier cholesterol levels than ever before. Plus, they're losing weight. This is a dramatic turnaround. I have a friend who is trying to get her cholesterol down. I keep telling her about Somersizing, but it's too much of a departure from her doctor's recommendations for lowering cholesterol. We were sharing a cup of coffee (mine was decaf), and she asked what I would like in my coffee. I happen to drink it black, but I watched as she poured fat-free, nondairy creamer into her coffee. The number one ingredient? Sugar! It's made with corn syrup and a load of unpronounceable words. And this is supposed to be a healthier choice than pure cream? Here is my friend banging her head against the wall as she watches every bit of fat and tries to exercise . . . but she's filling her meals with hidden sugars and starches that keep her insulin levels up. Raised insulin levels cause raised cholesterol levels. This is an undisputed medical fact. Some people just don't want to hear it.

Here is my message to people who just don't believe they can eat fat for health reasons: at least give up the sugar and the refined carbohydrates. If you are giving up fat and still not seeing your cholesterol drop, you must also try giving up the sugar and starches. When you see your cholesterol begin to drop, perhaps you will believe me that you can begin to eat fats and watch your numbers further improve. Then, my friend, you will thank me from here to kingdom come as you become one of the countless success stories of Somersizers who eat decadent foods while they lose weight and become healthier than ever. Please, won't you join me?

We are on the brink of a turnaround. I can feel it. Even the die-hard medical conservatives telling us to limit our fat intake and replace real fats with fat substitutes are coming around slowly. They are still adhering to the low-fat diet, but they are recognizing the need to limit sugar consumption as well.

I TOLD YOU SO

The questions raised by the plummeting health of our low-fat society have inspired several medical studies. More and more data is pouring in supporting the benefits of essential fats. The medical community does not trust testimonial letters, and they shouldn't. They only trust carefully monitored controlled studies. Teams of medical experts, out to prove the dangers of high-protein/low-carbohydrate weight loss programs, have recently completed these highly anticipated clinical trials to show

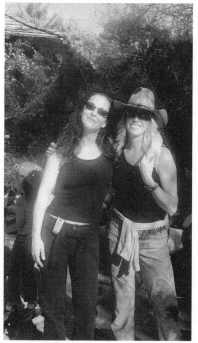

Caroline, my daughter and partner, and me.

the world the dangers of eating too much protein and fat.

The preliminary results were presented from a randomized controlled trial at the University of Pennsylvania, University of Colorado, and Washington University. The trial compared the Atkins Diet with a conventional low-fat, high-carbohydrate plan that restricted daily caloric intake to 1,200 to 1,500 calories for women and 1,500 to 1,800 calories for men. The Atkins group, after twelve weeks, lost twice as much weight as the low-cal/low-fat group, and had only 12 percent drop out of the program, compared to 30 percent of dropouts in the low-fat group. As for cholesterol? The low-fat group lowered their overall cholesterol and their LDL (the bad cholesterol), whereas the Atkins group, even though they had slightly higher total cholesterol, increased their HDL (good cholesterol) and improved their triglycerides and their overall cholesterol "ratio." Those enlightened in the medical field will tell you that the HDL to LDL ratio is more important than your total cholesterol number.

A similar study was held at Duke University. The researchers compared a low-carb diet with a low-fat/low-cal diet. At six months the low-carb group had lost considerably more weight and significantly more fat mass than the low-fat group. Similarly to the three-center study described earlier, the low-fat group lowered their total cholesterol and the low-carb group showed significant increases in their good cholesterol (HDL) and a significant decrease in cholesterol/HDL ratio. Both groups showed decreases in triglycerides.

It shocked the researchers that the high-protein program actually improved cholesterol, but it didn't shock me, or Dr. Schwarzbein, or Dr. Atkins, I'm sure. Never before have I wanted to say "I told you so!" more. (And just a quick note on Dr. Atkins, who recently suffered from a heart attack—his condition was diagnosed as a heart infection unrelated to cholesterol or hardening of the arteries.) Check out the additional medical studies listed in the back of the book. It's fascinating to read all this research and still hear doctors saying we should limit fats. Get the word out! Everyone should have this critical information.

Real fats are your friend and partner in good health. Your body cannot produce fats on its own; therefore, two important essential fatty acids must come from the food you eat. Let's look at two important essential fatty acids that we must include in our diets to enjoy health and longevity: omega-3 and omega-6. Omega-3 can be found in egg yolks, fish (salmon, tuna, herring, mackerel), nuts, soybeans, canola oil, and flaxseed oil. Omega-6 can be found in egg yolks, dark green leafy vegetables, whole grains, and seeds. (My doctor recommends a supplement called borage oil that is an excellent source of omega-6 and also helps tremendously to reduce the symptoms of PMS and menstrual cramps.)

Eggs are a wonderful food, a great source of protein and healthy fats. Omega-3 and omega-6 essential fatty acids are appropriately named "essential"! I eat as many eggs a week as I want. I often eat three eggs for breakfast and it really keeps me satisfied. It's as if my body is so happy with the nutrients

I have given it, that it is perfectly content until the next meal. Believe me, you don't feel that way when you eat a bowl of Frosted Flakes for breakfast. An hour or so later, you start craving more sugar or caffeine to make up for the dip in your blood sugar levels. Eat your eggs. The campaign does not lie; they are incredible and edible and a great way to get your protein and healthy fats.

Real fats are necessary for healthy cell reproduction. We need fats to make hormones, and hormones are essential for breaking down old cells and making new ones. "Why is healthy cell reproduction so important?" you ask. The human body is made up of cells. We must produce healthy cells to thrive. When we deny our bodies the nutrients they need for healthy cell reproduction, we will start producing abnormal cells. That's when disease sets in. You *should* care about healthy cells, because if you don't, your health is at risk. We must have sufficient hormones to make healthy cells, and we must have healthy cells to make more hormones. The health benefit comes from eating *real* fat in its natural state, like butter, oil, cheese, sour cream, eggs, or fat found in meat or fish.

HAPPY, HEALTHY CELLS

Dr. Schwarzbein explains that in the normal aging process, hormone levels will decline, causing the subsequent loss of healthy cells. Simply, aging results when our bodies break down more cells than they build up. Although there is no way to prevent *normal* metabolic aging, our society is on what Dr. Schwarzbein calls a frightening *accelerated* metabolic aging path. Bad eating habits, stress, caffeine, alcohol abuse, and inactivity can lead to extended periods of high-insulin levels that prematurely age our bodies on a cellular level. This aging process leads to disease.

In addition, when the hormone insulin is present at increased levels, it can disrupt every other hormonal system in the body, which can lead not only to excessive body fat, but to degenerative diseases of aging such as different types of cancer, cholesterol abnormalities, coronary artery disease, high blood pressure, osteoporosis, stroke, and Type II diabetes. *Hormonal imbalances always lead to disease.* We must control our insulin levels so as not to disrupt every other hormonal system in the body!

Furthermore, women who are already going through menopause are at extreme risk of disease. As women age, we naturally become more insulin resistant, which explains why it gets harder to stay slim as we get older. Adopting a high-carb diet exacerbates the problem because all those carbohydrates increase insulin resistance. The elevated amount of insulin in the blood increases testosterone levels, which further blunts the production of the female sex hormones, estrogen and progesterone. Compound the problem with a low-fat diet and you have even lower hormone production because we must consume dietary fat to create hormones. Besides the uncomfortable side effects of hot flashes, cramping, and mood swings, an imbalance of these sex hormones means we cannot produce healthy cells! It is at the critical stage of menopause that women become vulnerable to disease.

I hope I've made clear the connection between nutrition and health. Everything we put into our mouths, good or bad, has a direct effect on our health. We all know eating junk food is bad for us, yet I don't think we consider the consequences of the bad food choices we make. Years of poor eating habits cumulatively add up to damaged cells and our bodies' inability to produce new, healthy cells. When we eat poorly, we age faster, not only externally, but internally as well! And this accelerated metabolic aging process leaves us vulnerable to disease at an earlier age. Eating right isn't just about weight loss, but total health that will last us throughout our lives.

RADICAL, MAN

I've explained how important it is to eat real food and real fat to lose weight, but we need to stay away from processed foods and trans fats for another important health reason as well. Processed foods can also introduce free radicals into our systems. Free radicals are molecules that carry an extra electron. Since electrons need to be paired off, these free radicals roam through our system like little home wreckers, trying to steal electrons from healthy cells. This process damages our system on a cellular level. Antioxidants, such as Vitamin E, Vitamin A, and Vitamin C, help to neutralize free radicals. But when we replace real food (which includes natural vitamins) with processed food, we are not supplying our bodies with the natural antioxidants they need to fight the free radicals; instead, we are introducing more free radicals into our system! The damage that results over time accelerates the metabolic aging process and leads to insulin resistance, then disease and possible early death. Ironically, two of the most powerful antioxidants, Vitamin A and Vitamin E, are found in foods that contain fat.

Processed foods and trans fats aren't the only things compromising our health. Consider that the average American drinks 42 gallons of sugary soft drinks every year! Recent studies show that this consumption is a contributing factor to the startling rise in childhood obesity. We are literally killing ourselves with sugar and chemicals that break down our bodies on a cellular level. The sugar and caffeine in one cola wreak havoc on your body by spiking insulin levels. Think about it every time you consider having a can of soda. Imagine the insulin in your body looking unsuccessfully for places to store the abundance of glucose and visualize how the sugar then gets converted into fat because your cells just cannot accept any more sugar. Visualize the free radicals sweeping through your system, damaging your cells.

With diet drinks you don't have the sugar to contend with, but you have the additional free radicals from the artificial sweeteners and other ingredients. Many kids drink this poison regularly, and many adults drink diet sodas by the gallon. Imagine what it might be doing to your healthy cells. It's not worth it.

I know I've just thrown a lot of informa-

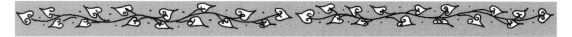

Dear Suzanne,

Somersizing is the best thing that has ever happened to me. I have been overweight my entire life, and I've tried just about every diet system out there. When I came off a particular program, I gained back what I had lost and then some. At one point I weighed 288 pounds because of this yo-yo effect.

Your plan was a revelation for me. I used to be the microwave queen. If it came frozen and said "low fat" on the carton, I bought it. I never realized it was the added sugar in those meals that was sabotaging my weight-loss efforts. Now, I only use my microwave to reheat the wonderful meals I am creating every day. The food is fabulous, easy to make, and the desserts are out of this world. Who would have thought I could eat dessert and not feel guilty!

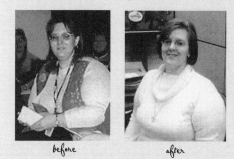

before   after

I have lost 20 pounds so far, and over 16 total body inches. I still have a way to go, but for the first time in my life, I feel confident that I will make my goal and stay there. I have no urge to go back to the unhealthy way I was eating before. This is for life—my life. And I can finally live it the way I always wanted.

Thank you so much,
Kathy Nichols

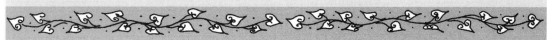

tion your way, but try looking at your body the way I look at mine—I visualize all my happy little cells. As I get older, I know some of them will die off and there is nothing I can do about that. But I imagine what happens when I am not giving my body the proper combination of nutritious foods, and I see the cells dying off at a rapid rate. When I give my body the protein, fat, and complex carbohydrates it needs, my cells thrive, and I feel empowered that I can stave off disease and aging for as long as possible. How wonderful to realize that Somersizing not only keeps me in control of my weight, but it also keeps me at my metabolic prime. I know the food I am eating is creating millions of happy cells that keep me youthful, slim, and healthy.

FIVE

Growing Family Problems: An Obesity Epidemic

Many centuries ago, being overweight was actually considered a status symbol. Kings, queens, dukes, and duchesses flaunted their protruding porcine bellies, their Rubenesque hips, and their corpulent thighs. Only the very wealthy could afford to gorge themselves enough to become overweight. Indeed, Princess Penelope would actually have been applauded for her pooch.

Today it's a different story. It seems every time I turn on the news I see another pro-

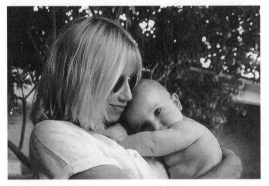

Grandchildren are a gift.

gram about a growing epidemic in our country . . . overweight individuals and obesity. The United States is the fattest nation in the world, and the statistics are overwhelming for adults and children alike. Absorb these statistics:

- 97.1 million Americans are overweight, meaning they have a Body Mass Index of 25 or greater. (BMI is a universally recognized cross-measure of weight for height and stature. A score of 25 indicates a body weight of 25 percent above an individual's ideal body weight.) As I cited earlier, overweight adults make up 54.9 percent of the U.S. population. More than half of us are clinically overweight!

- 39.8 million adults are obese (BMI of 30 or greater). That's an astonishing one-fifth of Americans. In fact, the prevalence of obesity has increased 61 percent between 1991 and 2000, with every single state in the nation showing a statistical increase.

We know the problem is lack of exercise and poor diet. We have become a nation with two staples: fast food and television. Only 22 percent of American adults meet recommended physical activity guidelines. Seventy percent do not exercise regularly and say they *never* engage in physical activity during their leisure time.

"So what?" you ask. "We are a nation obsessed with being thin and beautiful." If you think the cause for concern is vanity, you are sorely mistaken. Each year, 62.7 million doctor visits are related to obesity. Approximately 280,000 deaths are attributed to obesity each year, making it the second leading cause of preventable death next to cigarette smoking. We're talking about your life here. If you look around, you'll notice that you don't see old people who are obese. They simply don't live that long. The University of Colorado's James O. Hill, the dean of American obesity studies, says that if we don't get control of this nationwide problem, almost all Americans will be overweight within a few generations. As quoted in the *Arizona Republic,* he said, "Becoming obese is a normal response to the American environment."

And how about our kids? Super-scary statistics here. From 1980 to 1994, the prevalence of obesity among children has increased an alarming 100 percent. In 1998, the new U.S. Surgeon General, Dr. David Satcher, declared childhood obesity to be epidemic. Today, at least 25 percent of our kids under the age of nineteen are overweight or obese. Satcher told policymakers, "Today we see a nation of young people seriously at risk of starting out obese and dooming themselves to the difficult task of overcoming a tough illness."

If you think he's being dramatic calling the weight state of our union an "epidemic," I will tell you I don't think it's dramatic enough. Referring to obese children, William Dietz, the director of nutrition at the Centers for Disease Control, said, "This is an epidemic in the U.S. the likes of which we have not had before in chronic disease." The public health costs are predicted to run into the hundreds of billions by the year 2020. That's hundreds of *billions,* with a "B!" Economically, it could make the AIDS epidemic look like a case of the common cold.

Childhood obesity rates are particularly frightening for African American and Hispanic communities. In 1986 the rate of obesity for children ages 4 to 12 was 8 percent for African Americans, 10 percent for Hispanics, and 8 percent for Caucasians. By 1998 those figures jumped to an astonishing 22 percent for Blacks, 22 percent for Hispanics, and 12 percent for Whites. Yikes. Not only is this a major health scare, it takes an emotional toll as well. Children who are overweight or obese are subjected to teasing and severe cruelty from other kids. This can cause depression and even violence. Kids and insensitive adults alike can be so mean! Any overweight person knows the discrimination he or she is faced with on a daily basis. The problem is undisputed . . . but why the enormous increase in this deadly illness? Some say advanced technology is to blame. Simply, it takes less effort for us to get food. There is no hunting and gathering to speak of. We don't even have to get out of our cars to order our burger and fries. Oh, yes, and don't forget to Supersize it! That way you'll get twice as many fries and four times as much soda. As a consumer you think, "Heck, it's only 69 cents. Why not?" Lucky you, for under a buck you get a year's supply of extra insulin. Fast food is a nutrient zero; poor-quality meat or poultry, sugary sauces, and white flour buns. Add to that sugary, pressed potatoes fried in oil and a soft drink the size of a bucket. This is not real food. Why do you think you cannot duplicate the taste of a fast food hamburger at home?

When you Supersize your meal and drink your huge soda, what happens to all that insulin? By now you know the procedure: If your cells are filled with sugar, and will not accept any more, the pancreas will secrete more insulin to try to balance the blood sugar. Now your body is in a state of "hyperinsulinism." Since the cells are filled, the insulin will then carry the sugar to the fat cells where it will be stored for later use. This storage in the fat cells balances the blood sugar. This is how sugar can make us gain weight. And when you are eating sugar, the high calorie and fat content matter! Now that whole mass of food has the potential to be stored as fat.

The more serious problem occurs when the fat cells are also filled and will not accept the sugar. Now the insulin has nowhere to store the glucose and so the blood sugar remains elevated. This condition is known as Type II diabetes. Sixteen million Ameri-

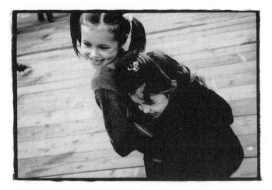

Could they be cuter?

cans suffer from Type II diabetes (often called adult onset diabetes), and yet one-third of them are unaware of their condition. The Super Big Gulp of today could lead to the amputated limbs, blindness, and even death associated with the more serious forms of diabetes.

The American Diabetes Association reports that between 8 and 45 percent of newly diagnosed cases of childhood diabetes are Type II, non-insulin dependent, which is usually associated with obesity and is caused by resistance to insulin and by the inability of the pancreas to keep up with the increased demand for insulin. I guess we can't just call it "adult onset" diabetes anymore. In 1990, the ADA reports, fewer than 4 percent of childhood diabetes cases were Type II; that number has risen to 20 percent! Eighty-five percent of children diagnosed with Type II diabetes are obese. The ADA attributes the increase in Type II diabetes to the fact that more children lead sedentary lives and overeat. I will add that our kids live on sugar and high-starch foods that lead to insulin overload. They don't have a chance unless we change these bad habits.

Unlike the royal feasts of the past where the rich got fat, today it's the poor who are the most prone to weight gain. Almost 66 percent of African American women and 56.5 percent of African American men are overweight. In the Mexican American community, it's 65.9 percent of women and 63.9 percent of men. The owners of fast-food chains prey on lower income consumers. In fact, one out of every four hamburgers at a leading fast food chain is sold to inner-city consumers who are predominantly young black men. The demand for inexpensive meals outside the home is the mainstay of fast-food chains.

If you think kids have so much energy that they'll just burn off all that extra sugar, you're wrong. Teenage kids today have cut their physical activity in half. When we were kids we used to play in the neighborhood. Our afternoons were filled with games of kick the can and running through parks and fields. These days we don't feel safe letting our kids run off as long as they show up at dinnertime. Many young people do not have access to safe parks and places to

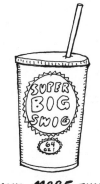

CONTAINS **MORE** THAN
1¼ CUPS OF SUGAR!

play. Today our kids watch TV, play video games, surf the Internet, and curl up with Game Boys. And many of us don't eat dinner together as a family. So the kids end up with a burger, fries, and cola that are twice the size they used to be, but their activity level is half the size of kids a generation ago. You do the math . . . it doesn't take a degree in nutrition to figure this one out.

SOFT-DRINK SUICIDE

I'm always shocked when I see people drinking a soft drink that is the size of a keg of beer. I have never been a fan of sodas. I'm not trying to be righteous—they just aren't my vice, but believe me, I have plenty of others. If you are drinking sugary soft drinks, you'll be astonished to know just how much sugar you are consuming in your "fat free" beverage. One 12-ounce can of Pepsi Cola has 41 grams of sugar. That's about ¼ cup of sugar. Next time you want a soft drink, sit yourself down and pour ¼ cup of sugar in a bowl and eat it with a spoon. I don't think you will ever drink another can again. And if you're someone who likes those 64-ounce Super Big Gulps, you are getting more than 1¼ cups of sugar just from your drink! If you allow your children to drink sugary sodas, the bowl of sugar and a spoon is a great way to get them off it as well. Talk to them about the effect sugar has on their teeth. Explain how junk food damages their healthy cells. Explain to them that eating too much sugar can make you gain weight. Let them know that sugar provides the body with no nutrients.

Sodas and other sugar-sweetened beverages are poison. They will keep your insulin levels spiking all day long. When your blood sugar drops between sodas you will become artificially tired or hungry. What happens when you are tired or hungry? You reach for a quick "pick me up" like a can of soda or junk-food snacks. If you drink caffeinated sodas, you double the problem. Caffeine causes even more of an insulin response and also blocks the hormone serotonin, which can throw your entire hormonal system off balance.

It's not just the sodas. Kool-Aid, Gatorade, fruit punch, Snapple . . . all of these sugar-sweetened drinks can lead to an overproduction of insulin. The U.S. Department of Agriculture has revealed that per capita soft drink consumption has increased by almost 500 percent over the past 50 years. Sixty-five percent of adolescent girls and 74 percent of adolescent boys drink a sugar-sweetened soft drink on a daily basis. A recent study performed in Boston, Massachusetts, from the Harvard School of Public Health, set out to examine the relationship between sugar-sweetened beverages and obesity in children. It was published in *The Lancet* in February 2001.

Approximately 550 ethnically diverse metropolitan kids in the Boston area, with an average age of 11.7, were enrolled in the study. A baseline examination measured the children for height, weight, and triceps-skinfold thickness. Nineteen months later, the children were measured again. The data showed that sugar-sweetened beverage consumption (soda, Hawaiian Punch, lemonade, Kool-Aid, iced tea, and other sweetened fruit drinks) is associated with

obesity in children. Those kids who increased their intake of these beverages had increased body weight. And, the odds for becoming obese among these children increased by 60 percent for each additional can or glass of soft drink that was consumed each day! They could actually show a correlation of how overweight the kids got based upon how many sugar-sweetened drinks they consumed each day. Of course, the National Soft Drink Association issued a statement saying that the study was wrong and that soft drinks do not cause childhood obesity. They claim their own research shows that soft drink consumption is not related to an increased body mass index in children. What do you think?

JUNKY JUNK FOOD

We all know the key to good health is eliminating junk food from our diets. Many examples of this kind of food are obvious: chips, candy bars, sodas, and fries. We know we shouldn't eat them, and we know we shouldn't feed them to our kids. But many foods are packaged to make us think they are healthy when actually they are filled with the same junk as their more obvious counterparts. How many of us reach for a muffin for breakfast? If it's a zucchini muffin or a banana muffin, or a bran muffin, then we really feel like we're doing something good for our bodies. Muffins are cake! White flour, butter, eggs, sugar, and a bit of zucchini, banana, or bran. Cake for breakfast—what a way to start out the day. How about breakfast bars—you know, the ones

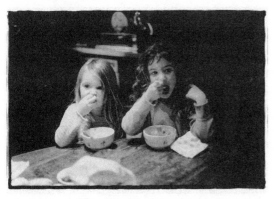

Go figure. They really like broccoli.

made with *real* fruit filling? Or protein bars? Many have as much sugar as a candy bar. Would you give your child a candy bar for breakfast? Then don't give him a breakfast bar. Breakfast cereals can be the worst culprit when they are made with white flour and sugar. It's a great recipe to start you on a sugar-binging cycle all day long. How about smoothies? Again, a seemingly healthy choice. Fruit smoothies made with all fruit are a great choice, but if you add sherbet or frozen yogurt, or sugar-sweetened juices, you are not doing your body any favors. It's now become a milkshake with added fruit. Be smart! Fat-free Entenmann's pastries are too good to be true. They may not have fat, but they have loads of white flour, sugar, starches, and chemicals. These are the foods many of us eat before we even leave the house. This is the fuel we are giving our kids before they head off for school.

How about mid-morning when we're ready for a snack? My granddaughter went to kindergarten this year. My son Bruce packs the lunches for the girls and tries to give them great-tasting nutritious snacks and lunches. My granddaughter came home from school absolutely thrilled because her friends had shared their Oreos and Cheetos with her at snack time. Bruce and his wife Caroline were stunned. The kids were eating cookies and chips at 10:00 A.M.

Lunchtime is no different. Yogurt? Healthy food, right? Not when it's Trix yogurt or Go-Gurt filled with artificial colors, flavors, and tons of sugar. No wonder kids won't eat the real stuff; they have become accustomed to the taste of overly sweetened, neon-colored, artificially flavored foods. Their lunches consist of peanut butter and jelly on white bread, lunch meat on white bread, bean burritos with white flour tortillas, Lunchables (chemicals and fat), white pasta or pizza. Their side dishes are crackers, chips, cookies, and Fruit Roll-Ups. (I don't need to tell you Fruit Roll-Ups are not actually a healthy fruit choice, do I? They are sugar, pure and simple.) They snack on Kudos bars and granola bars . . . you might as well give them a candy bar because these items have just as much sugar. (Okay, you get some nutrition from oats, but it's offset by the amount of sugar or honey.) They have fake butter spread that is colored blue! This is the food to which our kids have become accustomed. Why? Because that's what we give them! Then we wonder why our little boys and girls are getting plump bellies. No, it's not just genetics. Whether you are built long and lanky, or short and stout, we still each have an ideal body weight.

After-school snacks consist of cookies, granola bars, pretzels, or more little bags of chips. Sugar, sugar, and sugar. By the time the kids are hungry for dinner, we give them a plate of white pasta, macaroni and cheese, or chicken with mashed potatoes. How many of our kids eat vegetables? Not many. (P.S. Ketchup and french fries do not count as vegetables.) Even corn, potatoes, peas, and other kid favorites are actually more starches than they are vegetables. I'm always blown away when I look at kids' menus in restaurants and see that there are no vegetables anywhere in sight. Chicken nuggets with french fries, pizza, spaghetti with meat sauce, hamburgers, and macaroni and cheese. Most parents go right to these menus because it's the food their kids will eat, and it's less expensive. Our kids end up with the short end of the corn dog on a stick. Don't forget that these meals come with a soda or lemonade and a free dessert! Where is the real food? Where is the muscle-building food? Where is the brain food? Where is the bone-strengthening food?

Sadly, our adult diet is not much better; too many carbohydrates, too much sugar, and not enough fruit, vegetables, protein, and fat. Oh, we get plenty of fat, but we eat trans fats that are accompanied by sugar and starches, which make any kind of fat deadly. Our cells are dying at a rapid pace because we are not giving our bodies what they need to thrive. We are inviting extra pounds and disease by denying our bodies the foods they need.

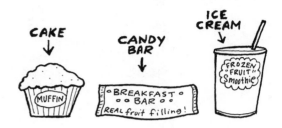

That's why it is vitally important to throw away the junk food, get rid of the fat-free snacks, stop drinking soda, and incorporate vegetables and real fats into your diet—it's the only way to end the obesity epidemic that is threatening adults and children all over the country. We often eat this junk food or feed it to our children because it's fast and easy and cheap to do so. In this book I will turn you on to real fast food, the kind that won't put on pounds or send your children into sugar shock. After you check out the recipes and different meal plans, you and your children will never be tempted to take shortcuts with fast food, junk food, and other snacks that may seem quick and easy at the time but will have dire consequences.

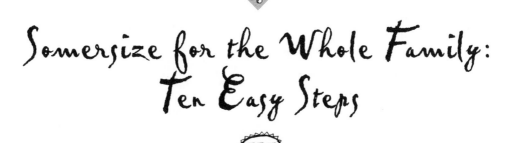

Somersize for the Whole Family: Ten Easy Steps

You obviously want to make a change in your life and in the lives of your family members, or you would not be reading this book right now. You are probably wondering whether you can handle this change and if your family can handle this change. I'm here to tell you, not only will you and your family handle it, but you will also embrace it. Most people tell me their families have never eaten better. I have women who say, "My husband thinks I am a great cook, now that I Somersize." I have men who say, "I do all the cooking in the house and my family loves all my Somersize recipes."

I'm not asking you to give your family food they will tolerate—this is food your family will love! I'm talking Tex Mex Pork Chops with a yummy cream sauce. I'm talking Somersize Mini–Pepperoni Pizzas! And Somersize Macaroni and Cheese made with egg noodles instead of white pasta. It's

inspired! It's Somersized! And you will not miss fast food burgers. When I want a burger, I make a Somersize Double Double Cheeseburger with Somersize Ketchup and Somersize Secret Sauce. I add tomato, pickle, and onion, wrap it in a lettuce cup, and serve it with Somersize Fast and Easy Onion Rings. Holy cow, it's great. The juice runs down my arms and I enjoy every bite. Insulin response? Next to nothing because it's made with acceptable Somersize proteins and fats and the condiments are made with Somer-Sweet instead of sugar.

TEN TRANSITIONS TO THE SOMERSIZE WAY OF LIFE

So how do you help your family make the transition from Insulin City to a Somersize Sanctuary? I'll give you ten steps that will help you and yours to adopt the Somersize way of eating. As an adult, I say, just dig in and start this very moment . . . cold turkey. Give up the sugar and the starches and begin the Level One guidelines of the program this minute. For those of you who want to help your whole family with this program, I think you need to ease them into it so that you do not receive any resistance. It's not easy giving up sugar and carbohydrates. Your body actually has a physiological craving for these foods, the same way an addict craves drugs. The more you eat, the more you crave. The weaning off can be tough, but once you heal your metabolism, you will not crave the sweets anymore.

STEP 1—WEIGH IN

The first step is admitting you need to lose weight, or get healthy—or admitting that your child needs to lose weight and get healthy. This probably will not be difficult for you to admit about yourself, but most parents are in serious denial that their children have a problem. It is much easier to convince yourself that your kid isn't really that fat, or that he actually eats healthy food and just is built a little large. It's easier to think that she eats the same as all the other kids, but she's just stockier. You convince yourself your child is physically active and doesn't eat that much junk food; she just has a little pot belly. You convince yourself because looking at the truth means you, as a parent, might be partially to blame. Do not feel guilty. Now you have the information and can turn the problem around. Remember the statistics about childhood obesity.

This problem is not getting any better. It's getting morbidly worse.

Without discussing this issue with your child, ask your pediatrician what the normal body weight is for your child's age and height. If you suspect your child might need to lose weight, he probably does.

STEP 2—DEATH TO THE WORD "DIET"

Don't ever use the word "diet." Delete it from your vocabulary. Diet is a dirty, four-letter word that drums up thoughts of deprivation. It creates a mind-set that makes you feel restricted and sets you up perfectly to rebel against those restrictions and fail. Dieting makes you obsess about food. We've seen this phenomenon over and over with the yo-yo dieters across the country.

Certainly, if adults are set up for failure with the word "diet," our kids will be even more susceptible. Simply tell your family that you've met with your doctor and you've decided how important it is to improve the way the family eats. Tell them you're going to be eating delicious food, but that you want to wean off the junk food and save those treats for special occasions.

STEP 3—MAKE IT A FAMILY AFFAIR

Studies show that the best chance kids have of getting control of their weight is when the whole family adopts a healthier lifestyle. Be a role model for your kids. You can't be downing Doritos and simultaneously wagging your finger at your kid to keep her hands out of the bag. Dr. Reginald Washington, chairman of the Sports Medicine and Fitness Committee for the American Academy of Pediatrics, remarks, "Almost always, when I see an obese child, one or both parents are obese. You must participate with your child." Remember, even if you don't have a weight problem, junk food will junk you up on the inside by killing off your healthy cells. When your healthy cells die off faster than they reproduce, you are inviting premature aging and disease. The whole family must join together.

STEP 4—CLEAN OUT THE CUPBOARDS

Get rid of all the junk. If you're feeling bad about wasting food, donate it to a shelter. Anything with unpronounceable ingredients should go. Cookies, cakes, crackers, chips, pretzels, sodas, punch, white pasta, white rice, and so on. Clean out the temptation and start fresh.

STEP 5—RESTOCK THE CUPBOARDS, FRIDGE, AND FREEZER

Take a trip to the grocery store. You'll notice that all the Somersize foods in the four food groups are on the perimeter of the market. Hit the produce section and stock up on plenty of fruits and fresh vegetables. Remember, fresh veggies will make up for the missing starches in your meals, so you'll want extra lettuce and salad goodies, and extra vegetable side dishes.

Then move to the dairy section and load your cart with eggs. They are inexpensive and are a great source of protein for meals and snacks. Load up on butter, cream, sour cream, olive oil, and mayonnaise—don't forget the cheese! String cheese is a great snack to keep on hand for you and the kids. You'll also want nonfat dairy products for your Carbo meals, like nonfat milk, nonfat yogurt, nonfat cottage cheese, and nonfat ricotta cheese. Then move to the meat department and get your favorite cuts of meat, fish, and poultry. Feel free to add bacon and sausage. Think about the items you can keep in the freezer to thaw out for a quick meal— ground beef, chicken breasts, pork chops, and more. Last, look for whole-grain carbohydrates as outlined in the specifics of Level One. You may need to go to a health-food store if your market does not carry these items. Whole-grain pastas, breads, and cereals must be made with whole grains like whole wheat, spelt, amaranth, or brown rice. Whole wheat flour is acceptable; wheat flour

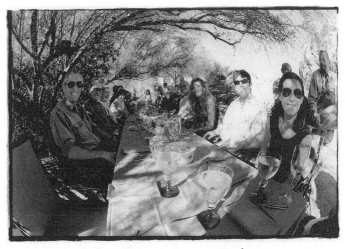

Family picnics are the best.

is not, nor are white flour or semolina flour. Make sure there are no sugars or hidden sugars like molasses, honey, raisin paste, or high fructose corn syrup.

Also, make a trip to SuzanneSomers.com to check our list of grocery items. Our Somersize list of foods is growing to help make Somersizing even faster and easier. For those of you who cannot locate certain products in your neighborhood, we have developed many Somersize items, such as Somersize Pasta and Sauce, Drink Mixes, and Dip Mixes. You'll find Salad Dressing Mixes and Bread Mixes so you can easily make Somersize meals at home. And you will definitely want to pick up some Somer-Sweet so you can eat desserts while you are losing weight. We also have SomerSweet Chocolates, like truffles and toffee. And SomerSweet desserts like Crème Brûlée, Chocolate Mousse, and fixings for Somersize Ice Cream Sundaes. And you were worried your kids wouldn't eat this way! I also have many, many products in development with new arrivals every month. Keep an eye out for my complete line of Somersize frozen foods. What could be faster and easier than that?

STEP 6—LIMIT TV AND COMPUTER TIME

This is a lesson for adults and kids. As much as it pains me, coming from television as I do, it's time to turn off the tube. If there's one thing all the experts agree upon, it's that our kids are watching too much TV. This type of inactivity is one of the most serious culprits in overweight and obese

kids. Only you can decide what is best for your child, but I think thirty minutes a day of television watching during the week is plenty, particularly *Three's Company* reruns. The computer is another physically inactive pastime that creates sedentary kids. Again, I would advise thirty minutes of non-homework-related computer time. Are there times when you should bend the rules? Definitely. Use these restrictions as guidelines, not hard-and-fast rules.

STEP 7—GET PHYSICAL

Getting active is much easier if the whole family participates. Again, don't make activity a penance: "Kids, you have to exercise!" Nothing will turn them off more quickly. Start taking walks after dinner. Take the stairs instead of the elevator. Get yourself and your kids involved in extracurricular sports. Most important . . . *play!* Nothing gets your heart rate going more than playing tag or hide and seek, shooting hoops, or jumping rope. It's a great way for you and your kids to connect and it's a great way to get active. You do not need to join a gym and commit all your time and money to exercising. Just find a way to get moving. Remember, physical activity releases stored sugar from your cells. As soon as that stored sugar is released, your body starts burning off your fat reserves. That's when "The Melt" begins and you are on your way to your ideal body weight. Eating the Somersize way will release this sugar on its own, but exercising will make it happen that much faster, and the benefits of physical activity are endless.

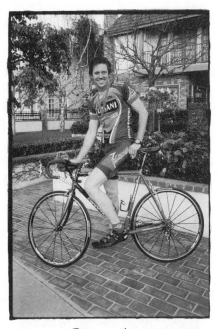

My son Bruce after winning the gold medal for the L. A. Circuit Cycling Race. Exercise is vital.

STEP 8—LISTEN TO YOUR TUMMY

One of the wonderful things about Somersizing is that you must eat to lose weight. Calorie-restrictive programs slow down your metabolism. Eating the Somersize way increases your metabolism . . . so when you're hungry, eat! If you do not eat when you are hungry, you may become over-hungry and then overeat. Since there are no portion sizes on this program, I advise you to eat until you are full. Listen to your tummy. Don't keep eating just because you may. Don't wait to feel stuffed. When you are comfortably full, stop eating. And know that if you feel hungry in an hour, you may eat again. You may eat all day if you are

truly hungry. That being said, once you clean out your system you will no longer get artificial hunger pangs from low blood sugar. Once you give your body the necessary proteins, fats, and carbohydrates it craves, it will stop asking you for food. If you eat junk food you can stay hungry all day long, munching and munching and never satisfying your body's need for nutrition. When you eat the Somersize way, your body receives the food it needs for growing healthy muscles, bones, and cells. When your body gets the nutrients it needs, it signals your brain that it is full. *Listen* . . . and teach your children to recognize these signals. It's a great feeling as a parent to know that you can help your child to lose weight and that you never have to say no if your child is still hungry.

STEP 9—A TIME TO CHEAT

You will lose weight more quickly if you do not cheat. That makes perfect sense. I advise you in the section on Level One to adhere strictly to the Level One guidelines while you are training your body to burn your fat reserves. However, for kids I think there are times when a little cheat can raise spirits and actually help keep them on the program longer. I have a whole book of desserts made with SomerSweet that are perfectly acceptable on Level One so they will feel like they're cheating even when they're not. You and your kids will love them. Now that we have SomerSweet, you can even have sweets while sticking to Level One.

What if your kid goes to a birthday party? Are you going to say, "Sorry, no cake for

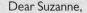

Dear Suzanne,

Since all other weight-loss programs meant terrible food or starvation, I had resigned myself to being fat. I just couldn't last on them. When I was hungry, I wasn't pleasant to be around. Then in February 2001, my mom recommended Somersizing to me. My first thoughts were, how could a weight-loss program be enjoyable? And what could TV's funny girl teach me about eating? Well, Suzanne, you taught me plenty!

Not really wanting to "diet," but needing to lose 180 pounds, I decided to Somersize. After discovering how the insulin response mechanism works and what improperly combined food and sugar does to the body, I knew I could NEVER eat the way I had been, ever again! I finally understood what had made me fat in the first place. Somersizing made perfect sense to me. I knew I could easily eat this way for life. Your recipes are delicious and satisfying. I never feel deprived. I don't miss sugar or caffeine. I never feel hungry like I did on low-calorie, low-fat diets. And SomerSweet is truly a dream come true.

In my first twelve months of Somersizing, I have lost a total of 75 pounds. I have every confidence in this program and that I will, for the first time in twenty years, be able to obtain my ideal weight and optimum health. Many of my family members now Somersize and all have enjoyed better health and weight loss, including my diabetic father-in-law, whose medications have actually been decreased since he started the program.

Thank you, Suzanne, from the bottom of my heart. Somersizing has given me my life back. With each pound I lose, I am discovering a new person both inside and out. For that, Suzanne, I am forever grateful. I am so glad that you were the messenger.

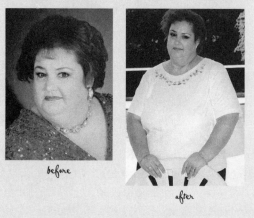

before

after

Sincerely,
Cheri Randall

you. You're on a diet."? Let your child decide. Let her know that she can choose when she wants to have a little cheat. Just make sure it's not a huge piece of cake and don't let her eat the bag of candy from the piñata along with the candy in the party favor. Help your child make the decision for herself. (Better yet, bring along a Somer-Sweet treat that she can enjoy while the others are eating cake.) For overweight kids, I think a cheat once or twice a week is perfectly acceptable. For obese kids, I think a cheat once a week is a good guideline. Just be careful and don't fall into the habit of cheating too much. If you start with a bit of sugar here and a bit of sugar there, you will increase your craving for sweets and carbo-hydrates.

For kids who do not need to lose weight, I think having one treat a day is a good guideline. That means one serving of chips, or one ice cream, or two to three cookies. It makes kids think about putting junk food into their mouths: "Hmm, do I really want these Oreos, or do I want to wait so I can have ice cream after dinner?" Again, these are not hard and fast rules. On some days the kids have more than one treat, but they have learned not to eat junk food with reckless abandon. They learn to monitor themselves without feeling like they have to sneak treats. There's nothing worse than setting up your kid to sneak treats! This will not accomplish your goal of helping your child learn to make smart food choices. You must make your child part of the equation. It takes education, and you must be the teacher, not the prison guard.

Step 10—Set Times for Meals and Snacks

Structure your meals and snacks as much as possible. Have breakfast in the morning. Don't skip this important meal. Make a smoothie for yourself and the kids. If you are using frozen fruit, it takes just minutes. And since we should all eat more fruits and vegetables, it's a delicious way to get a jump on that. Or have whole-grain cereal with nonfat milk. If you have more time, have eggs for breakfast. They really get you full and keep you going all morning long.

If your kids have a snack break in the morning, send them to school with cheese, hard-boiled eggs, or fruit as a snack. Kids usually have lunch at the same time each day. For lunch, I have included a whole section on "Brown Bagging It" with a week's worth of suggestions on what to pack for lunch or school. After school, kids are generally very hungry. This is the best time to get something healthy into their systems. Have cut-up fruit, or make tuna salad or egg salad with celery sticks, cut up veggies with dip, leftover chicken breasts from last night's dinner, or meat and cheese rolled up.

We are creatures of habit. If every time your child is in the car, you make sure he has something to snack on, he will always associate driving with snacking. Are you giving him snacks to keep him occupied? That's a mistake. Give him something to do. Snacks are for when we are hungry, a little something to get us through to the next meal. If your kids need a carpool snack, slice some apples. Better yet, give your child a snack when she arrives home from school. Better to sit and have a snack at home than to shovel something in while driving. Plus, you don't want the other parents responsible for what your child eats. She'll end up with more chips or pretzels. If the carpool snack is a must, have your child pack her own so she has fruit or cheese with a bottle of water or something healthy and Somersized. Also, don't associate snacking with watching TV. Many of us sit like zombies in front of the TV mechanically eating a whole box of crackers. Plus, watching TV ads makes us crave all the advertised junk food.

Most important, try to have dinner together as a family every night. I know you are thinking, "But that's not possible, our

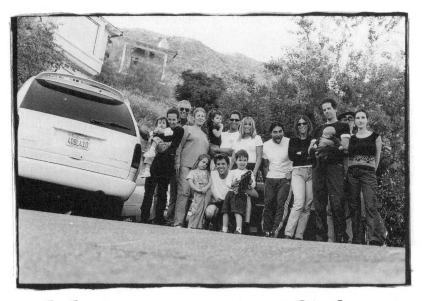

The Thanksgiving gang at our home in Palm Springs.

lives are too crazy with hectic work and after-school schedules." I will tell you this is the main reason for the increase in our country's weight. If you think you cannot have dinner as a family because your lifestyle doesn't allow it, I will contend that *our new chaotic lifestyle is exactly the reason adults and kids are gaining weight at a rapid pace.* The reason you can't sit and have a meal together as a family is because you don't make it a priority. We're always looking for a fast, inexpensive meal. We grab something to go, or we run out to a quick restaurant. Meals around the kitchen table are scarce, and our health is paying the price. Make it a priority. It takes some forethought, but you can make meals in minutes with just a little preparation. The recipes in this book are all geared toward people who don't have time to cook. Most can be made in under thirty minutes, and they are delicious! It takes minutes to prepare

Cheeseburger Pie, and it's a crowd pleaser. You can whip up Coq au Vin in minutes with a pressure cooker. You and your family will love this food. You may not find yourselves gathered around the table every night, but even a few nights a week would be an improvement for most of us.

These ten transitional steps will help you and your family get on track. Once you taste the delicious food, you will realize that Somersize is an improvement in the way you all eat, not a punishment. Adopting this new lifestyle will help you feel great from the inside out. And when you all start looking and feeling better from the effects of this way of eating, you will have renewed confidence to stick with it for life. Soon it will simply be the way you live and you will feel great knowing you and your family are on the road to a life of slim and healthy proportions.

❖

SEVEN

To Your Health! Supplements, Osteoporosis, and Serotonin

The next few sections of the book focus on the importance of our health. The most important part about finding your ideal body weight is to improve your health and longevity. You have a far better chance of warding off disease if you keep your body in great shape.

SUPPLEMENTS

One of the ways I have found to improve my health is by taking supplements. I have noticed such a turnaround in my health and immune system, that I frequently talk about my supplements. Now I get many requests for the lists of supplements I take. I am lucky to have as a dear friend Paul Schulick, the leading expert in the field. He is the president of New Chapter, a well-known manufacturer of supplements. Together we have developed a line of Somersize products

that provide a whole host of benefits, including supplements, protein shakes, and protein bars. In chapter 14 I will let you know how and when you can order them. I have asked Paul to write about what these supplements and herbs are and why they are so effective, and how they interact with a healthy diet and exercise to help us feel stronger.

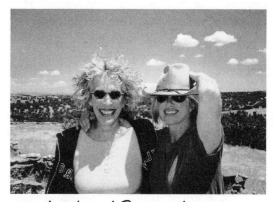

My dear friend Susie and me in New Mexico.

SUPPLEMENTS FOR A HEALTHY LIFE
BY PAUL SCHULICK

A healthy life. We all want one, especially one that lasts to a ripe old age filled with clarity, vigor, and strength. Conversely, two of the things we most fear are a short life or a long life with years of disease and physical or mental impairment. Pretty simple, actually, but what should we do to achieve the goal of a healthy long life?

You would think that would be *the* focus of the medical community, but doctors are often too busy handling emergencies and dealing with disease. In fact, that's what doctors are trained to do, and our "health care" system is perhaps better described as a "disease care" system. And that's a problem worldwide, for most countries have not, until recently, even bothered to keep track of their citizens' healthy life expectancy. That term, which measures both how long and how healthy a person's life is, was adopted only last year by the World Health Organization, and the statistics from 2001 are sobering for those of us in the United States. Our population does not even rank in the top twenty worldwide for healthy life expectancy, and we are far more "unhealthy" than our counterparts in nations such as Japan and France. Why?

First, let's review some of the simple causes of disease:

1. The stress of a poor diet
2. The stress of physical inactivity
3. The stress of obesity
4. The stress of age

What are people in nations such as Japan (number one in the world last year in healthy life expectancy) and France (number three) doing to add years of health to their lives and combat poor diet, lack of exercise, obesity, and lack of energy? What aren't people in America doing? Let's return to the four "stresses" as listed:

The Stress of a Poor Diet

Both in Japan and in France, people are, in general, eating foods that are more alive with nutrients. The French people are legendary for demanding the freshest, locally grown fruits and vegetables. They eat large quantities of fresh yogurt, and are, of course, obsessed with quality meats, cheeses, and wines. Each of those foods makes important contributions to a varied and nutritionally rich diet. In Japan, the population feasts on fresh fish, seaweeds, and cultured or "probiotic" foods like miso, which is fermented soy. Counterbalancing the pervasive air pollution and cigarette smoke in Japan are widely consumed antioxidant herbs and spices like green tea, ginger, and turmeric. By contrast, the American diet is full of processed and irradiated foods and chemical additives, flavorings, colorings, and preservatives. Unlike the array of fresh vegetables and fruits in France, we eat huge quantities of ketchup on french fries (our top two "vegetables"), and we do not regularly consume the living and powerful vitamins and nutrients that come from "probiotic" or cultured foods.

A poor diet seems like an easy problem to fix: just eat better! But it's not that simple. Our nation's food supply suffers from two serious problems that will take some time to fix. First, we don't grow a wide variety of fruits and vegetables. Instead of dozens of grains, we grow a monoculture of generic corn. Instead of hundreds of greens, we grow iceberg lettuce. I am oversimplifying, but the point is made every day in our grocery stores: we, as a rule, favor a few varieties of mass-produced foods, and we lose the nutrient diversity that comes from eating local foods harvested in season. We have chosen convenience and predictability over living in close harmony to the land, and that comes at a nutritional price. Worse yet, the land itself is not what it used to be. Not that I want to moan about the good old days, but the soil of today is lifeless compared to the sweetly nourishing soil of our forebears. Generations of chemical fertilizers and insecticides have made our soils basically dead. The indispensable soil bacteria, which digest the minerals in the soil and deliver them to the plants, have been eradicated along with insect pests. As a result, our soil is more like Styrofoam than loam, and the plants that are forced to grow in such lifeless dirt are severely lacking in spirit and substance. These are not simple problems with quick fixes. Quick fixes such as fertilizers and pesticides got us in this mess, and we need to slowly and intelligently rebuild our soil by returning to sustainable methods of agriculture. But until then, what do we do?

We could all move to France and Japan, but that's a stand-up comic's answer to the problem. We need a real diet solution that comes from eating living nutrients, probiotic foods, and an array of spices and herbs, and we need them now. I have formulated for Suzanne precisely such activated multivitamins and multiminerals. These activated multivitamins are made from nutrients that are probiotically cultured, much like the yogurt and wines of France and the miso of Japan. These activated multivitamins are easy to digest, even on an empty stomach, and activated multivitamins have been scientifically shown to be more powerful and effective than conventional vitamins made from isolates and synthetics. It may take us some time to heal the soil and repair our agricultural system, but until then the activated multivitamins will go a long way to fulfilling our requirements for probiotic nutrients, just like Mother Nature used to make.

The Stress of Physical Inactivity

Suzanne is one of the world's great champions of physical fitness, and she has made it simple and fun for millions to get back into shape. We all understand that we must exercise to stay in shape. Our bodies are high-performance engines, and the engines must be run and maintained or they will lose tone—and we could find ourselves in need of a serious tune-up. For example, our cardiovascular and bone health are in large part dependent upon regular and invigorating exercise, and many bodily processes work and feel better if we're moving our muscles and deeply breathing fresh air. But the journey to physical fitness starts with a first step, and how do we drag ourselves off the couch? We work

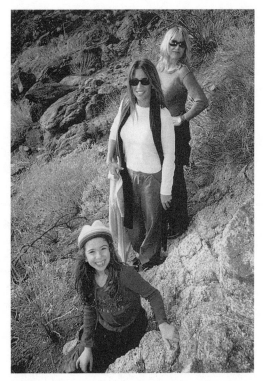

Three generations of healthy women. Me, my step-daughter Leslie, and my vibrant granddaughter.

Dear Suzanne,

I am writing this letter to thank you for all the work you did to come up with Somersizing. When I was in high school, I was a swimmer. I swam for two to three hours a day, five days a week, and was underweight at 5 feet 9 inches and 118 pounds. When I went to college, I quit swimming to focus on my classes and steadily gained weight. Of course, I did not eat anything healthy. Between work and classes, I was always on the run. I lived on jelly doughnuts and fast food. By the time I graduated, I weighed about 170. A couple years later, I was up to 225. I had tried all kinds of fad diets—cabbage soup, Dexatrim, you name it. Nothing worked for long, and I was always starved.

During the summer of 2001, a close friend got me to read your books, as well as many others on food combining. By this time, I was at about 274 pounds! We were sitting by the pool one afternoon, watching our sons swim, and she said, "I dare you to try it for a year and see if you can lose 100 pounds." I laughed at her, rolled my eyes, and said, "Okay, what have I got to lose? It won't work, but I'll try it." That was six and a half months ago, and now I weigh 65 pounds less than I did then. I am still in shock that it worked, but I believe completely in the program and look forward to reaching my ideal weight.

After about four months of Somersizing, I felt a strong urge to exercise. I started out slowly, and have worked up to walking 40 to 50 miles a month. I also use my Ultra Track about four times a week. My body is toning up and shaping up. I'm so very proud of what I have accomplished. With Somersizing, I have noticed that my body shape is changing dramatically. I am losing weight differently than I have before, in different places, so I know this is a great way of eating. I have never had so much energy or felt so good!

I have my whole family eating Somersized meals when we eat at home together. They eat whatever I eat, and they love the food too! My husband does not Somersize at work, but he has dropped some weight since we have been eating this way and looks great. My eight-year-old son seems to be a natural food combiner, for which I am thankful. He is thriving on this way of eating. Whenever he sees me with a Somersized snack, he steals some and is making better food choices.

It's a definite thrill to be able to make elegant, real food, and enjoy it rather than feeling guilty. SomerSweet has made it possible for me to not even feel the least bit guilty about eating dessert. At forty-one years old, I have also noticed that my mood swings have lessened. I have to say it must be due to Somersizing, as it's the only change I've made in my life at this point.

Thanks to you, Suzanne, I can now hike with my son, run with him, ice skate, rollerblade, and do all of the things I thought I would never do again. I've dropped four sizes so far, and too many inches to count! I know I will reach my goal, and I know I will be thin for the first time in my adult life, and it will happen soon. I can't wait!

Sincerely,
September Radecki

so hard all day, and with carpools and kids and shopping . . . there's just no time or energy. So we don't take that first step. Or maybe we try, but we are so out of shape, and our muscles ache, and we're exhausted, and then there's that latest television show we've been meaning to watch, and so we just sit there. We've lost the crucial balance between rest and activity, and we have no reserves of energy to sustain exercise or joy. This is when life becomes physically and emotionally flat, and we are overwhelmed by the stress of our circumstances.

There are many ways to jump start the exercise process and enable ourselves to react with greater balance to the stresses of our lives. There are meditation, yoga, and prayer, which are highly personal and are treasured by many. There is the supporting encouragement of a spouse or dear friend, which can inspire us to take that first step in the direction of physical fitness. And then there are herbal allies, key medicinal plants that have been used safely and effectively for thousands of years to support balanced energy.

Before explaining which herbs promote balanced energy, it's useful to set forth my formulation principles very clearly. First, humans have turned to many types of herbs over the course of human history. In fact, one could make the argument that human history is driven, in large part, by the search for herbs that provide some sort of advantage or unique pleasure. Just remember that tobacco, coffee, coca leaves, and opium poppies are all powerful herbs, and you get the idea. Those are controversial herbs, and I don't recommend them. Some herbs are clearly and unquestionably safe and highly effective, even when consumed daily and in large quantities. The premier examples of such herbs are green tea, ginger, turmeric, and holy basil. I prefer to deal with such time-tested and safe herbs.

Second, I talk about herbs, and not molecular pieces or chemical fragments of them. For example, when you take herbs such as white willow or meadowsweet and eliminate all their complex phytonutrients except salicylic acid, you are left with the chemical base for the drug aspirin. That process of "simplification" of the herb down to one chemical constituent is called "standardizing," and it basically converts a balanced and infinitely complex plant into a drug. I'm not opposed to drugs; they certainly have their place in our healthcare system. I simply believe that drug companies are better equipped and more likely to spend the hundreds of millions of dollars necessary to identify, isolate, research, and test a drug than are herbal companies. I also believe that herbs and drugs work differently, and I'm much more comfortable, long term, with the chorus of complex and harmonizing voices in an herb than in the loud shout of a one-molecule drug. We know, for example, from many thousands of years of experience with billions of daily consumers, that green tea has desirable and safe effects. We have no such depth of experience with consuming just one chemical out of green tea, such as isolated caffeine or one of the green tea catechins. The whole is more than the sum of its parts.

What all this means is that I believe that drugs (including ones in the guise of standardized herbs) can sometimes be safely taken over long periods, but the whole herbs and broad spectrum extracts that I use give us complete confidence that extended use is safe.

With those two formulation principles in mind (herbs time tested for safety and efficacy and using the whole herb, and not its isolated parts), I have created a Balanced Energy formulation for Suzanne that will promote sustained energy and help us get off the couch and back into shape. The key herbs are such treasures as green tea, American ginseng, cola nut, schizandra, rhodiola, eleuthero, ashwaganda, and a supporting cast of other herbs designed to support the full experience of active life. These herbs safely promote an increase in metabolic energy (often described as "thermogenic"), they assist the body's adaptation to stress, and they support immune system functioning. These herbs are (thankfully!) no substitute for physical activity, but they help to make that activity more energetic and pleasurable.

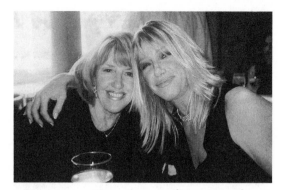

My sister Maureen and me, together forever.

The Stress of Obesity

Excessive heaviness of the body can contribute to a host of medical problems. The weight puts pressure on our joints, causing or contributing to the joint pain of osteoarthritis. With each pound our hearts have to work harder, and obesity is a major risk factor for adult-onset diabetes and a condition of insulin insensitivity called Syndrome X. With obesity also comes an excess of a stress hormone called cortisol, and elevated cortisol levels are associated with bone loss, tumor growth promotion, and a feeling of despair or depression.

So we want to lose weight, and we should. But like that first step off the couch and into an exercise program, the step toward a rational and lifelong weight-loss strategy is often challenging. Our bodies are chemically and hormonally accustomed to being overweight, and to suddenly change our eating and exercising habits in order to lose what has become our "normal" body can be stressful in and of itself. There is no substitute for a careful weight-loss program involving better dietary and exercise choices, but such a program is asking the body to change; and there is natural resistance to change. Certain herbs can help us make the transition to a new weight and new body less stressful, and can actually promote a normal appetite and normal

blood sugar. Suzanne asked that I create a Crave Control formula using those herbs, and the key herbal constituents are cinnamon, turmeric, holy basil, and chamomile. Together with other supporting herbs and two important activated minerals (probiotic chromium and vanadium), this formulation offers a dual approach to weight control. First, it promotes the normal sensitivity of cells to insulin, thus maximizing glucose/energy metabolism. For example, a USDA study identified cinnamon, cloves, turmeric and bay leaves (all in the formula) as potentiating insulin sensitivity by up to 300 percent. The USDA in 2000 demonstrated that cinnamon, green tea, cloves, brewer's yeast, and bay leaves (all in the formula) stimulate cellular glucose metabolism, with cinnamon showing the ability to increase glucose metabolism by upwards of twenty times. Second, botanicals in the formula reduce the effects of the stress hormone cortisol. Excessive cortisol is unwelcome for many reasons, including promoting the insulin resistance leading to obesity, sometimes referred to as Syndrome X. The Crave Control formula is not a faddish weight-loss formula, but is rather a sensible approach to making a smooth transition from the body you acquired to the body you desire.

The Stress of Age

One of the ironies of life today is that by living longer, we actually increase the chances of ending up with lingering disease and disability. I was in India recently, and I asked a physician escorting me through Bombay why the cancer rates in India were so much lower than in the United States. He answered immediately that cancers are "diseases of longevity, and people in India generally don't live long enough to get those diseases." Well, we who are in the Western world are cursed by the stress of old age, where the toxins that have built up over the decades have the greatest chance to work their mischief. Our very health successes thus expose us to new health problems as we age, and two of those health problems are the failure to digest or assimilate nutrients from foods and the incomplete elimination of waste or toxins. Those are gentle and scientific ways of describing "indigestion" and "constipation," and those complaints grow more frequent as we age. Two further ironies: if we don't properly digest or absorb our food, we hunger for more and more, eating more calories in search of energy and essential nutrients. And if we don't eliminate our body's waste, it builds up. If you eat more and eliminate less, you often gain weight, which for the elderly can lead to joint pain, diabetes, loss of mobility, and a downward spiral of ill health. Remember that people living in the United States are not even in the top twenty for healthy life expectancy, and widespread "indigestion" and "constipation" deserve some of the blame.

It's not only the elderly who are plagued by those conditions, for all of us, as we get older, lose some of the vitality of our digestive and eliminative systems. When we're twenty, we can eat fried foods and digest cold pizza, but as we hit forty and fifty, our digestive fires don't burn quite as hot and the same foods cause gastric rebellion.

Once again, herbs can come to our aid. For millennia, people have traveled the Silk Road seeking the riches of the Orient. It wasn't just silk that aristocrats craved: spices, most notably ginger, relieved their indigestion and made them feel better. That spice works for us as well. I wrote a book called *Ginger: Common Spice and Wonder Drug,* and Suzanne's long interest in ginger is what led to our first meeting many years ago. As my book describes, ginger is not only one of nature's best anti-inflammatories and cardio or heart tonics, but it is the king of digestive herbs. It also is a wonderful "probiotic" herb, supporting healthy intestinal flora and thus promoting the regular and complete elimination of wastes. With ginger, we all gain more nourishment from the foods we eat (thus needing to eat less), and we are more efficient in eliminating toxins. Eat less, burn more efficiently, eliminate more. That's a great recipe not only for maintaining proper weight but also for relieving some of the stresses of age that can diminish our senior years. Suzanne asked me to create an herbal formula, which she calls Digestive Complex, that brings together ginger and supporting herbs and nutrients to improve all aspects of digestion, whether of fat, protein, or carbohydrate, and then promote efficient and regular elimination of wastes. Some of the key supporting herbs are peppermint, celery seed, parsley seed, and more exotic botanicals like uva ursi and dandelion. Peppermint offers a wide range of benefits, most notably the strong support of the digestive system. Celery seed, parsley seed, and uva ursi promote normal kidney functioning and the elimination of toxins, and dandelion promotes normal bile flow, which is essential for proper fat digestion. The formula thus offers simple and natural support for digestion and elimination.

The stress of age is, to a certain extent, self-inflicted. We are often careless about our dietary choices, and over time we compromise our digestive and eliminative processes. This can lead to cravings, bingeing, and poor weight management as we get older, and in our senior years those burdens can have devastating effects. Ginger and the other complementary constituents in Digestive Complex can be of great assistance in supporting digestion and elimination, and thus form an important part of our strategy for living old, and living well.

To Life!

A healthy life. Yes, and a long one, too. Those are what we wish for ourselves and our friends and family. We are responsible for making dietary and lifestyle choices that can lead to a generous portion of good health; and there are herbs, properly selected and used, that can be of great support. It has been my joy to work with Suzanne in creating these herbal resources, and may you use them well in concert with following the dietary recommendations of the Somersize program. You may also want to take advantage of the delicious Somersize protein and energy bars and powders I've worked with Suzanne to create. They follow the Somersize program and contain the finest natural ingredients formulated to offer a range of both slow- and fast-acting proteins for optimal energy and lean muscle tone. The bars and powders use protein from eggs naturally rich in omega-3 fatty acids, which nourish and protect the heart and mind. In addition, we incorporate protein from whey, one of nature's best sources of strength for our immune systems. And unlike other nutrition bars and powders, the Somersize bars and powders do not include any artificial flavors or colors, added preservatives, or hydrogenated fats. Most of all, they are a great-tasting alternative to empty-calorie snack foods, and protein and energy have never been easier. Enjoy!

PAUL SCHULICK

DEM BONES

Have you ever considered how diet affects your bones? What would we be without our skeletons? A pile of jelly! The food we consume from childhood throughout our lives will directly affect our bone structure. At menopausal age we women start to worry about our bones. Our doctors tell us to have our bone-density tests done. Most of us have already experienced bone loss. We accept this; in fact, we expect this to be the case. But hear this—bone loss is not a condition that has to accompany middle to old age. Osteoporosis is insidious because you can't see or feel what is happening. Most people who have the disease don't know it. And then a bone breaks.

Each year 430,000 Americans wind up in the hospital because of fractures related to osteoporosis. Hip fractures, which represent about 300,000 of that total, are devastating. One victim in five dies within a year, and half are never able to live independently again. Most of us know someone who has suffered a hip fracture, but you may be surprised to learn that complications of this injury kill even more women every year than breast cancer. Preventing osteoporosis is really a life-and-death matter, like preventing cancer and heart disease.

Hip fractures are just the most obvious part of the problem. Millions of women suffer distressing symptoms that they don't connect to fragile bones. A woman may not realize that her chronic back pain comes from crush fractures in her spine. Fragile vertebrae may have crumbled under the ordinary stresses of everyday life. Osteoporosis can make a woman look old before her time, but she may have no idea that her slumped posture and protruding tummy are caused by fractures in her spine. As a woman, you have one-in-three odds of suffering from osteoporosis in your lifetime. You can beat those odds. Medical experts now consider osteoporosis a preventable disease.

Osteoporosis is treatable thanks to new findings about nutrition and exercise, as well as new medications. Somersizing provides the right kinds of nutrients to continue reproducing healthy cells, build bone mass, balance your hormones, keep your blood pressure at normal levels, and prevent heart disease. Remember, sugar is the body's greatest enemy, and Somersizing eliminates

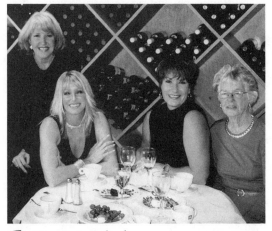

The Birthday Club; my sister Maureen, me, my sister-in-law Mardi, and my Auntie Helen.

sugar from your diet, replacing it with nutritious *real* food. This program helps you to protect yourself.

Even women in their twenties and thirties can get osteoporosis. Fortunately, this doesn't happen often, since most early victims of the disease have significant risk factors such as prolonged use of steroid medications or lengthy periods of eating disorders. Ironically, many of these women are dancers or athletes, who look healthy and fit. The bones we have later in life reflect what we did as kids, teens, and young adults. So in a very real sense, osteoporosis is a disease that starts in childhood. Consider this when you hear of a teenager who is struggling with anorexia. The immediate and long-term effects are devastating. This is why it is so important that our children eat healthy right from the start. What they put in their mouths now will affect not only whether they are overweight or obese later in life but also how healthy and strong their bones are.

If a woman is premenopausal or menopausal, extra calcium can help build strong bones. But simply upping calcium consumption has never been shown to increase bone density or prevent fractures in older women. Add Vitamin D to that calcium, and the effects are dramatic: bone density increases significantly and fractures are reduced by 50 percent. That's because Vitamin D is needed to absorb calcium and turn it into bone, and many postmenopausal women don't get enough.

Here's something you probably didn't realize: men also are prone to osteoporosis. An estimated two million men have this disease. In fact, a man is far more likely to suffer an osteoporosis-related fracture during his lifetime than he is to get prostate cancer. Yet men, and even their doctors, are largely unaware of this problem. Hormonal stimulation is just as important for men's bones as it is for women's. Low testosterone levels are responsible for about half the cases of osteoporosis in men. Usually, low testosterone is a consequence of aging, but certain medical conditions can lead to more rapid loss. Signs of low testosterone include the following: reduced libido or impotence, decreased facial and body hair and enlarged breasts (although there are many men who have low testosterone levels without any symptoms at all). A blood test can measure testosterone levels. If you are low in testosterone, ask your doctor about a bone density test.

Men with a light frame and low body weight and also men with eating disorders are particularly at risk for osteoporosis. Competitive athletes in sports with weight classifications especially suffer from the problem. Anyone who has been a yo-yo dieter or had anorexia or bulimia is at a higher risk for osteoporosis. Other risk factors for men and women are inactivity, a diet low in calcium and Vitamin D, high alcohol consumption, and smoking (current or past).

The good news is, if you are Somersizing, you are already on the right track for continued good health and strong healthy bones. But as you can see, poor nutrition and lack of exercise may already have caused problems. In addition to eating real foods and eliminating sugar from your diet, here's what else you can do to restore your body and your bones to good health.

1. Nutrition: Eat real foods and enough of them. Remember, food is fuel, which you need for energy, and real foods promote healthy cell reproduction. In addition, real foods promote strong healthy bones.

2. Physical activity: Be active. Weight training in particular promotes bone growth. Here's how. When you do weight training, the muscles tug against the bone, promoting and stimulating bone growth. The outward physical benefits are also apparent. Nothing is more beautiful than toned, defined, cut muscles. Your clothes will look better on you, but the inward effects are the most exciting benefit. You will be building bone, or in the case of bone loss, restoring bone.

3. Supplements: Take calcium, Vitamin D, and Fosamax, if necessary (depending on your bone loss). This, of course, should be discussed with your doctor.

I hope this has stimulated your interest in the importance of promoting healthy bone growth. Imagine the effect you can have on your children and your whole family by insisting upon proper eating and exercise. You are the one who generally shops for the groceries and provides the family meals. Keep sugar out of the house. Keep chemicals and trans fats, like potato chips, corn chips, or those cheesy things, and so on, out of the house. (I call these things cancer in a bag.)

How wonderful to say that because of

you, your family is developing sound nutritional patterns that can help lead to a healthier lifestyle. It's all about quality of life. Remember when your parents used to say "as long as you have your health"? Well, they were right! There is no quality of life if you are not healthy. It doesn't matter how much money you've earned, or how great a house you've built. If you are not healthy, the quality of your life diminishes. If you don't have strong healthy bones, it will be much harder to enjoy old age.

Remember, you are in control of your life. You can start now to build up your bone structure by Somersizing. Enjoy delicious meals, eat until you are full. Learn to enjoy those foods that have misguidedly been off your acceptable list for so long, like butter, cream, olive oil, sour cream. These foods are good for you because they are real fats. It's your body. It's your life. Life is what you make it. You should enjoy life to the fullest and provide the means to do so in the future too. Your children will thank you today, and down the road.

SEROTONIN — THE FEEL-GOOD HORMONE

What is serotonin and why should you care? Remember how we call insulin "the fat-storing hormone"? Serotonin is known as "the feel-good hormone." Once again, I refer to my dear friend and doctor, Diana Schwarzbein.

As Dr. Schwarzbein explained to me, serotonin is a hormone that is produced by the foods we eat. If there is no ongoing serotonin production in your body, your brain will cry out for carbohydrates. If you crave carbohydrates or stimulants, that means that your serotonin levels are low. Your brain will demand stimulants to raise your serotonin levels. Bingeing on carbohydrates will lead to reactive hypoglycemia or low blood sugar. When it feels as though your blood sugar levels have dropped below normal ranges, what you are actually experiencing is the side effect of the rising adrenaline levels. We have all had this experience when we feel depressed and crave comfort foods like mashed potatoes, macaroni and cheese, or chocolate. This is your body asking for carbohydrates so that it can "cure" your depression with a blast of serotonin.

There are no serotonin supplements you can buy at a health food store. Serotonin is only produced by your own body and by the foods you ingest. Serotonin plays a major role in how well people are able to adhere to a balanced diet. Without balanced serotonin levels, the brain sends powerful signals that can make willpower ineffective, no matter how much you want to change. Overconsuming carbohydrates creates a low serotonin state; similarly, no carbohydrates at all will eventually lead to a low serotonin state. This is where my program differs from other "high-protein" diets. My beliefs are based in science and on the premise that we require protein, fats, and carbohydrates for healthy cell reproduction. Balance is the key. The way to keep your serotonin balanced is to eat the right ratio of proteins, fats, and carbohydrates. For Somersizing purposes, we eat a variety of these foods throughout the day. Remember, fruits and vegetables are carbohydrates as well as the foods found in the Carbos group.

When we eat too few or too many carbohydrates, we may experience hypoglycemia (low blood sugar). The symptoms of hypoglycemia are nausea, shakiness, clamminess, sweating, lightheadedness, irritability, racing heart, anxiety, and carbohydrate craving. If you continue in a low serotonin state, you will keep craving carbohydrates. If you keep overconsuming carbohydrates, you will never lose the weight you desire, your insulin levels will remain elevated, the cravings for carbohydrates (sugar) will never go away, and the merry-go-round of your weight will continue.

To lose weight the Somersize way, it is necessary initially to only consume carbohydrates in their whole-grain form (complex carbohydrates). To lower your insulin levels, I ask that you eliminate sugar and all things that the body recognizes as sugar (simple carbohydrates). I also ask you to eat proteins and carbohydrates separately, because you do not want insulin present when you are consuming protein and fats. Plus, proteins and carbohydrates digest at different rates of speed, which slows down your metabolism. What we are trying to do is heal your metabolism and have it work at optimum. By consuming proteins and carbohydrates separately, you speed up your metabolism, which allows your body to shed the weight more quickly.

After you reach your goal weight, you then proceed to Level Two. Level Two is not as restrictive. We start to cheat by having a potato or your favorite high-starch veg-etable with your protein meals as often as your body can handle. If your waistline starts to thicken, you are overdoing it. When consumed in the right proportions, this new addition of carbohydrate to our protein meals is important.

A couple of years ago I had a new experience on Level Two. At one point, after Somersizing for a long time and maintaining a perfect weight, I began to notice that I was putting on some pounds. I went back to Level One and tried to stick exclusively to Pro/Fats and Veggies. I still had fruit in the morning, but I was eating almost no carbohydrates. The weight was still not coming off, and I couldn't understand it, because I wasn't aware that I had been cheating.

I called Dr. Schwarzbein and asked her what was happening. She explained to me that by eliminating the carbohydrates so severely and for such a long time, I had depleted my serotonin levels. Without knowing it, I was craving sugars in some form and cheating on the side. I asked her to prescribe some serotonin pills. She laughed and said, "No such thing exists. You can't buy serotonin; your body has to produce it, and the only way to produce it is to begin adding some kind of carbohydrate at every meal, like a small potato, whole grains, or another high-starch vegetable."

At first I resisted . . . a potato! The evil insulin raiser and master of all Funky Foods? It was so un-Somersized I couldn't accept it. Of course, I am also an Irish girl at heart, and the idea of bringing potatoes back into my meals was secretly thrilling. I had long talks with Diana about this and she tutored me on the importance of the entire hormonal system being in balance. If one hormone is depleted, the entire hormonal system can be disrupted. Sure enough, as soon as I added some carbohydrate to my Pro/Fats meals (even an occasional small potato!), my weight gradually returned to normal.

A truly balanced diet must include protein, fats, and carbohydrates at every meal. In the beginning, while you are overweight and still craving carbohydrates and sugars, having carbohydrates with your meals increases your desire for more. Also, your cells are filled with sugar, so you must eliminate the Funky Foods until the stored sugar is cleaned out. In the Somersize Pro/Fats and Veggies meal we get our carbohydrates in the form of vegetables, which have small amounts of carbs that help keep your system balanced but won't send your insulin soaring.

When you reach your goal weight, you have cleaned out your cells of the stored sugar. You have healed your ailing metabolism, and you are most likely not craving the carbs and the sweets anymore. At this point, you will want to reintroduce a small portion of carbohydrates in their whole-grain form, or in the form of a high-starch vegetable, for reasons of health. This new proportion of protein, fats, and a small amount of carbs produces a balanced serotonin state. When your serotonin state is balanced, you will not crave carbohydrates; thus, you will be getting what you need for healthy cell reproduction, without gaining any weight. And oh, how wonderful it is to have a small potato with your meals again. Be sure to have them with butter and/or sour cream, because now that you have healed your

metabolism you can handle this without gaining any weight.

Here is the warning: Don't overdo this. After you have graduated from Level One, and have maintained your weight on Level Two for a significant period of time, then you can move on to add small amounts of carbohydrates with your protein meals. The proteins, fats, and vegetables need to be the largest portion on your plate, with a small portion of whole-grain carbohydrates. Have about a half-cup of whole-grain pasta or brown rice. Or feel free to include a small potato a couple of times a week, or half a sweet potato. Your system is now balanced and you need to keep it that way; otherwise, you will create a low serotonin state and the weight may start coming back. Use your common sense. Carbohydrates are essential

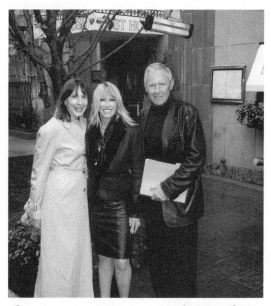

Sandi Mendelson, my publicist, Alan, and me, right after the "Today Show" in New York City.

to your health, but they must never be the largest part of your diet. If so, you will become fat or depleted metabolically. If this happens, a whole host of other problems will arise. Don't blow all this work for nothing.

Somersizing is the one program you can happily stay on for life. It will give you everything you need, but you have to be sensible about it. Focus on what you can have, not what you can't have. Enjoy your fats—eat steak, chicken, or fish, with beautiful butter or wine sauces, slather your vegetables with butter or olive oil, and when you have your waistline back (which means you have lowered your insulin levels), then you can start adding that small potato with your meals.

EIGHT

❧

Commitment: It's All Up to You

Rarely does a day go by that someone doesn't come up to me and say, "I want to lose weight." My response is always the same, "Well, that is exactly what you will get . . . wanting." Wanting is not enough to motivate and get results. Wanting is desire; what you want is conviction. In other words, you must *commit* instead of wanting. Commitment produces results. People call me on the air when I am appearing on HSN and tell me, "Tomorrow I'm going to start your program." I always tell them the same thing: "It'll never happen. The same excuse that you are using for not starting the program today is the same excuse you will have tomorrow, and the next day and the next day." I don't mean to be harsh, but losing weight requires determination and a willingness to make this the most important project of your life.

The reason losing this weight is the most important thing you can do for your life is because weight determines the quality of your life. It's not about being the thinnest person in the room; it's about finding, as Dr. Schwarzbein calls it, your "ideal body composition." When you do find the weight your body was intended to be, your body operates at optimum. What does that mean relative to the quality of your life? It means that your system will run smoothly, you will have more energy and vitality, you will think more clearly, you will have balanced hormones and an increased sexual drive. When your body is operating at optimum, the diseases of aging are measurably decreased. Genetics plays a role, but even genetic predispositions to diseases are lower when you are at your ideal body weight.

How do you know if you are at your ideal body composition? Stand in front of the mirror naked. It doesn't matter if you are thin or heavyset; if your body is not at its ideal weight and you are thick or soft through the middle area, you have had an elevated insulin level. Why should you care about this? Balanced insulin levels are a key component for good health. All of the processes leading to hardening of the arteries (built-up plaque) are caused by overproduction of insulin. Also, the older we get, the more chance we have of developing heart disease. This is because we become more insulin resistant with age. This thickness around our middle section means that our cells, which are made up of protein, fat, and carbohydrates, are loaded with all the stored sugar they can tolerate, and from that moment on any sugars you ingest have the potential to be stored as fat. Our magnificent bodies are talking to us saying, "Hey, there's no room here for all the sugars and carbohydrates you are eating, so if you keep on consuming these things I have no choice but to store this food as fat." Next, our hips get bigger, then the stomach, buttocks, and thighs. Once these storage areas are loaded up, the next storage spaces are the neck, arms, face, chest, and back.

Now you are overweight, all because you

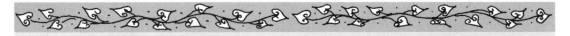

Dear Suzanne,

I wanted to take a moment to personally tell you how much I enjoy Somersizing. I have followed the plan for almost a year now and have been so happy with my results. The recipes in your books and the ones I have swapped with fellow Somersizers are fabulous. The variety of foods that I can eat and the wonderful desserts keep me faithful to the plan.

I have always loved to cook, but rarely took the time to make gourmet meals. Now I have the energy to cook that way every night, in spite of the fact that I work full time and have an active toddler; as a result, everyone in my house enjoys healthy meals. The drastic change in my eating habits—I've eliminated white flour, sugar, and processed foods—helped me to lose 20 pounds in three months, even with the occasional cheats. When I realized that this plan really worked, I made the commitment to follow the plan to the letter and quickly lost another 10 pounds in just three weeks.

This is a plan I can stick to for life. Thank you, Suzanne. I am eternally grateful!

Warm regards,
Erika Hindes

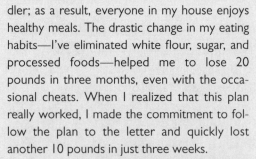

before   *after*

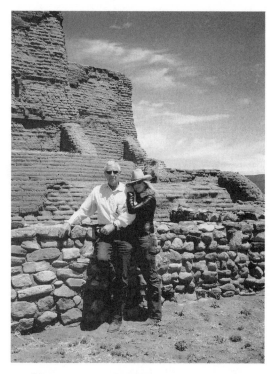

Alan and me in one of my favorite places on earth, New Mexico.

Weight creeps in on little cat feet: a pound here, a pound there. It all adds up, just like food. A piece of cake here, a candy bar there, and pretty soon those favorite pants are hard to button. When your insulin levels are elevated, you have passed the point of no return. You have to make some changes or your weight and health will spin out of control. That means you have to take this seriously, because now that you are thick through the middle, even a carrot (which the body accepts as sugar) will be stored as fat.

Insulin plays a major factor in your good health. Dr. Schwarzbein says, "High insulin levels result in high blood pressure. Insulin causes an abnormal increase of salt retention at the kidney level. Increased salt in the system increases water retention. More overall fluid means higher blood pressure. Also, insulin overstimulates the nervous system, which increases blood pressure. The amount of blood pumped out by each contraction of the heart is increased, and the artery wall becomes stiffer."

Being sedentary contributes to heart attacks because overall insulin levels are higher when you don't exercise. Exercise lowers insulin levels. It's that car analogy again—you can have a brand-new car sitting in your garage, but if you never drive it, even though it is brand new and in good shape, it won't run properly because of lack of use. Your body is the same: it doesn't matter how new it is or how old; if you don't use it and move it you are at greater risk for health problems. You are at greater risk for elevated insulin levels and all the negative effects from that.

For you smokers, nicotine in tobacco

didn't understand the early warning signs and because you didn't listen to your body. It's not the weight that is the problem; it's the resultant negative effects on our health. We all think it will never happen to us. Yeah, you're carrying around a little extra weight, but you know you are going to get rid of it . . . tomorrow, right? The problem is that you put it off and put it off, and one day you are sitting in the doctor's office, he is telling you about a variety of health problems you are now experiencing or facing, and you wonder how this happened to you. Sound familiar? When you were young you didn't have digestive problems or gas or bloating, did you? What happened?

stimulates the release of insulin, leading to insulin resistance. Studies have shown that smokers have an increased risk of developing Type II diabetes. Type II diabetics have the highest risk of heart disease because of prolonged high insulin levels. Think about that next time you reach for that cigarette or that piece of candy.

You want to keep your arteries free of plaque. Plaque-free arteries are your best insurance against heart attack or stroke. You can do it by eating balanced meals and by eating sufficient amounts of protein, fats (real fats), and nonstarchy vegetables and by including whole-grain carbohydrates in your diet as outlined in my Somersize program. As I explained in the last chapter, in Level Two, you will see how you can even add the occasional starchy vegetable like a potato, or yam, especially if exercise is a part of your routine.

I hope after you read this I will have given you the motivation to commit to losing weight. Knowing the harmful effects of all sugars and hidden sugars will have even more impact than the fact that you don't like the way you look in your clothes. Granted, we all possess a moderate amount of vanity. I know when I feel my clothes getting the slightest bit tight, I walk by the mirror and feel disgusted, but I think the disgust comes from a deeper place than it once did. I now know that this weight signals an increase in my insulin level. That means I have been neglectful, or arrogant, or weak, and that those desserts I talked myself into when I was last traveling not only have had a negative effect on my appearance, but also, and more important,

those pounds indicate that I have chosen to accelerate my internal metabolic aging process.

Aging happens when you break down more cells than you build up. Life is about healthy cell division. Having already had breast cancer, I now know that I am not invincible. But I cannot tell you how happy I was, knowing when I was diagnosed that for the last ten years I have done everything in my power to keep my insulin levels in check, exercised, and worked toward relieving the stress in my life. I believe my cancer had to do with the stress of my childhood, and poor eating habits in my youth, plus drinking caffeine and alcohol, and eating chemicals, mainly in the form of margarine and processed foods. My lifestyle and eating habits those years broke down my cells rather than built them up. I feel that my chances of complete recovery are definitely on the plus side, because I value my life and my health, and I eat for wellness, which translates to a slim figure.

I can eat the most sumptuous meals, like chicken with a beautiful rich sauce, or steak, or vegetables smothered in butter, or salads with my favorite dressings, and still be healthy. My desserts are almost always made with SomerSweet, which keeps me on the plan. Believe me, it is not difficult to Somersize. In fact, I eat more and better food than I ever did with my old patterns.

You can have the body you've always wanted. You can have good health. You do not have to accept growing older with disease. It takes a shift in your thinking, and most of all, it takes *commitment!* Commit today. Your life will change, your body will change, and you will have the opportunity to change whatever bad eating habits your family has acquired. What an incredible gift to give your family. To start your children with good eating habits at an early age is one of the most important gifts you can give them. You can't start tomorrow. You must start right now. Do it! Make a roast chicken with roasted vegetables, and a beautiful salad with your favorite dressing. Make them some Somersize Ice Cream for dessert. Believe me, your family will appreciate this simple meal much more than another trip to a fast-food joint.

It's up to you. You can have it all, or you can condemn yourself to a life of aches, pains, sluggishness, a stopped-up system, poor body shape, elevated insulin levels, and diseases that result from ingesting bad food. Somersizing is something you can do for the rest of your life. Imagine eating great food, never experiencing hunger, never counting anything, and having improved health, better-looking skin, more energy, and that confidence that comes with knowing you are taking superb care not only of yourself, but of your whole family as well. Or you can drive to the nearest fast-food drive-in and order a carcinogenic, insulin-building meal made up of questionable foods and chemicals. Which would you rather have?

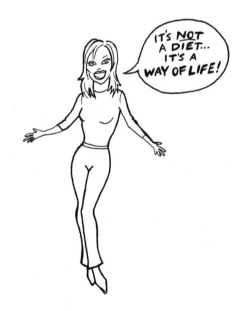

Part Two

EVERYTHING

YOU NEED TO KNOW

ABOUT

SOMERSIZING

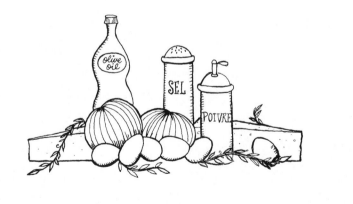

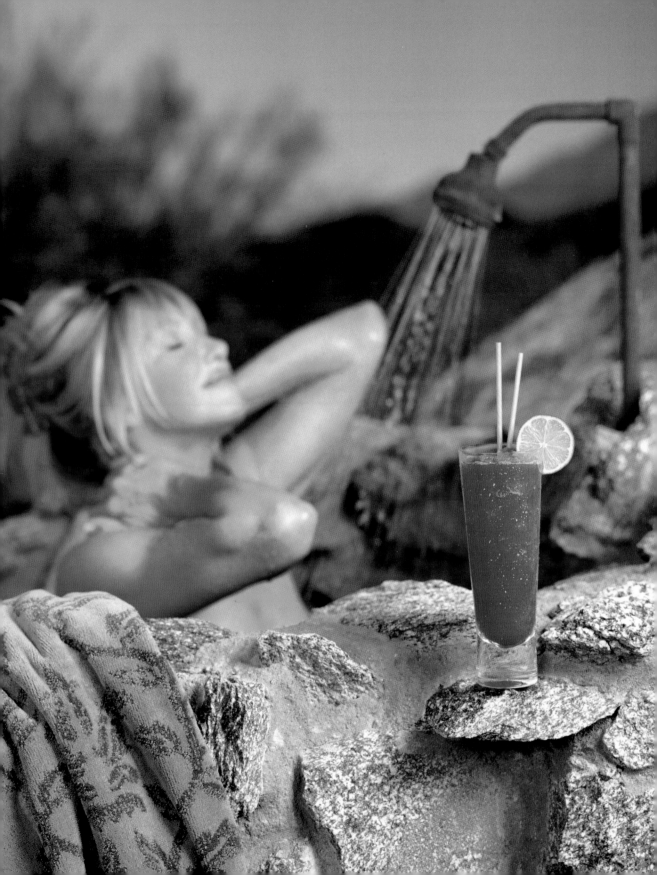

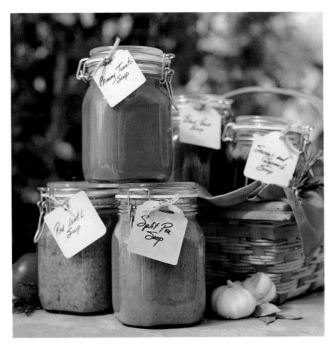

Previous page: My morning outdoor shower and a Watermelon Icy. What could start the day better?

Left: Red Lentil Cumin Soup, Chicken Sausage and Spinach Soup, Eight-Minute Creamy Tomato Soup, Split Pea Soup, and Tex Mex Black Bean Soup

Below: Easy Eggs Florentine with Easy Blender Béarnaise Sauce

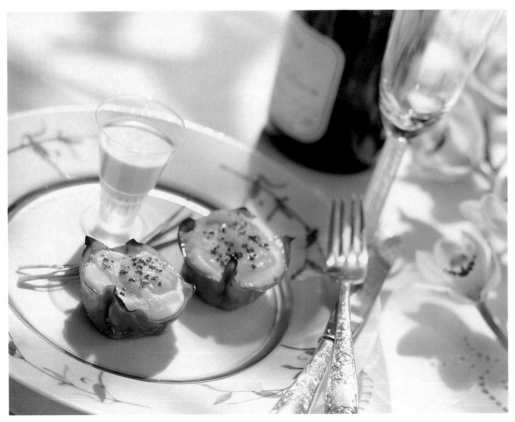

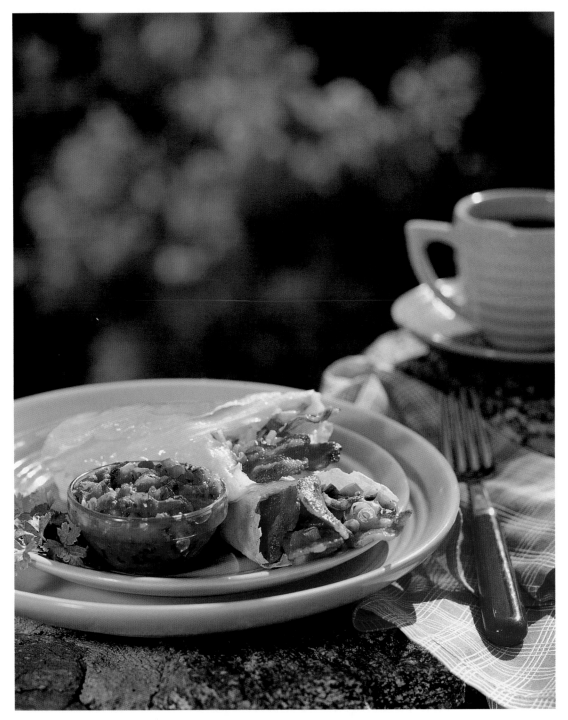

Breakfast Burrito with salsa

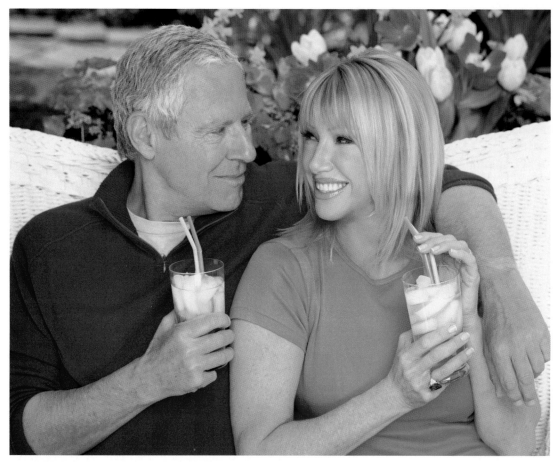

My husband, my pal, Al and me enjoying Somersize Lemon-Lime Flavor Drink Mix.

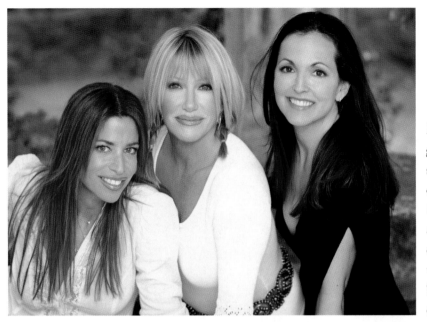

Me and my beautiful girls. Leslie, my stepdaughter and designer/book illustrator, me, and Caroline, my daughter-in-law, who oversees the Somersize food division.

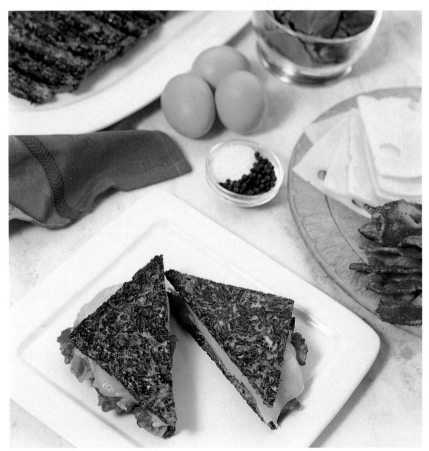

Green Eggs and Ham Sandwiches!

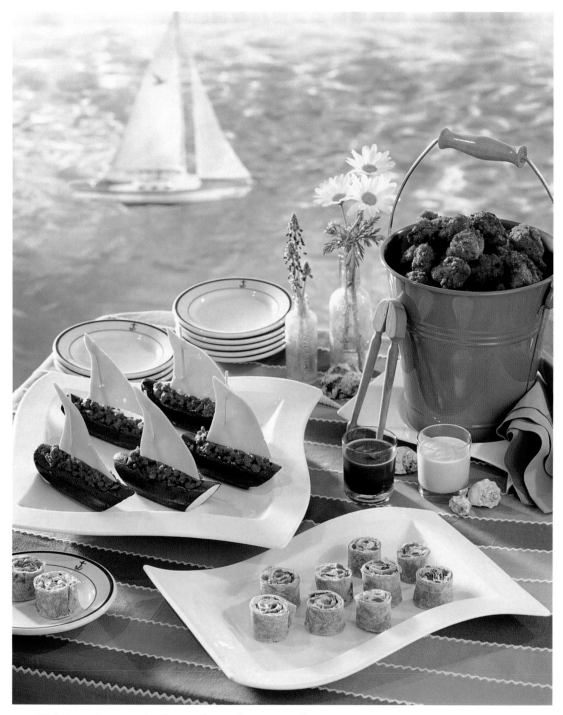

Kids love these foods: SomerSails, Somersize Chicken Nuggets, and Pinwheels. Yum!

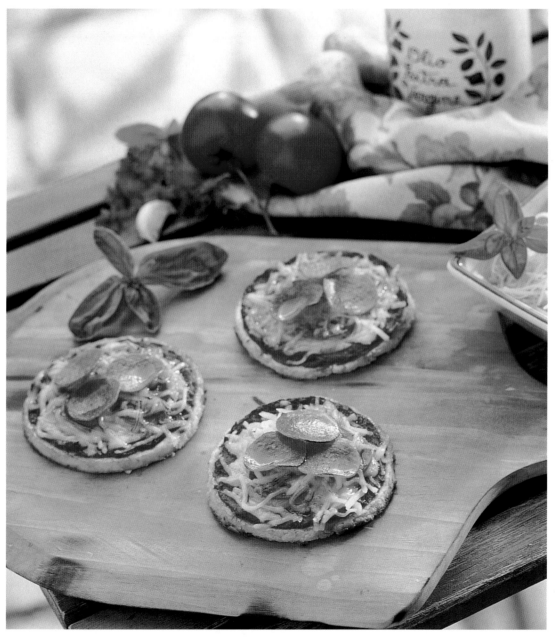

"Legal" Mini-Pepperoni Pizzas

Following page: A Family Feast! Fennel, Red Onion, and Hearts of Palm Salad with
Pink Goddess Salad Dressing, Lemony Artichokes with Artichoke and Onion Dip,
Warm Steak and Arugula Salad with Parmesan Shavings, and Chicken Kiev.

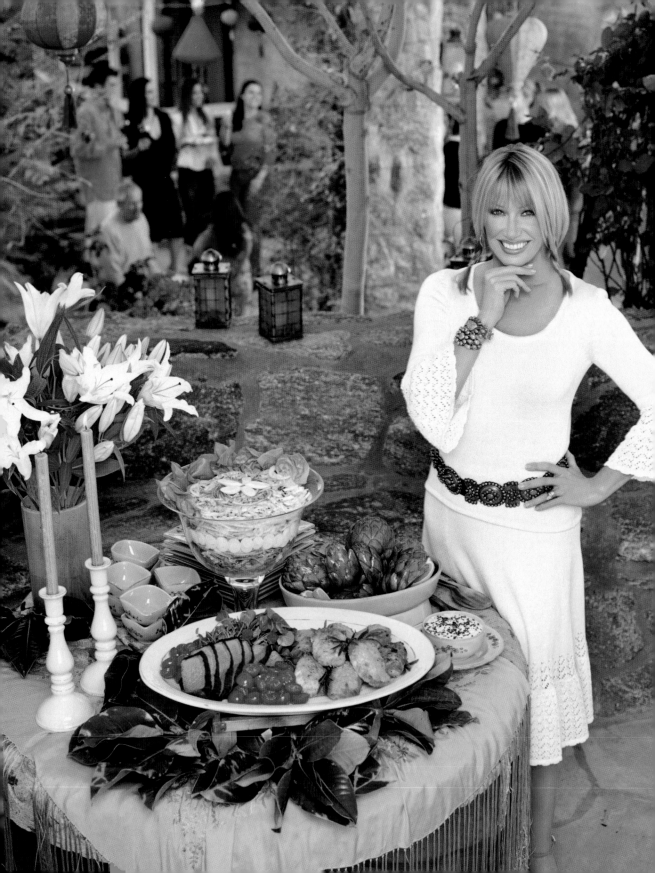

N I N E

The Program

Now that we've covered why Somersizing works and you understand how crucial it is to balance your hormones, let's get down to the nuts and bolts of what you eat on a day-to-day basis.

ELIMINATE

As we've discussed, the most important foods to eliminate are the ones that cause our blood sugar to fluctuate too much. In addition to sugar and white flour, I have made a list of Funky Foods that cause similar problems.

The first group of Funky Foods is made up of sugar sources. Some are natural and some are refined, but natural or not, they're still sugar and I avoid them completely when I'm trying to lose weight.

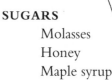

SUGARS

White sugar	Molasses
Brown sugar	Honey
Raw sugar	Maple syrup
Corn syrup	Beets
Sucrose	Carrots

I know it seems weird to eliminate carrots, which have many nutritional qualities, including essential beta-carotene and Vitamin A, but carrots are very high in sugar. We get plenty of beta-carotene from broccoli and kale, and Vitamin A is found in cantaloupe, peaches, and apricots.

Also, a word about fructose. Fructose is a low-glycemic sugar that causes low to moderate rises in your blood sugar. My Somer-

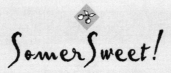

SomerSweet!

She's sweet—five times sweeter than sugar. She's delicious, with no unpleasant aftertaste. She's blended with natural, sweet fiber—fiber your body needs. She bakes; in fact, she cooks like a dream. What more could you ask for . . . SomerSweet is here!

Now you can have something sweet while you Somersize down to your goal weight. This is truly the most exciting product I have ever developed. You can enjoy fabulous, guilt-free treats made with SomerSweet, with no unpleasant aftertaste—just a clean, sweet taste that is perfect for sweetening coffee or tea. SomerSweet is approximately five times sweeter than sugar. A little goes a long way. There are 150 servings per can, which is like getting 1½ pounds of sugar. SomerSweet is also available in convenient individual packets for when you're on the go.

Controlling your sugar and carbohydrate intake is the key to my Somersize weight-loss program. Now it's even easier to stay on the program because you can have something sweet without having refined sugar. With less than 1 gram of carbohydrate per serving and zero sugars per serving, it's a great choice for anyone who understands the health benefits of a low-sugar diet.

SomerSweet has been specially formulated for individuals who want to control their sugar intake and maintain normal blood sugar levels. SomerSweet is a delicious blend of oligofructose, inulin, fructose, sprouted mung bean extract, and acesulfame K. Let me tell you about these wonderful ingredients. Oligofructose and inulin are sweet fibers derived from chicory. The bit of fructose is naturally occurring in these sweet fibers; we do not add it to the blend and it's such a small amount that our nutrition label boasts zero sugars per serving under the FDA guidelines for labeling. Acesulfame K is a nonnutritive sweetener that is fed to a mung bean plant along with water. When the mung bean plant sprouts, the leaves become sweet with only a touch of the acesulfame K in the sweet extract that is used in the finished product. This incredible combination of ingredients adds up to a product that tastes amazing, that bakes beautifully, and that you can feel good about using.

In my last book, *Eat, Cheat, and Melt the Fat Away,* I described SomerSweet as an all-natural pure crystalline fructose from the Lo Han Kuo fruit. After the book went to press, I continued my testing with Lo Han Kuo and found that I was getting an aftertaste in baking. That's when I started working on the delicious blend that we now know as SomerSweet, a blend that bakes and even caramelizes! It was too late to change the text in the book, but I felt it was important to put out the very best SomerSweet. The overall combination of health benefits from the sweet fibers, the delicious taste profile, and the superior baking ability of SomerSweet make it a winner beyond any other product on the market.

I get many questions from diabetics asking if SomerSweet is safe for them. If you are diabetic, please check with your doctor to see if SomerSweet is right for you. We have many diabetics who use the product and love it, but it takes millions of dollars of clinical studies to say that a product is safe for diabetics. Please put your health before your taste buds and make sure SomerSweet is approved by your doctor.

I've developed many incredible desserts using SomerSweet. Believe me, you will not miss the sugar. In fact, you'll feel like you're cheating. There are several delicious recipes in this book like Boston Cream Pie Cake and Coffee Toffee Ice Cream, and for serious dessert lovers, check out *Somersize Desserts* with thirty mouthwatering desserts all made with SomerSweet. Imagine, Dark Chocolate Mousse, Raspberry Sorbet, and Hot Fudge Sundaes while you're losing weight! Finally, Somersize Desserts made exclusively with SomerSweet. You really can have your cake and eat it, too!

SomerSweet is available in cans, in packets, and by the case at SuzanneSomers.com.

 Sweet contains a small amount of fructose that is naturally occurring in the sweet fiber. I do not add any fructose to the blend. Plus, SomerSweet is concentrated (it's five times sweeter than sugar); you get only a very small amount. Each 1-gram serving has so little fructose that by FDA standards, SomerSweet is considered sugar-free, with less than .5 grams of sugar per serving. If you are freely using fructose to sweeten your foods, those sugars can add up and upset your balance. Some Somersizers are able to use moderate amounts of fructose without disrupting their weight loss. Others report that when they started to use fructose they gained weight.

The next group of Funky 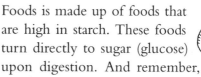 Foods is made up of foods that are high in starch. These foods turn directly to sugar (glucose) upon digestion. And remember, we don't need to give our bodies extra sugar because we can burn our fat reserves for energy instead.

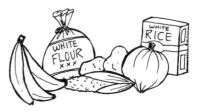

STARCHES

Acorn squash	Potatoes
Bananas	Pumpkin
Butternut squash	Sweet potatoes
Corn	White flour
Hubbard squash	White rice
Parsnips	Yams

There are so many wonderful alternatives to white flour: whole wheat, pumpernickel, rye, amaranth, spelt, and kamut, to name a few. White rice can be replaced with brown rice, which has a wonderful earthy flavor, or better yet, wild rice, which has even less starch. As for corn and potatoes, you will be eating greater amounts of green vegetables rather than filling up on starchy vegetables, which cause a sugar surge and extra pounds. Think about the fact that corn and potatoes are most often used to fatten up our livestock and then maybe it won't be so hard to resist that plate of fries! And I know you will be shocked when I tell you to eliminate

bananas—how about all that potassium? Sorry, but bananas are very high in sugar, and with all the other fruits you can eat, you won't miss them.

The third group of Funky Foods doesn't seem to fit into any of our four Somersize Food Groups because these foods contain protein or fat *and* carbohydrates. Take nuts: they are a protein, they do have fat, *and* they are rich in carbohydrates. That makes them a no-no for Level One Somersizing purposes. Of all the Funky Foods, the foods on this list are the least of your problems. When you graduate to Level Two these are the first foods you may incorporate back

SOMERSIZING FOR VEGETARIANS

Many people ask me if you can Somersize if you are a vegetarian. The answer really depends on how strict you are. If you are the type of person who simply does not eat red meat, you will have no problem following the Level One guidelines. You can get plenty of protein and fat sources from poultry, fish, eggs, and dairy products.

If you do not eat any animal products, you will have a difficult time on Level One, because the only foods left in the Pro/Fats group are vegetable-based oils. This means you will be eating predominantly Carbos. Since Carbos are not eaten with fats on Level One, I worry you will not get the essential fatty acids you needs. Therefore, if you do not eat animal products, you should Somersize on Level Two. This way you can enjoy fats with your Carbos and Veggies. This is probably how you eat anyway, but you will eliminate the sugar and high-starch vegetables, and you will replace white flour, rice, bread, and pasta with their whole-grain counterparts. Anyone will benefit from making that simple change.

In addition, if you are a strict vegetarian and you need additional protein sources, I do make an exception regarding soy. Although tofu has protein, fat, and carbohydrates, I recommend you include it in your meals, either as a Pro/Fat or a Carbo since it has protein, fat, and carbohydrate. As for soy milk, buy fat-free soy milk and treat it as a Carbo with the other nonfat dairy products.

into your meals. In fact, many eat olives, avocados, and soy products on Level One and still enjoy all the effects of losing weight and feeling great. I regularly eat soy beans (edamame) without any problems. They are a great source of protein and fat, and even though they have a little carbohydrate, I find that eating them does not disrupt my weight loss. Plus, they are so good for you!

BAD COMBO FOODS

Avocados	Nuts
Coconuts	Olives
Liver	Soy
Low-fat or whole milk	

The last group of Funky Foods is made up of caffeine and alcohol. Just like other Funky Foods, caffeine can cause highs and lows in your blood sugar, which leads to insulin resistance. I'd hate to see you eat a perfectly combined meal and then blow it with one cup of coffee. Feel free to drink decaffeinated coffee (try Starbuck's delicious Guatemalan decaf) and herbal teas, especially decaf green tea. And don't worry; when you combine correctly, you'll have a steady source of energy to get you through the day, rather than experiencing the highs and lows that keep us reaching for caffeine or sweets. As for alcohol, everyone knows it makes you fat, especially beer and hard liquor. Now that you understand the connection between insulin and weight gain around the midsection, a "beer belly" makes perfect sense. Red wine has recently been found to have beneficial effects, and we will incorporate it later on when we are maintaining our weight, but during Level

One we will steer clear of all alcohol. I do, however, make an exception with regard to cooking. If you are doing well on Level One you may use wine in some of my recipes because the alcohol burns off and it leaves a delicious flavor in your cooking.

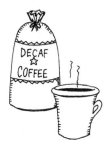

CAFFEINE AND ALCOHOL

Beer	Coffee
Caffeinated teas	Hard alcohol
Caffeinated sodas	Wine
Cocoa	

I know it seems like a strange list of foods to eliminate, but soon it will become second nature. Sugar, starches, bad combo foods, caffeine, and alcohol are all avoided *completely* on Level One. But don't worry, you don't have to say good-bye to these foods forever. They'll be back in moderation when we reach our goal weight and advance to Level Two, the maintenance portion of Somersizing.

SEPARATE

In order to learn how to combine our foods in a way that maximizes our digestion, we must first separate foods into our four Somersize categories: Proteins/Fats, Carbos,

THE CONNECTION BETWEEN CAFFEINE AND COMFORT FOODS

When we drink caffeine, we increase our adrenaline. Oh, how we love that caffeine rush in the morning, at lunchtime, or during that afternoon dip. But increased adrenaline blocks estrogen receptors and increases insulin levels. Since insulin is the fat-storing hormone, we don't want to drink caffeine with a meal because the insulin released could send the whole meal to the fat reserves. Also, caffeine initially increases serotonin, the feel-good hormone, but then makes it lower over time. Low serotonin levels can trigger us to crave "comfort foods." Comfort foods vary from person to person, but usually they are high in carbohydrates (mashed potatoes, macaroni and cheese, cookies, cake, and so on). These comfort foods cause spikes in our insulin, and by now we all know the ill effects of raised insulin levels. Plus, caffeine raises adrenaline, and adrenaline breaks down lean body tissue. Lean body tissue is proportional to our metabolism. The less lean body mass, the lower our metabolism, which leaves us open to weight gain. It's hard to kick the habit at first, but I tell you, decaffeinated coffee is the way to go.

Veggies, and Fruits. Although many foods are made up of a combination of protein, fat, and carbohydrate, we have grouped them by their predominant feature to help simplify the program. For instance, *all* the foods found in the Carbos, Veggies, and Fruit groups contain carbohydrates, but the carbohydrate levels vary greatly, which is why I have broken them down into different groups. I have briefly described each group here and have included complete lists of these foods in the Appendix, which you'll find at the back of the book.

PRO/FATS

The first Somersize group is made up of foods high in protein and/or fat. I put these two food groups together because many of the foods that contain protein also contain fat. Meat, poultry, fish, eggs, cheese, butter, and cream are just a few of the Pro/Fats you'll enjoy.

Proteins are made up of organic compounds called amino acids. These amino acids are the building blocks for the human body. Proteins play a role in virtually every cellular function: they regulate muscle contraction, antibody production, and blood vessel expansion and contraction to maintain normal blood pressure. Protein is a critically important part of the diet because it supplies us with new amino acids that are needed to make these different proteins.

By now you understand the virtues of fat and know that completely eliminating fat from your diet is unhealthy. Fats provide a major storage form of metabolic fuel. When they break down they provide us with energy. Fats also help to facilitate the use of essential fat-soluble vitamins like A, D, E, and K. Vitamin A is necessary for healthy eyes and skin; Vitamin D helps to absorb calcium; Vitamin E prevents cholesterol deposits; and Vitamin K contributes to healthy blood clotting. Fat also helps to stabilize blood sugar. And fat is the body's fuel source that causes the lowest insulin response. Essential fatty acids cannot be manufactured by our bodies on their own; they, too, must be included in our daily meals. Unsaturated fats, like olive oil, canola oil, and fish oils, help to lower cholesterol levels and should be included in our meals.

Any of the foods in the Pro/Fats group can be eaten together, or in combination with Veggies. (See the complete list of Pro/Fats on page 315.)

CARBOS

Carbohydrates are mostly derived from plant sources, rather than from animal sources. Carbos are the primary metabolic fuel in our Westernized diets. As I explained earlier, carbos break down into glucose, which is one of the body's main sources of energy. (The other is fat.) Since we have other mechanisms in our bodies to produce glucose, carbos are the one nutrient that is not absolutely essential in our diet. However, completely eliminating carbohydrates from our diet is dangerous. On the Somersize system we eliminate *refined* carbohydrates like sugar, white flour, and white rice, but we do enjoy complex carbohydrates, like whole-grain pastas and cereals, which still have many essential vitamins and nutrients intact. In addition, complex carbohydrates provide fiber and roughage necessary for the digestive process.

On an emotional level, carbohydrates cause a release of serotonin—the feel-good hormone. If you are prone to depression, completely eliminating carbohydrates causes a halt in serotonin levels, which can lead to depression and weight gain. Be careful, however, of loading up on the wrong kinds of carbohydrates if you are depressed and looking for a serotonin fix. Comfort foods, like macaroni and cheese or a turkey pot pie, loaded with white flour, may give you the serotonin release, but they also bring the ill effects of poorly combined, high-starch meals. Stick to the reasonable amounts of the foods listed in the Carbos group and you shouldn't have a problem.

Any of the foods in the Carbos group can be eaten together, or in combination with Veggies. (See the complete list of Carbos on page 316.)

VEGGIES

All vegetables are technically carbohydrates, but those found in this Somersize category have been chosen because they are low in starch and cause only a minute rise in the blood sugar. These include green beans, broccoli, cauliflower, artichokes, tomatoes, peppers, onions, and more. Vegetables are packed with vitamins and minerals and provide essential roughage for proper elimina-

ASPARAGUS—THE ALKALINE VEGETABLE

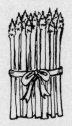

Many health-care professionals feel that we are facing the most dangerous crisis in history. There have been numerous studies linking illness and disease to overacidity in our bodies. We want our bodies to be alkaline, not acidic. Unfortunately, we breathe polluted air, our food and water supply are filled with chemicals, and our stress levels are through the roof. All of these factors cause our bodies to overproduce acid wastes, which can upset the delicate alkaline/acid balance.

For more information on this serious health issue, I highly recommend you read Dr.

Theodore A. Baroody's book Alkalize or Die. *It gives important guidelines for evaluating your alkaline/acid situation, and how to fix it. One great way to reduce the acid in your body is to eat asparagus! Baroody cites asparagus as a powerful acid reducer and a known therapy for cancer. Its high ammonia content literally plummets your body into alkalinity in a short period of time. And it tastes great, too!*

Now when I go to pick my vegetables for my meals, I choose asparagus several times a week. I especially like it steamed and dipped in Lemon Dill Mayonnaise.

---

tion. I implore you, fill up on vegetables! They are an essential part of your daily diet.

Any of the foods in the Veggies group can be eaten together. And since Veggies can easily be digested with either Pro/Fats *or* Carbos, you may eat them with either group. (See the complete list of Veggies on page 317.)

FRUITS

Fruits are also technically carbohydrates, but because of their unique sugar content, fruit must always be eaten alone. Fruits are a great source of fiber and help to keep the digestive track moving. They are loaded

with nutrients and vitamins, but if you mix fruit with other foods, it can lose its nutritional benefits and upset the digestive process. Fruit turns to acid when combined with other food groups and spoils in the stomach, causing gas and that horrible bloated feeling. Fruit as a supposedly "healthy" option for dessert can ruin a perfectly combined meal. Not only will it make you feel uncomfortable, it can trap the energy of other foods and cause unnecessary storage of fat. So eat fruit . . . please eat fruit. But eat it alone to get the maximum benefits.

As far as fruit juice is concerned, most of the vital nutrients have been pressed out of the fruit by the time it is turned into juice. The remaining juice is mostly fruit sugar. Therefore, I recommend you eat the whole fruit to receive the fiber and drink fruit juice sparingly. Concentrated fruit juice is often used as a sugar substitute. Unfortunately, your body reacts exactly the same to fruit sugar as it does to regular sugar, because it makes your insulin spike. Every now and then I may have an all-fruit-juice-sweetened sorbet or ice pop (on Level One), but not with great frequency, because on Level One we are trying to heal our insulin resistance. The same goes for dried fruit; the sugar concentration becomes far more intense with dried fruits. I eat them rarely, if at all, on Level One.

Here are some guidelines on how you can eat delicious and nutritious fresh fruit and gain all the benefits without creating digestion problems.

Eat Fruit on an empty stomach.

Eat Fruit alone, then wait twenty minutes, and you may follow up with a Carbos meal. (The twenty-minute lead time gets the digestion of the fruit going and eliminates problem combinations.)

Eat fruit alone, then wait one hour, and you may follow up with a Pro/Fat meal.

If you want Fruit for a snack or for dessert, you must wait two hours after your last meal to avoid any problems.

Any of the foods in the Fruit group can be eaten together. (See the complete list of Fruit on page 317.)

FREE FOODS

There are a few items that may be combined with Pro/Fats, Veggies, or Carbos because they do not conflict with any of the food groups. These include soy sauce, vinegar, mustard, herbs, and spices. In addition, lemons and limes, though technically fruits, are very low in sugar and therefore may be used to flavor any of the four food groups. Of course, the most exciting Free Food of all . . . SomerSweet!

THE GLYCEMIC INDEX

All carbohydrates will break down into sugar upon digestion. But as we've discussed, some carbohydrates create a much greater insulin response than others.

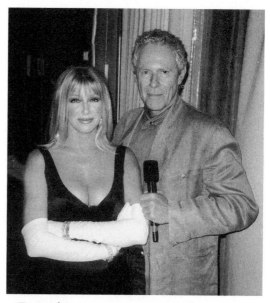

Right before going onstage. Alan always announces me.

Although I do not ask you to calculate calories, fat grams, sugars, or even carbohydrates as part of the Somersize program, I am including this chart, called the Glycemic Index, to assist you in seeing the effects of various kinds of carbohydrates. The glycemic index rises corresponding to the level of hyperglycemia caused by eating carbohydrates. The higher the glycemic index, the higher the level of hyperglycemia.

You will notice that foods in their natural state have a lower glycemic index than foods that have been processed. Whole-wheat bread breaks down into less glucose than its processed counterpart, white bread. Brown rice has a lower glycemic index than its refined counterpart, white rice. This is largely due to the fiber content of foods. The greater the fiber, the lower the glycemic index.

Fruits and vegetables are also carbohydrates, with varying degrees of glucose potential. Seeing how they rate on the glycemic index will help to explain how I divided all food into my four Somersize Food Groups. Those vegetables with the highest glycemic index, such as potatoes, beets, and carrots, have been labeled Funky Foods and eliminated altogether. Whole grains, beans, and dairy products have a moderate glycemic index and have been categorized in the Somersize Carbos group. And nonstarchy vegetables with the lowest glycemic index have been categorized in the Somersize Veggies group. You'll also notice that SomerSweet has a glycemic index in the same range as low-starch green vegetables.

GLYCEMIC INDEX CHART

Beer	110
Sugar	100
White bread	95
Instant potatoes	95
Honey	90
Jam	90
Cornflakes	85
Popcorn	85
Carrots	85
Potatoes	70
Pasta (from white flour)	65
Bananas	60
Dried fruit	60
Brown rice	50
Whole-wheat bread	50
Whole-wheat pasta	45
Fresh white beans	40
Oatmeal	40
Whole rye bread	40
Green peas	40
Whole cereals	35
Dairy products	35
Wild rice	35
Fresh fruits	35
Dried beans	30
Dark chocolate	22
Fructose	20
Soy	15
Green vegetables	Less than 15
SomerSweet	approx. 5

WHAT'S THE DEAL WITH DAIRY?

Many people, including me, get confused about dairy products with regard to Somersizing. When you're having a Pro/Fats meal, you may eat all the cheese you want and you may add cream to your sauce, but you can't use a splash of milk in your decaf coffee. When you're having a Carbos meal you can eat nonfat yogurt, but you can't use nonfat yogurt with a Pro/Fats meal. What's the deal? Let me help to clarify this issue.

Milk has protein and carbohydrates, whether it's nonfat, low-fat, or whole milk. Yogurt has protein and carbohydrates, whether it's nonfat, low-fat, or whole-milk yogurt. When we eat proteins or fats, we do not eat foods that contain carbohydrates; therefore, we cannot include any kind of milk or yogurt in the Pro/Fats meal. When we eat a Carbos meal, we can include products with protein, as long as they do not contain any fat. Therefore, we can include nonfat milk and nonfat yogurt. Low-fat and whole milk or yogurt are grouped as Funky Foods because they have fat and carbohydrates.

What about cream, butter, cheese, sour cream, and the like? These "milk" products have a very different quality than their plain milk or yogurt cousins. In the process of making cream, butter, or cheese, all the carbohydrates are processed out of these dairy products, leaving only the protein and fat. That is the reason why these dairy products without *carbohydrates are included in the Pro/Fats group, while the milk products with carbohydrates are grouped in the Carbos group.*

Get it? If not, read it again.

DAIRY PRODUCTS

PRO/FATS—DAIRY PRODUCTS WITHOUT CARBOHYDRATES	CARBOS—DAIRY PRODUCTS WITH CARBOHYDRATES AND NO FAT	FUNKY FOODS—DAIRY PRODUCTS WITH CARBOHYDRATES AND FAT
Butter	Nonfat milk	Low-fat milk
Cream	Nonfat yogurt	Whole milk
Cheese	Nonfat cheese	Low-fat yogurt
Sour cream	Nonfat soy milk	Whole-milk yogurt
Crème fraîche	Nonfat rice milk	Buttermilk
	Nonfat cottage cheese	Low-fat or whole soymilk
		Low-fat or whole rice milk

TEN

❧

Level One and Almost Level One

Now that you have a basic understanding of what foods to eliminate and how to categorize the rest of foods into our four Somersize groups, you can get started on your new lifestyle. Let me walk you through each meal so you can see how easy it is to Somersize at every meal.

BREAKFAST

Each meal is an opportunity to eat something great, even on Level One when you're trying to lose weight. Let's talk about all the delicious breakfast options. I love breakfast! Cereal, toast, fruit, eggs, bacon, sausage . . . bring them on! As long as you follow the Somersize combinations, you may eat *any* of those foods for breakfast, just not in the same sitting. Here are your choices.

Breakfast #1—Fruit Meal
Breakfast #2—Carbos Meal
Breakfast #3—Fruit, wait twenty
   minutes, then Carbos meal
Breakfast #4—Pro/Fats and Veggies
   meal

BREAKFAST #1—FRUIT MEAL

Start your day off with a couple of plums, an orange, or half a cantaloupe. Or combine your favorite fruits in a blender with some juice and a few ice cubes for a frosty fruit smoothie. Or dice some mangoes, pineapple, papaya, and grapes for a tasty fruit salad.

Remember, you may eat any kind of fruit, except bananas, which are a Funky Food. Fruit is best in the morning when eaten on an empty stomach. Fruit keeps you regular and is loaded with vitamins, nutrients, and a natural source of energy.

Examples of Breakfast #1—Fruit Meal
- Fruit smoothie with peaches, raspberries, strawberries, and fruit juice
- Fruit smoothie with pineapple chunks, papaya, and orange juice
- Fruit salad of melon, grapes, and oranges
- An apple
- A bowl of fresh cherries
- A slice of watermelon

To DRINK: Decaf coffee or tea, black (or sweetened with SomerSweet)

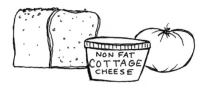

BREAKFAST #2—CARBOS MEAL

Morning is the best time of the day to eat your Carbos so you can use the natural energy they supply throughout the day. There are a number of wonderful options to satisfy your hunger. I like whole-grain toast with nonfat cottage cheese or yogurt. Or I like hot or cold whole-grain cereal with nonfat milk. Since we cannot combine any fat with our Carbos, this is the only time we choose fat-free products, specifically nonfat dairy products. I guard against choosing

processed fat-free dairy products, like some fat-free cream cheeses, because they are often loaded with starches, fillers, and chemicals.

Check your labels. Focus on the ingredient list, rather than the nutritional panel. If all the ingredients are acceptable Carbos, without any Funky Foods, you may eat the food. Do not look at the number of carbohydrates, proteins, or fats listed in the panel. If they are unpronounceable ingredients, you are better off avoiding that product.

And remember, you may have Veggies with your Carbos, so feel free to top your toast with tomato and basil or a slice of red onion, if you like.

Examples of Breakfast #2— Carbos Meal
- Whole-wheat toast with nonfat cottage cheese and tomato
- Rye bagel with nonfat ricotta cheese
- Fat-free wheat tortilla with black beans and salsa
- Nonfat yogurt sprinkled with Grape-Nuts
- Shredded Wheat with nonfat milk
- Oatmeal with nonfat milk

To DRINK: Decaf coffee or tea, black or with nonfat milk (and/or sweetened with SomerSweet)

BREAKFAST #3—FRUIT, WAIT TWENTY MINUTES, THEN CARBOS MEAL

Fruit, then Carbos is my favorite choice for breakfast because these foods provide me with necessary fiber and a whole host of vitamins and nutrients. Besides that, they just taste good! Alan is the master breakfast maker in our home. Usually he brings me a great fruit smoothie in the morning. Then I do my morning workout. Afterward, we have toast or cereal with decaf coffee. Morning is the best time to eat your Fruit and Carbos so that you have plenty of time to burn off the natural sources of energy they provide.

Here are a few more examples of Fruit and Carbos.

Examples of Breakfast #3—Fruit, then Carbos Meal

- Melon. Wait twenty minutes.
  Oatmeal with nonfat milk.
- Fruit smoothie with cantaloupe, raspberries, and grapefruit juice. Wait twenty minutes.
  Whole-grain toast with nonfat cottage cheese and a sprinkle of cinnamon.
- A couple of oranges. Wait twenty minutes.
  Puffed Wheat cereal with nonfat milk.
- Pineapple slices. Wait twenty minutes.
  Toasted rye bagel and a bowl of non-fat yogurt sweetened with vanilla extract and SomerSweet.
- Fruit salad. Wait twenty minutes.
  Oatmeal with nonfat milk.

TO DRINK: Decaf coffee or tea, black or with nonfat milk (and/or sweetened with SomerSweet)

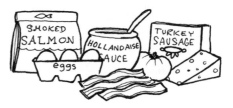

BREAKFAST #3—PRO/FATS AND VEGGIES MEAL

In a Pro/Fats and Veggies breakfast, you may have anything from the Pro/Fats group with anything from the Veggies group. You have so many choices with this breakfast. The "incredible egg" can be scrambled, fried, boiled, poached, or made into an omelette or a frittata. Don't be afraid of eggs! Have as many as you like. Cook them up in butter or oil and serve them with sausage or bacon (I look for brands with no nitrates). Try my Breakfast Burritos made with Egg Crêpes (p. 188). For additional flavor, you can even cook your eggs in the bacon fat or sausage fat. Some diet, huh? You can have meat, fish, or poultry including chicken, shrimp, crab, lox, and smoked fish. Feel free to add some cheese to that omelette! And don't forget your Veggies, like onions, tomatoes, zucchini, spinach, mushrooms, asparagus, and more.

Here are just a few examples of what you might create for a Pro/Fats and Veggies breakfast.

- Omelette with zucchini, Swiss cheese, mushrooms, and sour cream.
  Side of turkey sausage.
- Fried eggs with bacon.
  Side of tomatoes.
- Scrambled eggs with smoked salmon, asparagus, and sour cream.

- Huevos rancheros—fried eggs with caramelized onions, cheddar cheese, salsa, and sour cream. (Hold the tortilla).
- Poached eggs on a bed of spinach with Canadian bacon and hollandaise sauce. Side of green beans.
- Eggs Florentine with ham, cheese, and spinach.

TO DRINK: Decaf coffee or tea, black or with cream (and/or sweetened with SomerSweet)

Any of these foods would make up a perfectly combined Somersize breakfast, so you may eat until you are full. This is a great breakfast option when you're eating out because there are so few restrictions. Just stay away from toast, jelly, potatoes, and fruit with your Pro/Fats and Veggies breakfast.

If you want to start this meal with Fruit, you must wait one hour until you have your Pro/Fats and Veggies.

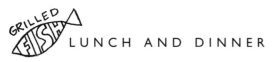 LUNCH AND DINNER

For lunch and dinner you may have salads, soups, sandwiches, chicken, steak, fish, pasta, and more! You just have to decide which food group you feel like and then design a meal in the proper Somersize combination. Here are your choices.

Lunch or Dinner #1—
    Pro/Fats and Veggies Meal
Lunch or Dinner #2—
    Carbos and Veggies Meal
Lunch or Dinner #3—
    Single Food Group Meal

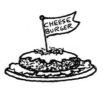

LUNCH OR DINNER #1— PRO/FATS AND VEGGIES MEAL

Flavor, flavor, flavor! That's what you can look forward to with every Pro/Fats and Veggies meal. Order from any restaurant menu with the Pro/Fats and Veggies meal: meat, poultry, or fish can be grilled, broiled, baked, roasted, or fried (no flour) and served with plenty of fresh vegetables, raw, steamed, sautéed, or grilled. It is important to balance your meals with vegetables because they give your body the small amount of carbohydrates it needs to stay balanced and to produce serotonin. Enjoy cooking with oil or butter and don't forget to add the cheese! Preparing meals for yourself at home or eating in a restaurant is a pleasure with the Pro/Fats and Veggies meal.

Examples of Lunch or Dinner #1— Pro/Fats and Veggies Meal

- Cobb salad with lettuce, chicken, bacon, egg, tomato, blue cheese, and green onions with full-fat sugar-free dressing of your choice. (Hold the avocado.)
- Taco salad with lettuce, shredded beef, tomatoes, cheddar cheese, salsa, onions, and sour cream. (Hold the beans and chips.)
- Grilled fish with lemon-butter sauce. Snow peas tossed in butter. Green salad with full-fat sugar-free dressing of your choice.
- Caesar salad (hold the croutons) with grilled chicken breast. Grilled red peppers, zucchini, and fennel.

- Hamburger patty with melted jack cheese and a pile of onions.
  Green salad with cherry tomatoes and blue cheese dressing.
- Egg salad tossed with celery, green onions, and mayonnaise, served in lettuce cups with tomato slices and alfalfa sprouts.
- Rotisserie-style chicken.
  Steamed broccoli and cauliflower covered with cheese.
- Steamed crab legs and grilled filet mignon.
  Steamed artichoke with butter or mayonnaise dip.
  Butter lettuce salad with zucchini and Parmesan cheese.
- Turkey cutlet served over sautéed Swiss chard with a butter-wine sauce.
  Green salad with goat cheese and candied tomatoes.
- Grilled lamb chops with lemon and olive oil.
  Greek salad with tomatoes, cucumber, red onion, feta cheese, and olive oil.
- Stir-fried shrimp with napa cabbage, celery, broccoli, yellow peppers, Italian squash, bamboo shoots.
- Chopped salad with salami, roasted peppers, tomatoes, onions, and provolone cheese.
  Fresh raw vegetables with dip.
- Steak with peppercorn cream sauce and sautéed mushrooms.
  Steamed green beans tossed in butter.
  Radicchio and endive salad with blue cheese and tomato.

TO DRINK: Water, mineral water, Somer-Sweet drinks, decaf coffee or tea with cream (and/or sweetened with SomerSweet).

Your Pro/Fats and Veggies meals will range from the incredibly simple to the luxuriously extravagant. With so much to choose from, you won't ever get bored eating the same old thing. In fact, your food will taste better than ever as you trim your way down to your ideal body weight.

LUNCH OR DINNER #2— CARBOS AND VEGGIES MEAL

I choose this option with very little frequency, because I prefer to eat my Carbos only in the morning when I'm trying to lose weight. But every now and then you just need a Carbo fix at lunch or dinner, and it really hits the spot. You can have any whole grains or beans with nonfat dairy products and any of the vegetables in the Veggies list. Be careful when you look for whole-wheat products . . . many manufacturers are now listing "wheat-flour" for regular white flour. It must say *"whole*-wheat flour" to really be a whole grain. In general, if it looks too white to be whole wheat, it probably isn't.

You might have brown rice with peas or black bean chili with fresh tomato salsa and whole-wheat tortillas or whole-grain pasta with tomato basil sauce or whole-wheat pita bread with hummus, baba ghanoush, and fresh vegetables. With any of these meals you could have a green salad. Try my Somersize Pasta and Somersize Sauces (with no fat) for a perfectly Somersized Carbos meal. The key to the Carbos and Veggies meal is to make sure there is absolutely no fat.

Examples of Lunch or Dinner #2— Carbos and Veggies Meal

- Brown rice with soy sauce and steamed vegetables.
  Green salad with a splash of vinegar.
- Whole-wheat pita bread with nonfat ricotta cheese, roasted peppers, and eggplant.
  Grilled zucchini and yellow squash.
- Whole-wheat pasta with tomato, basil, and garlic sauce.
  An artichoke with a squeeze of lemon.
- A bowl of black beans with whole-wheat tortillas and fresh salsa.
- Whole-wheat pita bread with hummus, baba ghanoush, lettuce, and tomato.
- Spinach whole-wheat pasta with fresh garden vegetables, peas, and stewed tomatoes.
- Whole-wheat cheeseless pizza with marinara sauce, mushrooms, onions, tomatoes, and artichoke hearts.
  Green salad with a squeeze of lemon.

To drink: Water, mineral water, Somersize drinks, decaf coffee or tea with nonfat milk (and/or sweetened with SomerSweet).

This is a very satisfying and healthy option with all the whole grains and fresh vegetables. It can be a little restrictive, however, because on Level One you can't have any fat with Carbos and you must watch for hidden sugars and Funky Foods. Because this meal is more difficult to obtain in a

restaurant, I normally prepare Carbos and Veggies at home.

LUNCH OR DINNER #3—SINGLE FOOD GROUP MEAL

Every now and then you might want to have a meal made up of only one food group, like the all Fruit meal or the all Veggies meal. Of course, this is perfectly fine on rare occasions, but I do not recommend it with any frequency.

FINDING A RHYTHM THAT WORKS

When I'm losing weight on Level One, I find that the fewer Carbos I eat, the more results I see. As I explained earlier, Carbos are an energy source, and if you're not giving your body many sources of energy, it will have to break down your fat reserves and use *them* as energy. But we don't want to cut out carbohydrates completely because they are an important source of fiber and help keep your system moving properly. And if you go too low with carbohydrates, your body will break down its protein, instead of its fat reserves, to be used as energy.

Here's what works best for me. I like to eat the Fruit, then Carbos breakfast. Because Carbos are a good energy source, it's best to eat them in the morning so that you can use that energy throughout the day. For lunch or dinner I find more options with Pro/Fats and plenty of Veggies. Don't forget to add your veggies! Eating proteins and fats alone, for any length of time, does not promote a healthy balance, so like Mom always says, "Eat your vegetables." Carbos meals for lunch and dinner are a little more restrictive because you can have absolutely no fat.

My recommendation is that for breakfast you have Breakfast #3—Fruit, then Carbos. For lunch and dinner I recommend Pro/Fats and Veggies as a rule with the Carbos and Veggies meal as the exception. If you eat too many carbohydrates, even the right kind of carbohydrates, they could get stored as fat for later use. (And if you're filling up on Carbos, you're probably not giving your body enough protein and fat.) Remember, you're giving your body the small amount of carbohydrates it needs because your Pro/Fats and Veggies meals include some carbohydrates in the form of the many vegetables you'll be enjoying. Make sure to include your vegetables. A meal of meat and cheese alone is not a good idea on a regular basis.

In fact, if you are eating plenty of vegetables, you could choose the Pro/Fats and Veggies meal at *every* meal and enjoy great health—it's a perfect combination of protein, fat, and carbohydrates (in the form of low-starch vegetables). (You know how I love my eggs with bacon and sliced tomatoes in the morning!) This combination gives your body all the essential building materials it needs to thrive. The Carbos and Veggies meal gives you some diversity now and then and, as I said, includes all that great fiber.

This is only a blueprint of how I divide my Pro/Fats and Carbos meals. For me, those Carbos tend to fatten me up like a corn-fed cow; especially at this age, when I am fighting even more hormonal imbalances. You may find, however, that your body can handle more carbohydrates and that you feel better eating mostly grains and vegetables. On the other hand, if you are eating mostly Pro/Fats, you must balance your meals with plenty of fresh vegetables. I cannot stress this enough. It is unwise to eat only meat and cheese without the fiber and nutrients added from vegetables. Also, this gives your body the essential serotonin it requires for balance.

COMMON SENSE

Last year I held a Somersize Recipe Contest on my website, SuzanneSomers.com. We had so many wonderful recipes from Somersizers around the globe, we published a book of all sixty winners and called it the Somersize Recipe Contest Cookbook. Everyone got so creative! (It's for sale on my website if you'd like to pick one up.)

One of the winners actually had several entries that I considered using. She is a great cook and has had wonderful success on the program. She was thrilled to hear she was one of our grand prize winners. When she was notified, she passed along a personal story as a warning to me and other Somersizers. While she was testing recipes for the contest, she really went to town on making desserts and other Pro/Fats meals. She spent the month testing and eating and testing and eating. Several times a day she was eating Chocolate Mousse Pie, Cheesecakes, Cream Cheese Pancakes, and so on.

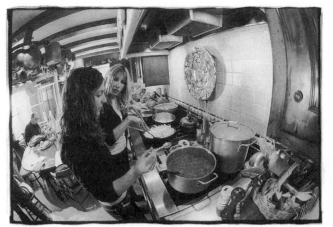

Caroline and me, where we connect best— cooking together.

After several days of eating nothing but Pro/Fats, she became sick. Yes, her body told her she'd had enough fats. Fortunately she was okay and got back on the program in a sensible manner.

Even though I stress throughout the books not to overdo it, sometimes we forget and push the envelope too far. Please use your common sense. Just because your cheesecake is made with SomerSweet, you should not eat the whole thing. One piece of cheesecake is plenty. Could you eat cheesecake for breakfast? Yes, technically you could because the ingredients are acceptable Pro/Fats, *but* that doesn't mean you should! (I was recently misquoted in a magazine on this issue. They took the beginning of my answer and deleted everything after "but.") Cheesecake is not breakfast food and I do not recommend it as such. You need to use your common sense.

There is no portion control, but please balance your meals with vegetables and enjoy some fruit for breakfast or snacks. I like to give you the freedom to eat without measuring or weighing your foods because it allows you to live your life and not obsess about everything that goes into your mouth. You know that eating a whole wheel of Brie is too much . . . so don't do it. Unlike other programs, you will always have enough to eat when you Somersize. The key is knowing when you are eating just for the sake of eating. So many of us are used to rigid diets that we gorge ourselves when we Somersize, just because we can. Once you realize that you will never again go hungry on this program, you will lose the urge to overdo it. Once you stop thinking and obsessing about food, food becomes your friend again. It no longer controls you. You sit in the driver's seat of your weight loss. You control the show.

To my friend who overdid it on fats, I thank you for sharing your story. It will help others and lead them down the proper Somersize path. And the next time you hear me say, "You can eat as much fat as you want" I'll remember to add, "But make sure not to overdo it!"

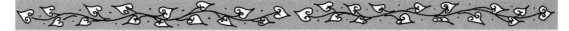

Dear Suzanne,

Thank you. I'm sure you hear that all the time, but I wanted you to know that I would not be alive if it weren't for your Somersizing program. Back in April 2001, my doctor told me I was in pretty bad shape. I weighed in at over 425 pounds, and am a heavy smoker with high blood pressure. I was told if something didn't change, I would not be here long after my next birthday. My doctor recommended Somersizing, so I went to the library and checked out *Eat Great, Lose Weight*. I read it, all the while thinking that I would not be able to stick to it. But on May 8, I began to Somersize in earnest. Within three days I was getting bursts of energy. By the fifth day a lot of my aches and pains that I had lived with for years were disappearing. I could feel the change in my body as I started to heal.

With the help and support of other Somersizers, by July I had dropped 43 pounds, adding years to my life with every meal. I could move better and was sleeping better than I had in the longest time. My doctor was thrilled with my progress and all my blood work was well within normal ranges. Best of all, my uncontrolled blood pressure was coming under control. By August, I was down 52 pounds and a wonderful thing happened to me. For years, I could not walk from room to room in my own home without having to stop and catch my breath. On August 4, I walked a football field without needing to stop. How remarkable and exciting that day was!

The best news however, happened yesterday. I weighed in again, and, after two months on plateau, reached 100 pounds gone! I am only one-third of the way to my goal, but nine months ago, I never thought I would even be here, let alone be this much lighter. My children, ten and fourteen, absolutely love all the great foods I am cooking and are grateful to have their real mommy back. And my husband is again looking to our future together. I now believe that in time, with Somersizing, I can be something I have never been . . . a normal size . . . and I will someday know my grandchildren. So thank you, Suzanne, from myself and all the people who love me and whom I love, for truly saving my life.

With much love and gratitude,
Barbara Ledgerwood

YOU'RE ONLY CHEATING YOURSELF

Cheating is not for Level One. Level One is when we first start the program and we are trying to unload the stored sugar from our cells and heal our metabolism. If you are finding little ways to cheat, you are only cheating yourself. I have a friend who is trying to lose weight and after a couple of weeks on the program, she called me to say she hadn't lost much. She was disappointed. I asked her if she was cheating and she told me she wasn't. Another week passed and I got another phone call. "I'm being so good, and this just isn't working for me." I asked her to take me through what she was eating and, sure enough, she was cheating! "Well, it was just a couple of bites of birthday cake . . . I didn't eat the whole thing." Or, "Well, this cereal doesn't have sugar; it just says cane juice." Those are cheats.

Sometimes we are so impressed that we have cut out the white bread and the potatoes and the alcohol and the caffeine that we reward ourselves with little treats here and there. This can really slow your progress. Cheating is a very personal decision. If you want to cheat, there is a sacrifice. You simply will not lose weight as quickly, and may not lose weight at all, if your cheating is throwing off your entire meal.

YOU CANNOT SOMERSIZE HALFHEARTEDLY ON LEVEL ONE!

Without the presence of insulin, the amount of calories and fat grams you eat does not matter (but there's no need to overdo it!). This scenario changes drastically when you add foods that create the presence of insulin, such as sugar and carbohydrates. If you are eating foods that create an insulin response, the entire mass of food has the potential to be stored as fat. Now the calories and fat grams *do* matter because there's simply more energy to be converted to fat. If you are going to cheat, cheat with an isolated food rather than adding it to a large meal. Let's take the birthday cake example. If you know you are going to have a piece of birthday cake, you do not want to eat a high-calorie high-fat meal right before-

hand. You would be better off having a light salad and vegetables if you know you are going to blow it on cake. The fiber in salad helps diminish the effects of the insulin. Plus, salad is low in calories and fat, so at least if you're going to send a meal to the fat reserves, it is only salad and cake. Now if you're *not* going to have the cake, you can eat mozzarella marinara and salad with full-fat dressing. You can eat the chicken with butter sauce, but if you add the cake, you now put a high-fat and high-calorie meal at risk of being converted to fat. Stay on Level One until you feel the full effects of "The Melt." When your cells are unloaded from the built-up sugar, you can cheat a little in what I call Almost Level One and still maintain your progress.

The moral of the story is . . . if you are not seeing results, you are probably cheating without even knowing it. Reexamine your meals, then reread all the food lists to make sure you are on track. If you are doing everything right and still not seeing results, you may be overeating. Yes, you can eat too much even when you Somersize. Listen to your tummy. Remember, eat until you are full, not stuffed. If you are a compulsive eater, you may be giving your body more food than it needs. Other reasons for slowed weight loss can be eating too much fruit and carbohydrates. My husband, Alan, got fat from eating too much fruit. He was eating fifteen to twenty servings of fruit a day, thinking he was doing his body good. It was too much sugar. It even made his cholesterol increase. Again, here's an example of someone pushing the envelope . . . and he lives with me, Queen Somersizer! If you are eating a lot of Fruit and Carbos meals, you should consider cutting back until your weight loss gets jump-started. That does not mean you should eliminate these foods completely. If you still do not see results, you may have a hormonal imbalance that requires hormone replacement therapy.

When you graduate to Level Two, your body will be able to handle a small amount of sugar because you have created room in your cells. Don't get cocky and overdo it! If you cheat too much, your cells will fill up with sugar and you'll have to go back to Level One until you correct the problem.

A SAMPLE WEEK ON LEVEL ONE

People always ask me, "Well, what do *you* eat?" I tell them that I may have a Carbos breakfast and then a Pro/Fats and Veggies lunch, but they want to know what I literally eat for every meal and snack.

I don't think about every meal with such detail because this way of eating has become second nature to me, but one week I did keep a food diary and have included here a whole week's worth of meals on Level One. I have not included portion size because, as you know, you simply eat until you are full. Your own meals can vary from mine tremendously, but perhaps this will give you some additional ideas for meal plans. (Many of these recipes can be found in this book, or in *Eat Great, Lose Weight; Get Skinny on Fabulous Food; Eat, Cheat, and Melt the Fat Away;* and *Somersize Desserts.*)

SUNDAY

9:00 Breakfast
Omelette with spinach, feta cheese, and tomatoes
Side of turkey sausage
Decaf coffee

1:00 Lunch at Home
Tuna salad with celery, onions, and mayo served in lettuce cups

4:00 Snack on the Beach
Two peaches

7:00 Family Dinner
Pot roast with onions and tomatoes
Steamed asparagus
Green salad with vinaigrette

MONDAY

Breakfast
(7:00) Fruit smoothie (peaches, raspberries, orange juice)
(7:30) Whole-wheat toast with nonfat cottage cheese
Decaf coffee

10:00 Snack
Apple

1:00 Lunch at a Restaurant
Grilled prawns with cayenne butter (appetizer)
Caesar salad with grilled chicken (no croutons)

4:00 Snack at the Studio
A hard-boiled egg

7:30 Dinner at Home
Fast and Easy Minestrone (no rice, potatoes, pasta, or carrots)
Salad with red leaf lettuce, tomatoes, fresh mozzarella, basil, and balsamic vinaigrette

TUESDAY

7:00 Breakfast
> Eggs Florentine (ham cups with spinach, eggs, and cheese)

1:00 Lunch in My Dressing Room
> Salad of iceberg lettuce with blue cheese dressing
>
> Grilled chicken breast with assorted grilled vegetables (zucchini, onions, peppers)

7:00 Dinner at Home
> Tex Mex Pork Chops with cream sauce
>
> Steamed broccoli and cauliflower with lemon garlic butter
>
> Butter lettuce salad with garlic vinaigrette

9:00 Snack
> A plum

WEDNESDAY

Breakfast
> (6:00) Honeydew melon
>
> (6:45) Decaf cappuccino with nonfat milk
>
> (9:00) Toasted whole-wheat bagel
>
> Nonfat yogurt

2:00 Lunch
> Baby greens with Parmesan cheese, sun-dried tomatoes, and chicken breast

6:00 Dinner at Restaurant
> Stuffed Bells (bell peppers stuffed with ground turkey, cheese, and vegetables)
>
> Radicchio, arugula, endive salad with Parmesan cheese

9:00 Snack
> A piece of cheddar cheese

THURSDAY

7:00 Breakfast
> Fried eggs with turkey sausage links
>
> Decaf coffee

10:00 Snack
> Piece of string cheese

1:00 Lunch
> Taco salad—romaine lettuce, ground beef, cheddar cheese, sour cream, and salsa (no beans, tortillas, or guacamole)

4:00 Snack
> Soft Whole-Wheat Pretzels (my no-fat recipe) with mustard

7:30 Dinner at Home
> Pan-fried halibut with lime butter
>
> Lemony Artichokes
>
> Green salad with Green Goddess dressing

9:30 Dessert
> Somersize Vanilla Ice Cream (made with cream and sweetened with SomerSweet)

FRIDAY

Breakfast
> (9:00) Papaya
>
> (9:30) Shredded Wheat with nonfat milk

12:30 Lunch
> Cobb salad—lettuce, blue cheese, turkey, bacon, tomato, scallions, hard-boiled egg, blue cheese dressing (no avocado)

3:00 Snack
> An orange

6:00 Dinner at Home
> Green salad with blue cheese and balsamic vinaigrette

Saltimbocca in Tarragon Butter Sauce
(chicken, ham, herbs, butter, chicken
stock)
Steamed asparagus

SATURDAY

Breakfast
(9:00) Mangoes and strawberries
(9:20) Decaf nonfat cappuccino

1:00 Lunch
Pinwheels (whole-wheat tortilla rolled
with Somersize Dip Mixes made
with nonfat dairy, red peppers, and
lettuce)
Vegetable sticks with hummus

6:30 Dinner
Flattened pork chops with pan drippings
Grilled zucchini and eggplant
Candied tomatoes
Green salad with Brie and red wine
vinaigrette

8:30 Dessert
Tangerines

ALMOST LEVEL ONE

For many years I have had two Somersize categories: Level One for weight loss and Level Two for maintenance. Simple enough, eh? Now we have a new category called Almost Level One. I love this category! Almost Level One allows you to have very small cheats while you are still losing weight.

I am a person who believes in rules. You have to have rules, and Level One has very clear guidelines. That being said, I also believe rules are meant to be bent when

there is no harm done by bending them. (How else could I have had any fun in Catholic school! No wonder the nuns never liked me.) Bending rules is how this category came to be. In Almost Level One we incorporate very small little cheats while we are still losing weight. For example, I have delicious SomerSweet Truffles made with high-quality Belgian chocolate. They are very low in sugar and carbohydrates. Now, I always tell you not to look at the nutrition facts, only to concentrate on the ingredients to determine if something is Somersized. If the ingredients contain no Funky Foods, and fall into the proper combinations, then you may eat that food. Technically my truffles would not be allowed on Level One because chocolate is a Funky Food (even unsweetened chocolate contains the bad combo of fats and carbohydrates). However, once you have begun to lose weight steadily, most people can incorporate one or two of these truffles per day without disrupting their weight loss. There is no reason that you should have to wait until you are down to your goal weight to enjoy these divine little treats! That's why we have Almost Level One, so you can feel good about enjoying the foods that only cause a minuscule imbalance while you are still losing.

When you first begin the program, stick to the Level One guidelines . . . all of them. I encourage you not to cheat. This is the best way to jump-start your weight loss. You need to be vigilant so that you train your body to unload your stored sugar and use your fat reserves as an energy source. This takes a different amount of time for each person. Some lose 10 pounds in the first week; for me, it took a couple of months before I started to see the weight loss. The speed of your weight loss may vary greatly depending upon how much healing your metabolism needs. Be patient. One day it hit me and "The Melt" began. It felt as if the pounds were literally melting off my body while I ate fabulous, rich foods.

Once you are steadily losing weight, you may begin to incorporate Almost Level One treats on occasion. How often? As often as your body can handle without disrupting your progress. For example, Somersizers often ask me if they can have berries with whipped cream on Level One. Again, the hard and fast rules say, "Eat fruit alone," but berries are the easiest fruit to combine with other foods because of their high fiber content. This is a perfect Almost Level One treat. Should you start out Somersizing eating berries with whipped cream after a Pro/Fats meal? No. Wait for "The Melt." When your weight loss is in full swing, then have your berries.

Your next question will be, "So how many Almost Level One treats can I have in a day?" I don't have a number for you . . . you're going to have to figure that out for yourself by using your own body as a guide. When I am losing weight on Level One and having little cheats on Almost Level One, a typical day might include a Level One breakfast, a Level One lunch, an Almost Level One treat in the afternoon, like a couple of squares of my SomerSweet Toffee, and a Level One dinner with an Almost Level One dessert, like Somersize Crème Brûlée or Somersize Chocolate Mousse.

I would not recommend eating desserts all day. A big part of this program is to help you eat like a normal person. Actually, I take that back—most "normal" people have horrible eating habits. A big part of this program is to help you eat like a *healthy* person—three meals a day, plus snacks when you want them. Real food. I cannot stress that enough. Eat real food, with treats in moderation. That is the true Somersize way. I have many Somersizers who will push the envelope and try to cram in as many desserts and treats as they can because "technically" these foods are allowed. Do yourself, your body, and your psyche a favor—eat sensibly. If you want this program to stick for life, you must change your lifestyle. Don't look at every meal as an opportunity to stuff your face with as much food as you possibly can, as long as you stay within the "rules."

I know you have questions about the guidelines of the program. I read them when they come in at SuzanneSomers.com. Sometimes when I sit down to answer them, I think to myself, "I wish you could let go of the worry and simply enjoy this luxurious way of eating. I wish you could not sweat the small stuff, and know that you are probably doing everything correctly, or at least close enough to see results. I wish you could relax and let go of your issues with food." I hope this explanation helps you do that. I have to have rules. Follow them, and bend them as you see fit. Embrace this way of eating. Don't push the envelope. Somersize sensibly. Once you do, you'll heal your metabolism, you'll be on your way to achieving your goal weight, and you will finally end your battle with weight.

ELEVEN

✦

Level Two—Or as I Call It, "Cheating"

When you stand naked in front of the mirror and you are thin through the middle, and you are feeling happy with the way you are looking, you can graduate to Level Two, which is the maintenance portion of Somersizing. Level Two is simply Level One with cheating. Look, we are human beings, and every once in a while that scrumptious dessert the restaurant is offering looks too good to pass up. Your insulin levels are balanced, which is evident by your beautiful new slim waistline, so you can afford to indulge every once in a while.

Everyone cheats in different ways. I find I rarely create an imbalance cheating on sugary desserts. Now that I have SomerSweet, I don't miss real sugar. The sugars I miss the most are a glass of wine once or twice a week. Wine is accepted by the body as sugar. When I drink a glass of wine or two, I know I have created a slight imbalance. As a result I will go back to Level One for the

next two or three meals. You have to be the judge how many times per week you can cheat. When your pants are feeling tight, or your waistband starts cutting into your skin, it is time to go back to Level One. I used to be able to cheat more without having any adverse effects on my body. Now I find that if I keep my cheating to a couple of times a week, I can maintain my figure. If I cheat any more than that, I find I start getting thick through the middle.

It's comforting to know that no foods are forbidden. Somersizing simply asks that you first lose the unwanted weight, and when you have reached your goal, you can begin to incorporate the sugars you miss the most in moderation. That is called cheating. You are your own policeman. You can't blow it. If you find that you have gotten off the Somersizing track, simply go back to Level One and resume eating delicious, flavorful foods, but be sure to eliminate all sugars, so you can give your body a chance to lower its insulin levels and efficiently metabolize the foods you are ingesting.

In general, I live on Level One for the most part. Level Two involves cheating to some degree or another, so I remain vigilant because I do not want to go back to struggling with my weight. I am in control of my weight by Somersizing. I have been eating this way for ten years. The reason I know I will eat this way for the rest of my life is that Somersizing recognizes how human we all are. If you are craving or missing certain foods, have them, and then return to Level One eating.

But don't slip back into bad habits. On Level One, by eliminating Funky Foods, you have trained your pancreas not to oversecrete insulin. And rather than filling up on empty carbohydrates that give your body a quick source of energy, you have trained your body to use your fat reserves as an energy source. You've conditioned your system to digest quickly and efficiently by cutting out bad combinations. You have released the stored sugar from your cells and healed your metabolism. Now your body is in great shape and can handle a few imbalances.

The last thing we want is for all your hard work to be thrown away by resuming old habits. Level Two is about helping you find a balance so you can enjoy previously forbidden foods in moderation, without completely throwing caution to the wind. On Level Two, *you* are the only person who can determine how much imbalance your body can handle. Some people have to stay very close to Level One guidelines, with a minor imbalance here and there, in order to main-

tain their weight. Other people find they can create quite a few imbalances and still maintain their weight. By using trial and error, you will soon know how many imbalances your body can handle. Listen to your body. I know I've created too much of an imbalance when I feel bloated after a meal. Another warning sign for me is if I feel tired an hour or two after a meal. These are signs that I have wavered too far from Level One and need to pull in the reins. Of course, the most obvious sign is if you start to gain weight. Then you know you need to cut back on the treats and get back to eating cheese!

There are specific guidelines necessary to lose weight on Level One, and if you've gotten down to your goal weight, you have followed them diligently. I wish I could give you specific guidelines for Level Two, but actually that's the beauty of it . . . there are no hard and fast rules for Level Two. You are in control of your body and you need to find a rhythm you can live with for the rest of your life.

The great thing is that no matter how large an imbalance you create, you can always find your equilibrium. Level Two is really an extension of Level One, with a few indulgences here and there. Of course, moderation is the key to maintaining your weight. I find that if I eat a Level One lunch, like a Cobb salad with chicken, cheese, bacon, scallions, and tomatoes, every now and then I can add a piece of whole-grain bread without upsetting my system too much. Or if I wanted to indulge myself a little more, I would hold the bread and maybe have a piece of flourless chocolate cake (made with SomerSweet, of course). Certainly, I would not have chocolate cake every day or it would catch up with me. And I would not eat the Cobb salad with the wheat bread *and* the cake because that would be more carbohydrates than I could handle. A Cobb salad with a *white* flour roll as well as the cake would make me Bloat City.

I also find on Level Two that I can handle a few more Carbos and Veggies meals. Whereas on Level One I almost exclusively eat my Carbos at breakfast, on Level Two I might incorporate an occasional lunch and dinner revolving around whole-wheat pasta or brown rice. Again, only you can determine how many of these Carbos meals you can eat without upsetting your system.

MIXING PRO/FATS AND CARBOS

As I detailed in the chapter on serotonin, now that your system is clean, you will find that your body can handle a small amount of carbohydrate *with* your Pro/Fats meal. In fact, your body will welcome it. Eating proteins, fats, and a small portion of carbohydrates at every meal will help keep your entire hormonal system balanced. On Level One, that small portion of carbohydrates comes from the low-starch vegetables we eat. Now that you are on Level Two, you may give your body those carbohydrates in higher starch forms without upsetting your maintenance. You may add one slice of buttered whole-wheat toast with your eggs. You may add half a cup of brown rice with your turkey soup. You may have about half a cup

of whole-wheat pasta with your steak and broccoli. You may add one slice of whole-grain bread with your salad. You may even have a small buttered potato—yes, a potato!—with your chicken and asparagus. I add these carbohydrates to my meals a couple of times a week. Just make sure that the carbohydrate is not the main portion of the meal. It should be a small side dish within a Pro/Fats and Veggies meal. Your body can now handle the moderate insulin release and will enjoy the benefits of the release of serotonin it gets from ingesting carbohydrates.

Remember, if we deplete our system of carbohydrates for too long, we can lower our serotonin levels. Eating too many carbohydrates, or not eating enough, can throw off our hormonal balance. When our serotonin levels are low, we will crave carbohydrates and sugar. That's when we become prone to cheating and we pig out on a gigantic chocolate bar. Adding these little carbohydrate treats on Level Two keeps our hormones balanced, and therefore keeps those sugar cravings away.

When you combine carbohydrates with Pro/Fats, don't go overboard. For instance, you might have one slice of buttered whole-wheat toast with your eggs in the morning, but a stack of pancakes made from white flour would be overdoing it. Or you could have a tuna melt on one slice of whole-grain bread for lunch, but white bread would not be advised. For dinner you might have a small portion of wild rice with your chicken and vegetables, but a side of white pasta would be a bit much.

Every now and then you may really want those pancakes, white bread, or pasta. Just make sure the imbalance is really worth it to you. Then go back and eat a few strict Level One meals for a while until you get your system back in balance. That's how Level Two works; you eat mostly on Level One and decide when you want to treat yourself. Sometimes I stay close to Level One with frequent but small little treats here and there, like a little olive oil on my pasta or some wild rice in my chicken soup. Other times I stay strictly on Level One for a series of meals and then have a big treat, like french fries. (I eat them with a salad. The fiber helps to minimize the effects of the insulin.)

Generally, I find that on Level Two I can eat a few more Carbos meals without a problem and I can add a little bit of fat. Sometimes I have whole-grain pasta or brown rice for lunch with vegetables. On Level One I have no oil with this meal, but on Level Two I can sauté the vegetables in some oil and have a more flavorful stir-fry without causing a significant imbalance. But adding protein to a Carbos meal is a little tricky. If I want to have meat with my pasta or brown rice, I would make the meal predominantly a Pro/Fats meal with a small portion of pasta or rice (about a half cup or so), rather than have a big bowl of pasta with a few pieces of meat. For me, the protein in combination with a significant amount of Carbos is harder on my body than a little fat in combination with the Carbos.

If I'm going to have a sandwich, I usually still have a vegetarian sandwich on whole-grain bread, but every now and then I add some avocado. The avocado has fat in it, but as long as I don't add meat as well, I generally find I do not have a problem. I also might add a little mayonnaise or olive oil depending on the sandwich. And if I feel like a meat or tuna fish sandwich, then I usually stick to Level One and use lettuce cups instead of bread. (If I were to eat bread with meat or tuna fish, I would use only one slice and it would definitely be whole-grain bread.)

MIXING FRUIT

I still try to eat the Fruit group completely separately. The only fruit I play around with is berries, because berries are easier to digest than other fruits. They have a very high fiber content and give me very little trouble when I combine them with other foods. On Level Two I do not even think twice about eating fresh berries with whipped cream after a Pro/Fats and Veggies meal. Also, when I get tired of toast with nonfat cottage cheese or nonfat yogurt, I use SomerSweet Jam on my toast in the morning. And if I just have to have blueberry pancakes, there's no need to cheat because I can use my Somersize Pancake and Waffle Mix, which is made with whole grains. Then I top it with Somersize Syrup. Regular pancakes with butter and maple syrup would create a huge imbalance, whereas these whole-wheat or multigrain pancakes create less of an imbalance and still satisfy my craving. Or you might try the delicious Cream Cheese Pancakes on page 180 for Level One. I also like to use berries in tarts and pies made with whole-wheat crusts; certainly not Level One fare, but easier on your system than an apple tart or a pumpkin pie. And for breakfast or a snack in the afternoon, I like to have fresh berries with nonfat yogurt.

I also may add a few products that are sweetened with fruit juice. At health food stores I found a few cereals made from spelt and amaranth and kamut, flakes that are sweetened with a little fruit juice. They provide a nice change in the morning. Fruit juice, like sugar, creates an insulin response, but your body can handle it now in moderation because your cells are not overloaded with sugar.

ADDING A LITTLE SUGAR AND FUNKY FOODS

As far as sugar goes, I loosen the reins a little. I'm not quite as diligent about hunting for sugar in sauces and salad dressings. If I'm at a restaurant, I don't worry about eating a prepared blue cheese dressing on my salad, even if it has a little sugar in it. It's not enough to cause a problem for me on Level Two as long as I'm not having any Carbos. I continue to avoid gravy made with white flour and very sweet sauces, like barbecue sauce. And watch out for those thick Chinese sauces made with sugar and cornstarch. Most restaurants are happy to prepare your food without these ingredients.

I also find I can have moderate amounts of the foods on the Bad Combo list such as nuts, olives, liver, avocado, and tofu. These are the easiest foods on your system to bring back because they are all real foods and they have incredible health benefits. Now your body can handle the small amount of carbos naturally occurring with the proteins and fats.

And how about desserts? With SomerSweet, I enjoy Level One desserts a few times

a week. Almost Level One desserts can be eaten as frequently as you can handle. It depends on your system. As a rule, I still try to stay away from desserts made with sugar. Take a look at the sugar content in my beloved favorite—birthday cake! Just how much sugar is in a double layer white cake with lemon filling and buttercream frosting? Two cups of sugar in the cake, a half cup in the lemon filling, plus one more cup in the frosting. Three and a half cups of sugar! Add the copious amounts of white flour, which is a Funky Food, and the butter and eggs, Pro/Fats, and you have a poorly combined Pro/Fat–Carbo–Funky Food concoction sure to send your system into mayhem.

Check out some of my recipes for desserts made with SomerSweet. Chocolate Cupcakes with Whipped Cream Filling! They're made with unsweetened chocolate, eggs, cream, and SomerSweet. They are a delicious Almost Level One treat. For additional dessert recipes, buy my book *Somersize Desserts*. The beauty of this program is that if you really want it, you can have white cake with lemon filling and buttercream frosting—you'll just have to live back on Level One for longer.

Another good dessert option after a Pro/Fat meal is Somersize Ice Cream with Somersize Triple Hot Fudge. Even regular ice cream is often lower in sugar than other desserts and is made mostly of Pro/Fats, (eggs and cream). If you can't make your own Somersize Ice Cream, make sure to buy the best-quality ice cream, because you want it to have more cream than milk (remember, milk has carbohydrates; cream does not). Pudding, crème brûlée, and chocolate mousse are generally lower in sugar than most other desserts and do not include white flour as many other pastries do. My Somersize versions of these products are made completely with SomerSweet. And as I mentioned, flourless chocolate cake is a great option on Level Two, or Chocolate Dipped Strawberries with freshly whipped cream!

You really can eat these desserts and maintain your weight if you are Somersizing properly. Check out my recipes for Level One, Almost Level One, and Level Two desserts. You'll be knocked out by how great they are. They are all made with SomerSweet. The Almost Level One and Level Two desserts contain whole-wheat pastry flour instead of white flour and unsweetened chocolate. With SomerSweet, we can enjoy many more desserts the Somersize way.

YOU'RE IN CONTROL

As far as Level Two goes, you are in control. Maybe you don't miss the sweets as much as you miss the bread. Then save your treats for a great baguette or a chewy sourdough roll. Or if it's white pasta you're craving, eat mostly Level One meals and then indulge yourself with a little pasta fix. It's up to you. For me, the whole-grain pasta is so good, I don't ever feel deprived eating it instead of white pasta. Sometimes I even bring it to my favorite Italian restaurants and ask the kitchen to use it, instead of white pasta. They never seem to mind, as long as I pay full price for my dish. I still stay away from meat sauce with my whole-grain pasta because the combination makes me bloat.

How you choose your imbalances depends on many factors. How many imbalances have you had today and how big were they? How many big imbalances have you had this week? Don't get cocky with your new figure! The pounds can creep back onto your body if you're not careful.

Beware of the slipups. It usually starts with one dessert, which leads to another, and then another. Before you know it, you've started adding bad combinations and a little white flour here and there. Your body will signal you with warning signs. Learn to listen to them! If you start craving sugar and carbohydrates, it means you are eating too much of them. That's what happens; the more sugar you eat, the more you crave. Then come the energy dips, the extra pounds, and don't forget about the damage you're doing on the inside to your healthy cells. And remember, the best way to take away a sugar craving is to eat a Pro/Fat because Pro/Fats help to stabilize blood sugar. So next time you have a craving for sugar or carbohydrates, eat a piece of cheese and it should help. All in all, if you notice signs that your body is starting to crave sugar again, go back to Level One until you get rid of the problem. Stay on top of the new you. Take care of your body.

I also want to mention a few words about portion control. On Level One you may eat as much as you want as long as you are following *all* the Level One guidelines. (That means technically you can eat until you are full and not gain weight. I'm sure you learned not to overeat, because your appetite was fully satisfied with wholesome, nutritious foods.) On Level Two, you must consider limiting your portions when you are creating imbalances. You can't have it both ways—the bonus of Level One is that you can eat as much as you want. The bonus of Level Two is that you have more variety, but you must limit your portions moderately now that you are adding foods that will create moderate amounts of insulin. Your cells are clean . . . let's keep them that way!

WINE AND CHOCOLATE

Recent studies have shown that red wine has been proven to have beneficial effects on the heart by helping to keep your arteries clear. I have incorporated it, in moderation, in Level Two. Remember, your body accepts wine as sugar, so don't overdo it. Some people find they can enjoy a glass or two of wine with their meals without having any problems. However, wine combined with other imbalances can add up to too much sugar. Keep those insulin levels intact or you'll end up back where you started. I drink wine a couple times a week, and I freely use it in many of my recipes. It creates only a slight imbalance because most of the alcohol is cooked off in the process. In fact, I even cook with wine on Level One because it wonderfully enhances the flavor of my meals and does not seem to disrupt my system. If you are doing well on Level One, you should not have a problem doing the same.

Now for chocolate . . . my great love! I can't seem to live without chocolate, and I don't have to. SomerSweet Chocolate is a perfect treat. I enjoy it several times a week. Even regular dark chocolate (made with more than 60 percent cocoa) is relatively low in sugar and does not create a huge imbalance. The best time to eat chocolate is on an empty stomach, perhaps a couple of squares in the afternoon. And I have many sinful desserts made from dark chocolate that are perfect for Almost Level One and Level Two.

You will continue to use all of the recipes in Level One for Level Two. I have included a few recipes specific to Level Two for your enjoyment. In addition, check out all the great recipes in *Eat Great, Lose Weight* and *Get Skinny on Fabulous Food; Eat, Cheat, and Melt the Fat Away;* and *Somersize Desserts.* Good luck in this new phase. You have such freedom on Level Two; I just know you will love it. Any questions you have will be answered by your own body as you experiment with Level Two. Also, check my list of Frequently Asked Questions in chapter 13. Eating this way is truly a pleasure and I'm sure you will be the envy of all of your friends who can't believe what wonderful foods you eat and still manage to keep your beautiful figure.

MEAL PLANS, LEVEL TWO

From week to week my meal plans will vary greatly on Level Two. I am sharing this particular week of meals with you because it was a good model week for me in terms of balancing my Pro/Fats and Carbos and getting plenty of Fruits and Veggies. You will see that there is a combination of Level One meals and Level Two meals. Remember, your body may be able to handle more or less imbalance depending on your unique metabolism. I can handle about this many imbalances and still maintain my weight. To help you see how I choose my treats, I have put an asterisk next to the items that are Level Two with a brief explanation regarding the imbalance.

SUNDAY

9:00 Breakfast
Spinach and Parmesan cheese frittata
Decaf coffee

1:00 Lunch
Sliced gyros served over lettuce with tomato and garlic cucumber sauce
1 piece of whole-wheat pita bread★
(★I combined whole-wheat pita with a Pro/Fats and Veggies meal)

4:00 Snack
A hard-boiled egg

7:00 Dinner
Grilled chicken breast
Steamed broccoli and cauliflower tossed in garlic vinaigrette
Small buttered potato★
Green salad with garlic vinaigrette
A glass of red wine★
Somersize Chocolate Mousse★
(★Wine, a Funky potato, and the Almost Level One Chocolate Mousse)

MONDAY

Breakfast
(9:00) Mango
(9:30) Rye toast with SomerSweet berry jam★
Decaf coffee
(★Berry jam creates a slight imbalance with my toast)

1:30 Lunch
Warm goat cheese salad with chicken,
pine nuts, and sun-dried tomatoes★
(★I added pine nuts to my salad)

4:30
SomerSweet English-style butter toffee (two pieces)

7:30 Dinner
Pan-Fried Pork Tenderloin
Celery Root Purée
Steamed green beans
Butter lettuce salad with balsamic vinaigrette

TUESDAY

Breakfast
(7:30) Cantaloupe
(7:50) Decaf coffee

12:00 Lunch
Stir-fried vegetables with brown rice★
(★I combined oil with a Carbos and Veggies meal)

3:00 Snack
A piece of cheddar cheese

7:00 Dinner
Roasted yellow pepper soup
Green salad with zucchini and shaved parmesan
Braised lamb shank
Whole-wheat couscous★
(★I added the Carbo, whole-wheat couscous, to my Pro/Fats meal)

WEDNESDAY

7:30 Breakfast
Omelette with sausage and cheese
One slice whole-grain toast with butter★
Decaf coffee
(★I added a whole grain to my Pro/Fats meal)

1:00 *Lunch*
Somersize Barbecue Ribs
Crunchy Coleslaw
Steamed green beans

4:00 *Snack*
Deviled eggs

7:30 *Dinner*
Turkey chili topped with cheddar
cheese, sour cream, and cilantro★
Green salad with red wine vinaigrette
Whipped cream with fresh berries★
(★I added a few garbanzo beans and
navy beans to the chili. Dessert was
barely an imbalance at all because I
did not sweeten the whipped cream
and the berries are fine for Level
Two.)

THURSDAY

7:30 *Breakfast*
Whole-wheat toast with tomatoes and
basil★
(★I put a little olive oil on my toast in
this Carbos and Veggies meal)

10:00 *Snack*
An orange

12:30 *Lunch*
Whole-grain pasta with pesto★
Green salad with romaine, red cabbage,
celery, and red wine vinaigrette
A glass of red wine★
(★I combined oil, pine nuts, and cheese
with my Carbos and Veggies, plus a
glass of wine)

6:30 *Dinner*
Chicken Paillard with Lemon Parsley
Butter

Sautéed spinach with garlic, lemon, and
olive oil
Steamed asparagus
Somersize Crème Brûlée

FRIDAY

7:00 *Breakfast*
Somersize Cinnamon Pancakes
Decaf coffee

1:00 *Lunch*
Rotisserie chicken
Caesar salad (no croutons)

4:00 *Snack*
Two SomerSweet Chocolate Truffles

6:30 *Dinner*
Fried shrimp with cocktail sauce
Broccoli and cauliflower
Salad with creamy tarragon dressing

SATURDAY

8:00 *Breakfast*
Fruit smoothie

(8:30)
Whole-grain toast with berry jam★
(★Berry jam creates a slight imbalance
with my Carbos)

1:00 *Lunch*
Somersize Double Double Cheese-
burger (no bun)
Somersize Fast and Easy Onion Rings
(not breaded)
Green salad with vinaigrette

7:00 *Dinner*
Grilled chicken breast salad
A glass of red wine★
Somersize Ice Cream Sundae★
(★The wine, and the minor imbalance
of the Somersize Hot Fudge)

As my son, Bruce, says, "Level Two is just eating." And he's right. You don't ever have to deny yourself anything. I can't indulge myself *every* time I have a craving, but I do it often enough so that I never feel deprived.

With your new figure and your improved health come a renewed sense of self-confidence. You set out to achieve a goal and you have attained it. You should be proud of yourself. Enjoy your meals, enjoy your new body, and enjoy knowing that you are giving your body the nutritious foods it needs to thrive and to ward off disease. Somersizing has truly been a liberating experience for me. I am finally in control of my weight rather than my weight being in control of me. I hope that in sharing my program with you, your life has been enhanced in some way; either through losing a few pounds, learning some new tricks in the kitchen, or helping your family to embrace this healthy, delicious way of eating. Enjoy!

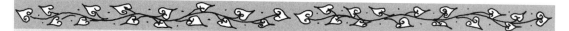

Dear Suzanne,

I wanted to let you know about the success my husband John and I have had with your Somersize program.

I have been very overweight for many years. Every time I would try to lose weight I would become shaky and hungry on low-fat diets. One day, I saw you on TV and thought your program looked interesting. At least if I didn't lose weight, your recipes looked yummy.

The first week of Somersizing I lost 8 pounds. I was so excited. It was not easy coming off sugar and refined carbs, but I never felt deprived with all the food I could eat. After a couple of months, my husband was amazed with how great I was looking and feeling. He would Somersize at dinner with me and loved the meals, but didn't want to give up his ice cream, chocolates, and sugar cereals. Then he read your books, and decided to try it 100 percent. He switched his cereals to whole grain, and I made his lunches. His coworkers always ask him what he is having because it smells so good!

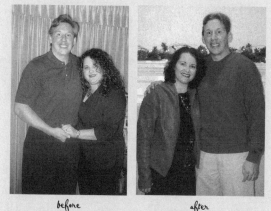

before   after

We have both lost weight and no longer have that puffy look anymore. I have lost 50 pounds and John has lost 37 pounds. I have been Somersizing for over a year now. It has become so natural to eat this way. Now I love to cook, where before I was too tired. John and I have a lot of fun trying new recipes and creating our own. We are so much healthier and happier.

Thank you, Suzanne, for your wonderful program. It has changed our lives in the most wonderful and positive way.

Sincerely, Gina and John Wood

⚜

TWELVE

Somersizing Tips: Fast Food, Brown Bagging It, and Much More

I realize this program may seem a bit overwhelming at first, but soon you will discover how simple Somersizing can be. Whenever my friends and family first start the program, they frequently call me with questions. And since I can't give my home phone number to everyone, I have compiled some helpful tips for dining out, eating at fast-food restaurants, eating at home, brown bagging it, and more.

TIPS FOR DINING OUT

So many people tell me, "I eat two to three of my meals each day in restaurants; it's impossible to lose weight." Once you understand Somersizing, eating in any restaurant is truly easy. First I scan the menu and decide if I want to choose a Pro/Fats and Veggies meal or a Carbos and Veggies meal. Ninety-five percent of the time I'll

choose a Pro/Fats meal, which might be a green salad with dressing of my choice, a chicken, meat, or fish entrée with a lovely sauce, and plenty of steamed, sautéed, or grilled vegetables. On the rare occasion that I choose to have a Carbos and Veggies meal, I might order a vegetarian sandwich on whole-grain bread or brown rice with steamed vegetables and soy sauce.

The key to the Pro/Fats meal is no bread, pasta, potatoes, or rice. We are accustomed to beginning every meal in a restaurant by emptying a basket of bread into our bellies before we even order! Then we eat a meal of meat with potatoes, or a turkey sandwich, or a Chinese chicken salad piled high with fried rice noodles and wontons. Add a couple of glasses of caffeine, like iced tea or diet cola, and you have a recipe for metabolic disaster. These are the things that throw your system into chaos.

You'll be surprised at how quickly you'll

get over missing the starch. Make sure to watch for hidden sugars or starches in the salad dressings or sauces. Drill your server a little to get the information you need; ask the kitchen to substitute extra vegetables or salad for the starchy side dish. Just make sure all the vegetables are on the Veggies list. It does you no good to get a big side dish of sautéed carrots—and it's a terrible waste of food to be served items you know you cannot eat.

You will also have to get over that feeling of being overstuffed when you finish a meal. I used to think I was not full until my stomach became distended and I could not consider putting another bite in my mouth. When you Somersize, you will not get that overstuffed feeling because your body is not fighting with bad food combinations that cause digestive problems. Your system becomes cleansed and you become accustomed to feeling satisfied without feeling stuffed.

The Level One Carbos meal is much more restrictive when you're eating out. It must be fat free so that all those carbohy-

drates are burned off rather than stored as fat. Also, watch out for sugars and hidden Funky Foods, and avoid anything from the Pro/Fats group; meat and cheese on that sandwich would throw your system into a tizzy. Even mayonnaise, oil, and avocado on a sandwich are not okay on Level One.

With minimal effort, you can enjoy any restaurant and still lose weight. And it's worth it! Try and judge for yourself. I guarantee you'll like the way you feel when you Somersize. No bloating or gas, improved elimination, and more energy than ever before.

FAST-FOOD FIX

I am not a fast-food junkie, but there are times when you are on the road and there's just not much else to eat, or the kids are really demanding a fast-food meal because that's what kids do. While the purpose of this book is to make it easier to incorporate Somersizing into your life, occasionally you are going to find yourself resorting to a fast-food meal. How can we stick to the program when our choices for sustenance are so limited? You can still Somersize at fast-food restaurants. Here are a few tips.

If you like burgers, it's not too tough to Somersize. Just don't eat the bun! My favorite burger joint in Palm Springs is Tyler's. They have a Somersize Burger on the menu. It comes with a cheeseburger, lettuce, tomato, pickle, and grilled onions. Yum. As far as fast-food chains? My choice is In 'n' Out Burger. I believe they are only located on the West Coast. They also understand the wave of high-protein pro-

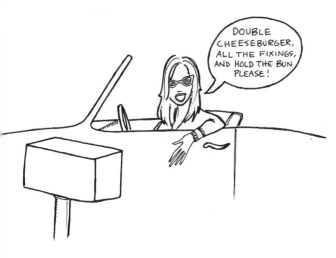

DOUBLE CHEESEBURGER, ALL THE FIXINGS, AND HOLD THE BUN PLEASE!

grams and now are offering a Protein Burger. It's not on the menu, but if you ask for it, they know just what you're talking about. They simply take the hamburger and wrap it with all the fixings in lettuce leaves. I get a Double Double Cheeseburger, with lettuce, tomato, pickle, onion, and Secret Sauce. The secret sauce has some sugar, I'm sure, so that makes it Almost Level One. The key is resisting the french fries. Even without the bun, the Double Double mixed with fries will wreak havoc on your metabolism. Save that treat for when you're going to blow it a couple of times a year.

Other well-known chains? How about Carl's Jr.—they have a salad bar, so you can add a salad to your bunless burger. They also serve a couple of sandwiches with chicken breasts, like the BBQ Chicken Sandwich and the Southwest Chicken Sandwich. You can pull out the chicken and scrape off the sauce and top your salad with it. (I'm sure the BBQ sauce has sugar in it.) The chicken stars are breaded and fried, so you'll want to stay away from them.

Jack in the Box—you're pretty much stuck with the burger with no bun. They also have Teriyaki Bowls, but they're covered in sugary sauces and not a good option. Their chicken is breaded, so don't go there. At McDonald's I would stick to a Big 'n' Tasty, or a Quarter Pounder with Cheese, and leave off the bun. They also have salads, like Chef's Salad, a Garden Salad, and a Grilled Caesar (leave off the croutons). Watch out for the dressings. They all have sugar, but the Ranch has the fewest carbohydrates of the bunch, so if you are venturing into a little cheat, that's your best bet.

There are breakfast items that you can work around, as well. Take the English muffin off the Egg McMuffin and you can have the eggs, bacon, and cheese. Wendy's has a salad bar, and a few new salads that can be Somersized by plucking out a few Funky Foods. Plus, you can do the burger thing. They also have chili, but you have to pick around the beans. At Subway you may have a vegetarian sandwich on whole-wheat bread with mustard (no mayo or fats). You can also have a salad topped with all the meat, cheese, and veggies you want. Read labels for the dressings to watch for sugars. As for Mexican, go for the taco salad, just leave off the beans and guacamole, and don't eat the shell. Del Taco has the Deluxe Taco Salad and Taco Bell also has a good taco salad.

In fact, a few years ago I was filming a television movie in a remote part of Arizona. The shooting days are very long for TV movies. We were housed in a very modest hotel that did not have a restaurant or room service. There was not a single decent restaurant in the vicinity. After a long day of shooting I just wanted to get some food into my belly and get to bed. How I wished for a nice bowl of hot soup and a salad, but it was not to be found.

So what do you do when you just can't find a decent meal at a decent restaurant? You find a decent meal at a not-so-decent restaurant. We became Taco Bell junkies. Taco Bell was one of the only "restaurants" nearby. I found I could actually Somersize quite well at Taco Bell. I would order two taco salads with no beans, and extra sour cream. The taco salads come in a large tortilla shell. I didn't eat that part. I just ate the lettuce, meat, cheese, sour cream, and salsa. It was actually really good. It filled me up and tasted great.

When you're in a pinch, you can still stay on the Somersize plan and eat at fast-food restaurants. Try not to make it a habit, because you'll find better-quality food in your grocery store, or at nicer restaurants, but when you need a quick, fast, and inexpensive meal, you can still Somersize!

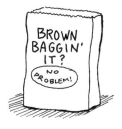

BROWN BAGGIN' IT

Many, many people eat lunch at work or school during the week and they need to bring their lunch with them. The most common question I get is, "What suggestions do you have for those of us brown baggin' it?"

When we think of lunch-box food, we associate it with a sandwich, chips, cookies, crackers, and maybe an apple. No more! You must rethink your lunch box for you and the kids. The most important word in your Somersize lunch box . . . Tupperware! Anything you would eat at home can be brought to work or school in plastic containers with lids. The best and easiest lunch is to make enough dinner the night before so that you have extra for lunches.

As I mentioned, my son Bruce makes the lunches for his daughters. Caroline usually cooks dinner and Bruce does the dishes and packs the lunches. When dinner is over, Caroline takes the kids to bathe, and instead of putting away the food, Bruce takes the leftovers and packs them into small containers for the kids. He cuts up bites of chicken, pork, or other meat. He adds leftover steamed vegetables like broccoli, cauliflower, and green beans. Then he adds a small container of wild rice, brown rice, or whole-grain pasta (Level Two!). For snacks he packs cubes of melon, sliced apples with a sprinkle of cinnamon, applesauce, or yogurt. The kids love it. In fact, my granddaughter in kindergarten has the option to eat the school's hot lunch two days of the week. They serve pizza, teriyaki bowls, burritos, hamburgers, spaghetti, salads, and the like. It comes with a dessert, like a big cookie, or Rice Krispies treat, or brownie. Plus, they get a bottle of water and sliced celery and carrots. My granddaughter thought the food was marginal, at best, and asked if she could bring her own lunch every day.

Finding healthy options that your kids will eat is always a challenge. Then you need to rotate your foods with enough variety to keep them satisfied. It's not easy! If you give your kids foods that they don't like, they won't eat them. They'll end up eating junk food from their friends. And believe me, they'll be exposed to everything at school. In her first week of school Bruce and Caroline's daughter came home with a whole new set of taste sensations . . . "Mommy, I had something called Cheetos today! Have you ever had a Cheeto? They're so good."

How do you help your child make smart food choices when her friends are eating treats in the morning?

First of all, talk to your child's school about a "no-sharing" rule. Many schools have adopted this policy to protect children with allergies. Serious allergies are dangerous business, and the school could be liable if a child is endangered from sharing food. On a less serious note, but still a very important one, how can parents guide what their kids eat if all the kids share with one another? This is especially important for kids who are obese or overweight. If you can't convince your school to have a no-sharing policy, you need to talk to your kids. Just like any other issue they will face, you need to empower them to make smart choices on their own.

What Bruce and Caroline found is that they have a better chance of keeping their kids eating their own lunches if they occasionally include treats for them. That way they can choose healthier treats, like cookies made with whole-wheat flour and Somer-Sweet. They're not Somersized, but they are a better option than cookies made with white flour and refined sugar, and perfectly suitable for Level Two.

Here is a whole host of ideas for your lunch box and for your kids' lunches. When you are preparing your food, make enough for a few days to lighten the load for the week. Also, keep your eyes peeled for my new products that will make your Somersize lunch a snap.

PRO/FATS AND VEGGIE LUNCHES
- Rotisserie chicken with side of vegetables
- Chicken salad with iceberg lettuce cups
- Egg salad with celery sticks
- Tuna salad with romaine lettuce leaves
- BLT served in lettuce cups
- Chicken breast with broccoli and cauliflower
- Sliced steak over salad greens with Parmesan cheese
- Sliced turkey, Swiss cheese and mayo, rolled then secured with a toothpick. Cut-up vegetables and Somersize Dip.
- Sliced roast beef, provolone, and mustard, rolled then secured with a toothpick. Salad with dressing of your choice.
- Sliced ham with Cheddar, mustard, and mayo, rolled then secured with a toothpick. Side of steamed broccoli.
- Greek salad
- Chicken Caesar salad with no croutons
- Cobb salad

For Level Two, feel free to add some whole grains. Add one slice of whole-wheat bread

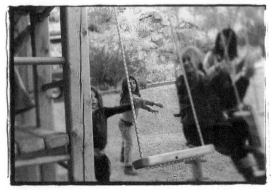

I'm the Big Kid.

to your meat roll-ups. Have some brown rice with your chicken. Add some whole-wheat pasta to your Pro/Fats.

CARBOS AND VEGGIES LUNCHES
- Whole-wheat tortilla pinwheel rolled with Somersize Dip (made with non-fat dairy) and fresh vegetables.
- Soba noodles, soy sauce, and steamed vegetables
- Whole-wheat pita sandwich with nonfat cheese and vegetables
- Brown rice and vegetables
- Lasagna made with whole-wheat pasta and fat-free sauce
- Vegetarian sandwich on whole-wheat bread (with lettuce, tomatoes, onion, sprouts, pickle, and mustard)

TIPS FOR EATING AT HOME

As far as eating at home, if you're used to eating prepared foods, you will need to make some adjustments. Most prepared foods are made with processed products like sugar, white flour, and a variety of unpronounceable ingredients. Say good-bye to Hamburger Helper! With a little preparation, you can learn to create fresh foods that taste much better and are far more nutritious. I keep my refrigerator stocked with ingredients that allow me to prepare meals quickly.

Everyone says, "I have no time to cook." Neither do I. I have seven careers and I travel quite a bit. Cooking happens to be what I like to do when I am relaxing, but I do not have the luxury of cooking dinner every night. I find that my odds of cooking at home increase dramatically if I do a small amount of preparation. Before I leave in the morning I take a package of meat or poultry out of the freezer to thaw. That way, if I get home in time to cook, I can whip up a quick meal. I always have fresh vegetables in the house, so making a salad and a steamed vegetable takes only a few minutes. The key is having your meat, fish, or poultry ready. If you don't have time to shop before dinner, you have to have the forethought to thaw something.

I get so happy when I realize we do not have to go out to eat. I usually pan-fry chops, chicken breasts, or fish fillets, and then deglaze the pan with broth, wine, and butter. It's the fast and easy way to cook . . . and it's delicious! This is a meal in minutes. When Alan and I sit down to dinner, we are so happy to be eating such great food at home.

This book is all about preparing meals at home quickly, and you will notice that some of the recipes call for using a slow cooker, or a pressure cooker, and other appliances. If you don't have these appliances, don't worry—there are plenty of recipes that don't require them—but using appliances like a bread maker, pressure cooker, or grill will really help you prepare meals in minutes. How about throwing a few items into a slow cooker in the morning and then coming home to a beautiful dinner that night? That's what a slow cooker can do for you. Or, how about arriving home at 6:00 P.M., throwing a few items into a pressure cooker, and having a meal in twenty minutes that tastes like it's

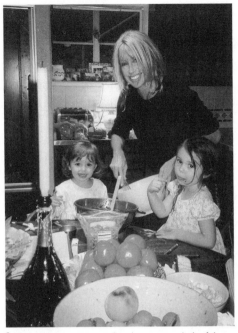

I love to cook with the grandchildren.

dilute your digestive juices, which slows down the digestive process. Your stomach acids are strongest right before you begin a new meal. When you eat, the acids break down the food quickly and pass it from the stomach. If you drink a big glass of water before your meal, these gastric juices become diluted and are less effective at breaking down the food. Therefore, if you must drink with your meal, eat a portion of your food before you drink anything so as not to dilute the strength of the gastric juices. It's best to drink your eight to ten glasses between meals. Besides water, you can also have decaffeinated coffee, teas, and even diet sodas, if you must. Personally, I stay away from soft drinks; they are loaded with things I don't want to put into my body. You would be doing your body a favor to eliminate them as well.

Many people ask me if the beverages they drink that are not pure water count toward their eight to ten glasses of water per day. Yes: decaf coffee, iced tea, Somersize Drinks, they all count. So drink up!

been braising for five hours? These appliances are great time savers and your food tastes delicious! It is an investment to purchase these appliances, but it's worth it.

In chapter 14 you can read more about the different appliances I have been developing that will help make meal preparation easier, as well as prepackaged foods that will make Somersize meals in minutes a reality.

WHAT TO DRINK?

If you have read my other books, you know that I highly recommend drinking eight to ten glasses of water a day. Water assists your metabolism in running at optimum speed. It is essential to weight loss. But try not to drink *with* your meals because water can

DON'T SKIP MEALS

Whether you're eating at home or dining in restaurants, make sure not to skip meals. Our mothers always told us that breakfast is the most important meal of the day, right? In many ways she was correct. Your body has been fasting while you sleep, so when you wake up in the morning you have gone for some eight to ten hours without food. If you skip breakfast and don't eat until lunch, your body has gone for twelve to fourteen hours without food. When you finally eat lunch, your body's survival instinct may kick in. If it's concerned about when you're going to feed it again, it may hang on to every morsel instead of properly processing the food. Remember to eat at least three meals a day—or eat several smaller meals throughout the day, if you prefer.

PORTION CONTROL

People often ask me about portion size because they are used to feeling deprived on diets. Somersizing does not require you to measure any of your foods. You simply eat until you are full. At first you may need to eat more food to feel satisfied because you

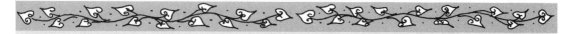

Dear Suzanne,

In February of 2000, I was desperate. I had an incurable autoimmune connective-tissue disease that made it almost impossible to exercise, and I was on three drugs that caused weight gain. The pain in my joints was crippling, and I really needed to lose weight, but it seemed impossible. I had tried every other diet and failed. I had decided it was better to give up the struggle and just stay fat. Then I saw you explaining the Somersizing program on TV. It inspired me to buy one of your books. I read it, and decided this was worth a try.

The first two to three days of detoxing felt great. I stayed away from sugar, caffeine, and alcohol and just ate plenty of luscious food. In the past when I had dieted, I felt starved, but with your way of eating, I felt completely satisfied. If I ever was hungry, I ate without counting calories or portion control, and still lost weight. Now, two years later, I am proud to say I have lost 81 pounds. I am able to swim 45 minutes five days a week. Plus I can now walk again without crippling pain. As an added bonus, I went from a tight size 20 to a size 10/12. I have succeeded beyond what I had dared to dream.

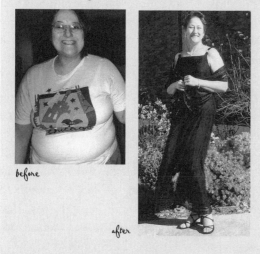

before

after

My "diet" food was also so good that the entire family wanted to eat it. My eldest daughter, Caroline, who is twenty-one, started Somersizing with me because it is such a healthy lifestyle. My eighteen-year-old son, Stephen, who is already tall and trim, just enjoys eating all the wonderful food, and my seven-year-old daughter, Rebecca, said to me the other day, "Sugar is yucky!" My husband, Frank, lets me know every day that he thinks I have done an amazing thing.

Thanks for all the good things Somersizing has brought to my entire family and me.

Sincerely,
Mary S. Barrett

are accustomed to having that "stuffed" feeling when you finish a meal. You will not feel stuffed or bloated when you eat in proper combinations. Most people do not have a problem overeating because it is difficult to overeat when you are eating only nutritious foods, and your body will signal you when it is satiated. (Certainly there are exceptions, like my friend in the recipe contest.) Overeating junk food, however, is a cinch because you can eat and eat and eat without ever giving your body what it needs to thrive! Your body may keep sending hunger messages until you give it the nutritious food it craves.

GET MOVING

Exercise is an important part of any weight-loss program. That doesn't mean you have to spend three hours a day taking aerobic classes. I realize that not everyone has the time or the money to join a gym and work out every day. I know with my busy schedule that it's hard to find the time to exercise regularly, but I do. You can make excuses from here to Timbuktu. Just do it. I stopped making excuses when I started reading about bone loss and muscle loss in women. The remedy? Eat right and exercise. I do not want to lose my muscle mass, and I do not want to start shrinking. I fight for every quarter inch of my body height! The last thing I want is to lose inches.

I work out for thirty minutes a day. My favorite activity is my Ultra Track. It's outside on the patio in our desert home, and I spend thirty minutes doing lunges and working my abdominal muscles while I look out at the red rocks and listen to the birds. What a difference it has made in my muscle tone! Just thirty minutes a day. I try to get my workout in every day, but I still feel good if I get at least three workouts a week. Thanks to my Ultra Track and my ThighMaster, my arms are no longer floppy, my tummy is tightening, my thighs are firm, and my backside is moving on up!

Somersizing helps me stay at the right weight. Exercising helps me keep the right shape. And it makes you feel great! Just make sure that you're giving your body the protein and fat it needs to build muscle while you're exercising. A low-fat, high-carbohydrate diet in combination with strenuous exercise is a recipe for disaster. Your muscles and bones can deteriorate without the proper nutrients to keep them healthy and strong.

Get yourself out and start moving. My motto is, "Be fit, not fanatic." On the days when you just cannot find time for a workout, take a walk, just a twenty-minute walk, in the morning or the afternoon. Play tag with your kids. Take the stairs instead of the elevator. Take an active look at your activity level. Exercise helps you build lean muscle mass, which is a key element in losing weight. Lean muscle mass helps you burn calories twenty-four hours a day. Plus, exercise is another way to keep insulin levels balanced. It helps us release the stored sugar from our cells so that we can get down to burning our fat reserves and losing that extra weight. So get out there and get moving. Find an activity that brings you enjoyment. It doesn't have to cost money—it just has to get you breathing a little harder.

BE DILIGENT!

As long as you are following *all* the Level One guidelines, you may eat until you are full and still lose weight. Be diligent! You cannot Somersize half heartedly. Your body is in the process of healing as it unloads years of stored-away sugar in its cells. In order to retrain your body to burn your fat reserves, you must not confuse it by slipping up with bad combinations or Funky Foods. Besides, you have so many choices, there is no need to slip up. You will love eating this way and seeing the amazing results. Some people see results immediately and lose five or more pounds in the first week. Others don't see results until the second, third, or even fourth week. Be patient! Your body is detoxifying from all the sugar and chemicals and bad combinations to which it has become accustomed. You *will* see results, and once it begins, you'll start to melt away down to your ideal body weight. Best of all, you'll love eating this way!

I have synthesized all the information you need to know for Level One in the Reference Guide, which you'll find in the back of the book. Use this guide as a reminder of which foods belong in what category. In no time, you will get the hang of Somersizing and it will all become second nature.

SEND ME YOUR STORIES

My favorite part about putting these books together is reading all the success stories from people just like you. I can't tell you how gratifying it is for me to hear about the weight you've lost and about how you've learned to cook some fabulous new recipes. We have a section on my website to post your testimonials and also a photo album if you'd like to share your pictures. You may also write to me at Crown Publishers and let me know how you are doing on the program. I would love to hear from you. And if you like, pass along any good recipes of your own!

Suzanne Somers
c/o Crown Publishers
1745 Broadway
New York, NY 10019

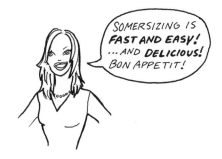

SUZANNESOMERS.COM

At www.SuzanneSomers.com you can join our community of Somersizers. Share information with others who are following this way of eating. Check our extensive FAQ section. Chat with others about the program, or anything you're interested in. Get free e-mail! And don't forget to check out all of our Somersize and SomerSweet foods, appliances, supplements, shakes, and protein bars to help you along with this way of eating. They are quick and delicious! Straight from my kitchen to yours. Make sure you register so I can send you updates about exciting new developments. See you there.

THIRTEEN

❧

Frequently Asked Somersize Questions: A Handy Reference

In my last book, I included a chapter of questions I had received from Somersizers and my answers to them. Since then, I have been inundated with even more questions from devoted Somersizers on my website. I have gone through them and put together an extensive section divided up by category, so you can easily find the answer to whatever questions you have about the program. You will also find some good tips here about creative ways to eat well and stay Somersized!

ALCOHOL

I am young, so I often go out with my friends drinking. I know you cannot support alcohol, but if it was a must, which combo would you recommend it be mixed with? Carbs and no fat?

You're right, I can't support alcohol. And as you know, alcohol is not allowed on Level One. I always say that if you are going to create an imbalance with alcohol, a Pro/Fats meal with red wine is your best bet. As far as your meal is concerned, you should be careful about portion size. You cannot eat unlimited portions if you are creating an imbalance. Your alcohol intake will spike your insulin, so your meal is in danger of getting stored as fat. Here's an idea—club soda with lime!

I have always used port wine in my spaghetti sauce to cut the acid and provide the sweetness. Also, I use marsala wine with veal and chicken skillet dishes. Do these wines contain sugars? Also, will simmering the wine in sauces for a few hours eliminate the alcohol?

I use wine freely in my recipes on Level One. I find that the modest imbalance does not disrupt my weight loss. You are correct that most of the alcohol cooks off in the process.

I heard someone talking about only having wine in combination with a little cheese to mitigate the sugar content of the wine.

I'm sure there are some theories behind this, but they are not Somersize theories. Some feel that fat slows down the insulin response. That may be true, but whenever insulin is present, the food you are eating has the potential to be stored as fat. A piece of cheese on its own will not cause your body to release insulin and, therefore, will not be converted to fat. Wine causes an insulin response, so if you eat it with cheese, both now have the potential to be stored as fat. Add a cracker and you have even more insulin and more potential for this food to be stored as fat. That being said, I love a piece of cheese with a glass of wine. This is a lovely Level Two combination.

I know you say it's okay to cook with wine because it burns off, but what about cooking with beer?

Beer has an extremely high sugar content. In fact, on the glycemic index, it rates higher than pure glucose! I would avoid using beer in any way on Level One.

I really enjoy good wine! I find it relaxing and enjoyable before dinner. If I treat a glass of wine as I would fruit, drinking it half an hour before dinner or between meals, would that modify its negative effect on the diet?

Sorry, wine is not permitted on Level One because of its sugar content. You can add it back, in moderation, on Level Two. If you are going to have it on Level One, you might lessen the effect by following the fruit guidelines, but you will still slow your progress.

I'm craving a beer! Is it possible to enjoy an alcohol-free beer? Also, I can't find a reference to capers, which I love with my beer! Are capers a goodie or a baddie?

First, the capers. They are a "goodie"! They're considered a vegetable. But an alcohol-free beer will still cause an imbalance, though it won't be as much as a beer with alcohol. The lack of alcohol doesn't make it a free food, and it should be used in moderation. Me? I'll take ice cream over an alcohol-free beer if I'm going to cheat!

Is it okay to drink red wine that has no carbs on Level One?

Technically, we eliminate all alcohol on Level One. However, if you're going to create an imbalance with alcohol, red wine is your best choice. If you find that incorporating a little red wine on Level One doesn't affect your progress, enjoy in moderation!

What can I substitute for wine in recipes? No one in my family drinks.

Try substituting chicken, vegetable, or beef stock.

What type of wine should I cook with?

When using wine, cook with something that tastes good enough to drink. If you use sour wine, you'll get sour sauce. As far as brands? Whatever you can afford. There are hundreds and hundreds from which to choose, at all price levels.

BREAD, GRAIN, OATS, CEREAL, YEAST, STARCH, WHEAT

What is the best type of flour to look for when Somersizing?

Barley flour has the lowest glycemic index of all the whole-grain flours, but anything in its whole-grain form is okay. That includes whole wheat, spelt, amaranth, kamut, and brown rice flour.

Are bialys made with high-gluten flour permitted on Level One?

High-gluten flour is white flour. Sorry, no bialys. If you can find them made with whole-grain flour, then they are okay. I have had good luck with whole-wheat bagels.

Are pumpernickel bagels okay to eat? If so, what can I have on them?

Most pumpernickel products are made with flour and molasses. There is pumpernickel flour, but you don't see it very often. Read the ingredients on the bagel packaging to make sure they have not added any sugar or white flour. If they are made from pumpernickel flour, they are fine for a Carbos meal, but on Level One do not use cream cheese or butter. Try nonfat cottage cheese, nonfat ricotta cheese, sliced tomatoes, onions, and fresh basil. Many people use nonfat cream cheese, but make sure to look for brands that are not filled with starches and chemicals.

Can arrowroot be used as a thickener instead of cornstarch? If not, can you suggest a thickener for gravies?

Arrowroot is a common name for a variety of starches obtained from roots of certain plants growing in tropical countries. Although it is the most easily digested starch, it is still a starch and is, therefore, not allowed on Level One. Look at the recipes in the Somersize books for naturally reduced sauces without any thickeners. They are delicious!

Can I have a sandwich with whole-wheat bread?

You can have a pile of vegetables on whole-wheat bread with mustard. Sometimes I get a vegetable sandwich with mustard, lettuce, tomato, peppers, onions, and pickles.

Can I have oatmeal for breakfast on Level One?

Yes! Oatmeal is a Carbo and can be enjoyed with nonfat milk. Feel free to sprinkle it with SomerSweet or your favorite artificial sweetener.

Can I have whole-wheat pancakes with sugar-free syrup? Do you have a recipe?

I have a recipe for Oatmeal Pancakes in *Get Skinny.* I serve them with blueberry sauce for a Level Two breakfast. In this book, see the Irish Oatmeal Pancakes with Raspberry Sauce. I also have Somersize Pancake and Waffle Mix plus syrup made with SomerSweet! You can get it at SuzanneSomers.com.

Can I use kasha, which is made of buckwheat? It says it's protein and not carb.

Look on the ingredients list. If it's made of buckwheat with no added fat, it is a whole grain and, therefore, placed in the Carbos group. It may contain protein, but that does not affect its grouping as a Carbo. If the ingredient list has buckwheat and added fat, it would be considered a Funky Food and you should wait until Level Two. On the nutritional panel sometimes you will see a couple grams of fat that occur naturally in whole grains. Do not worry about trace amounts of fat in the nutritional panel if there are no added fats in the ingredients list.

Can you please offer some help to people with wheat allergies?

Try kamut, amaranth, spelt, and brown rice.

How about cooking oatmeal in caffeine-free cinnamon apple spice tea instead of plain water, and, of course, adding some skim milk and SomerSweet.

Sounds like a delicious Level One Carbos breakfast!

I am a Mexican-American woman and throughout my entire life I have eaten tortillas for breakfast, lunch, and dinner. Can I eat tortillas if I am Somersizing?

You can have nonfat whole-wheat tortillas as a Carbo. You may have beans, brown rice, and salsa with these tortillas, as long as there is no fat. If you are going to have whole-wheat tortillas, don't mix them with any Pro/Fats. Sorry, but no corn tortillas.

I found a bread that has yeast but no fats or sugar. Would that be okay?

Yeast is not a problem. As long as the bread is whole-grain it sounds fine.

I have been unable to locate any whole-wheat pasta, cereal, or bread that does not have some fat. Even Grape-Nuts has $^1/_5$ gram of fat.

Don't worry about the fat content listed per serving. Look at the ingredients list and make sure there is no added fat. Many grains have minimal amounts of fat that will not create a problem. Grape-Nuts are perfect for Somersizing. As for bread, let your own body guide you. If it is not absolutely free of fat and sugar, limit your intake to reduce the effect. You may also purchase Somersize Pasta and Bread Mixes at SuzanneSomers.com.

I have found that almost all the whole-wheat breads have molasses or honey in them. Is there a certain brand you recommend? Will the amounts of molasses and honey in these breads throw me off track?

Unfortunately, most whole-wheat breads in standard grocery stores have sugar of some form or another. If you have a bakery in your city, ask them for a multigrain bread that has no sugar, molasses, honey, or any other form of sugar. Or use Ezekiel bread in the orange wrapper if you can get it. It might cost a little more, but the flavor is so much better and more delicious, I'm sure you'll find that it's worth it. And don't forget we have Somersize Bread Mixes to help out. There is another bread that a Somersizer told us about. It is called Ryvita Snackbread (the high-fiber one—don't choose the one made with enriched white flour). The ingredients are: whole-grain wheat flour, wheat bran, and salt.

I know that oatmeal is allowed, but what about the flavored oatmeal?

You must read the ingredients. I believe that some or all of the flavored oatmeals have sugar listed in the ingredients.

I noticed that oatmeal has fat. Is this okay? Or is there a specific brand I should be looking for?

Oats have a minimal amount of natural fat. As long as your oatmeal is 100 percent natural oats, you are okay. Check the list of ingredients to make sure.

In many dressings and whole-grain breads, high fructose corn syrup is listed as an ingredient. I have never seen these products without this ingredient. Is this an okay food to have?

High fructose corn syrup is not okay. It will spike your insulin levels. Once you've started losing weight steadily, you may be able to incorporate a small amount and still continue losing weight. In the beginning, it's important not to eat any sugar of any kind. Try making your own breads and salad dressings. There are some great recipes in my books. You can make these items ahead of time, freeze them, and enjoy without worrying about hidden sugars!

Is bulgur wheat allowed? It consists of wheat kernels that have been steamed, dried, and crushed.

Bulgur wheat is a whole grain and is included in the Carbos group.

Is it okay to have Malt-O-Meal for breakfast?

Malt-O-Meal is made from the "farina" of the wheat, meaning that the wheat bran and the wheat germ have been milled out of the grain. This is not a whole grain, so I'm afraid Malt-O-Meal is a Funky Food. If you want to eat it on Level Two, I would do so with nonfat milk, as it is a Carbo.

You said that Malt-O-Meal would be a Funky Food because it is wheat farina, so then why is Cream of Wheat okay?

Originally, I had listed farina as an acceptable whole grain. Since then, we have discovered that, like durum, farina is the name of a grain that has already been removed from its husk, making it a processed grain, and, therefore, a Funky Food. Now that we've got all the facts, both Malt-O-Meal and Cream of Wheat are Funky Foods.

Since water chestnuts are legal, is starch made from them fine to eat?

Just because a vegetable is included in the Veggies group does not mean that any *derivative* of that vegetable is allowed. What happens with water chestnut starch is that they extract all the starch from the water chestnut and concentrate it. Obviously, this yields a lot more starch than one would get from just eating a few water chestnuts. All vegetables have some carbohydrates, but if we take out all the other elements of the vegetable and reduce it just to its core carbs, it is no longer Somersized.

What about wheat flour?

Many people see wheat flour on an ingredient list and assume it is whole-wheat flour.

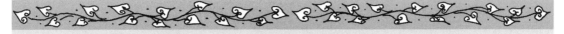

Dear Suzanne,

I have been struggling with my weight for much of my life. As a teenager, image was very important to me. I longed to be thin like many of my peers. I became obsessed with my weight and suffered from anorexia for almost ten years. When I was a high school senior, I saw you on *Oprah* promoting your very first Somersize book. I found *Eat Great, Lose Weight* at a local bookstore and thought I might give it a try. For some reason, I had difficulty leaving my old ways. Perhaps it had

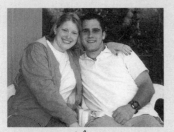

something to do with the low-cal/low-fat "brainwashing" that led me to anorexia in the first place. It wasn't until *Eat, Cheat, and Melt the Fat Away* that I made an honest attempt to make a change in my life.

In August 2001, I committed myself to Somersizing 100 percent. At that point, I was twenty-three years old, 5 feet 5 inches, and 182 pounds. After one month I lost 20 pounds. I could not believe the results I was seeing. After six months, I am now down 35 pounds.

before

While I would like to lose 10 more, I see this change as a way of life. I know that I will reach my goal before long. The greatest feeling is that for the first time in my life I can say that I love the way I look. I feel good about what I am doing for my body. My problems with asthma have also greatly decreased, and now I can participate in activities that I have not been able to in the past.

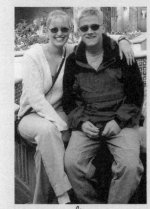

Since I began Somersizing, I have shared my success with those around me. My husband, Christopher, Somersizes with me at Level Two and has been so supportive. My parents have lost 40 pounds between them thus far and love the delicious recipes.

This program has changed my life. Suzanne, I can't thank you enough.

Much love,
Rachel Harwood

after

This is incorrect. While flour can originate as wheat flour; it has just been stripped of its nutrients and its color. You must look for whole-wheat flour, whole wheat, cracked whole-wheat, or stone-ground whole wheat. You may also have other whole-grain pastas and breads (remember, no fat or sugar added). They include amaranth, barley, bran, brown rice, buckwheat, kamut, millet, oats, pumpernickel, rye, spelt, or lavash bread (or any combination of the above). Semolina is not included in this group because it is "the purified middlings of hard wheat (as durum) used for pasta (as macaroni or spaghetti)." When something has been "purified," it is usually bleached as in "bleached wheat flour"—white flour. So, when the label says "durum wheat semolina" or "durum semolina," they mean the bleached inner part of what used to be whole wheat.

What can I substitute for honey or molasses when I make bread in my bread machine?

I use SomerSweet in my bread mixes and recipes.

What category is quinoa?

Quinoa is a grain and would fall in the Carbos group.

What cereals can I have?

Regular Grape-Nuts, Puffed Wheat, and Shredded Wheat are fine. Grape-Nuts Flakes have added sugar so you need to avoid them. Don't get confused by reading the grams of sugar on the nutritional panel. For instance, Grape-Nuts and Grape-Nuts Flakes show the same sugar content in the nutritional panel, but regular Grape-Nuts' sugar comes from malted barley and Grape-Nuts Flakes have added sugar, so no Flakes. Rule of thumb: read the ingredients list for added sugars and fats. Cheerios have added sugar and modified cornstarch, but very little, so I enjoy them in Level Two without a problem.

What do you suggest as a spread on toast?

You may have whole-wheat toast with nonfat cottage cheese and a sprinkling of cinnamon, if you like. You may also top your toast with tomatoes or a slice of red onion or nonfat ricotta cheese. On Level Two you may use a little berry jam (sweet-

ened only with fruit juice). Also, look for my SomerSweet Jams on my website, SuzanneSomers.com.

Would flax meal be considered a Carbo or Pro/Fat?

I am not familiar with flax meal. Look at the ingredients list and compare the ingredients with your Somersize Food Groups to determine whether it is a Carbo, a Pro/Fat, or a combination of both, which would make it a Funky Food. My instinct tells me it's probably a Funky Food because flaxseed has carbohydrate and fat. Regardless of the specifics, it probably does not create a great imbalance. If you are doing well on Level One, you should be able to incorporate it without a problem.

You say tabbouleh is a Carbo, but the dressing includes olive oil. Is it only allowed on Level Two?

You're right. Cracked bulgur wheat is a Carbo, which is fine for Level One with Veggies and no fat. Tabbouleh is a salad made of the bulgur wheat, mint, parsley, tomato, cucumber, scallions, and olive oil. It's fine for Level Two. Remove the olive oil, and you can eat it on Level One.

You stated that All-Bran cereal would be okay, but there is sugar and corn syrup in the bran cereal I have seen. Are you sure this is okay? If so, why can't we have Cheerios with only 1 gram of sugar?

Fiber helps counteract the negative effects of insulin. All-Bran is so full of fiber that it won't spike your insulin, even though it does contain a small amount of sugar. It is only for that reason that I make an exception for All-Bran. Cheerios are also low in sugar, but not as low as All-Bran. Cheerios are fine for Level Two.

GUM, CANDY, SWEETS

Are the SomerSweet Chocolate Truffles a Pro/Fat or a Carbo?

SomerSweet Truffles are made with chocolate, which is a Funky Food; therefore, the truffles do not fit neatly into the Pro/Fats or the Carbos. Even though they are made without sugar, you should not eat more than one or two a day while you are still losing weight. And if you are just starting to Somersize, wait until you are steadily losing before you incorporate this fabulous treat.

Can I have the sugar-free hard candies?

Technically, yes, but I don't recommend them. Real food is a better choice.

How about sugar-free chocolate candy?

This Almost Level One treat should be enjoyed in moderation.

I am craving sweets. What do you suggest?

Eat a piece of cheese to stop the craving. Also, you can try my supplement Crave Control, a blend of herbs proven to help stabilize blood sugar. And don't forget Somer-Sweet!

I'm starting to Somersize and wondered if the small amount of Nicorette gum I chew would have any effect on my progress.

Nicorette may have an effect on your weight loss, but it's better than smoking! I know several people who chew a modest amount and still have success Somersizing. Work your way off the gum as quickly as possible.

Is gum allowed? If so, what kind?

Sugar-free gum is allowed, but don't overdo it.

What are sugar-free gummy bears and hard candy considered, Pro/Fats or Carbos?

Sugar-free gummy bears and hard candies are considered neither, as they're made entirely from icky ingredients. If you must have them, eat them in moderation.

CARBOS MIXED WITH PRO/FATS

Can I add butter to brown rice and to broccoli?

You can't add butter to brown rice on Level One, as brown rice is a Carbo and may not be eaten with Pro/Fats (butter). You may add butter to broccoli and eat it alone or with a Pro/Fats meal. If you want to eat butter *and* brown rice *and* broccoli, you may do so only on Level Two.

Can I eat tuna fish with whole-wheat-flour bread on Level One?

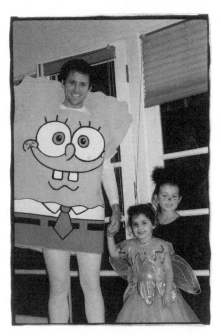

Bruce will do anything to make his gals happy.

No. Tuna is a protein and whole-wheat bread is a Carbo. We do not mix Pro/Fats and Carbos. This combo is acceptable in Level Two, though.

I am on Level One and was wondering if reduced-fat products such as mayo and cheese can be eaten if there are no additional sugars or carbohydrates?

If there are no sugars or carbohydrates added, you may eat reduced-fat products if that is your preference. Beware of reduced-fat products that replace the fat with sugars or starches because then the item becomes Funky with a combination of Pro/Fats and Carbos.

I heard that if you eat brown rice with black beans it is considered a protein, and therefore you can add other meats or cheeses to create a hearty meal. Is this true, and is it okay for Level One meals?

Brown rice and black beans both contain protein, but they are not Somersize Pro/Fats. Brown rice, black beans, and vegetables would be okay on Level One. Adding meat or cheese to this meal would also add fat and protein, which is not okay on Level One.

Is peanut butter acceptable to put on toast, because it's a legume, which you said you could mix with carbs? Is apple butter (without added sugar) okay though it's a fruit?

You cannot have peanut butter. Peanuts are a Funky Food on Level One because they have fats and carbohydrates. You must keep Pro/Fats separate from Carbos. You also may not have apple butter on toast. Remember, anything you put on toast must be fat free, and you cannot mix with fruit. Try nonfat cottage cheese or nonfat ricotta. You can add sliced tomatoes, or if you want something sweeter, you could add a little SomerSweet and some cinnamon.

CHEESE

Can I have fat-free cheese with my Carbos?

Technically, yes, but check the ingredients list because many of these products are filled with things your body does not want or need.

Can I have processed presliced cheese, or does the cheese have to come in blocks?

You may have processed cheese, but the unprocessed kind is healthier.

Can I have Velveeta cheese on Level One?

Velveeta is an American cheese, and as such we haven't technically ruled it out. However, it does contain enough preservatives to sit on a shelf unrefrigerated! Just remember that the closer you stay to whole, unprocessed foods, the better.

Can regular ricotta cheese be used with Pro/Fats or can we only use nonfat, which can only be combined with carbs?

Regular ricotta cheese has trace amounts of carbohydrates, but we have included it with our Pro/Fats group so as not to split hairs. You may eat regular ricotta cheese with Pro/Fats, or nonfat ricotta cheese with Carbos.

Can ricotta and mozzarella cheeses be eaten with veggies like eggplant and tomato sauce as in eggplant rollatini, or must they be nonfat?

Yes! I have several recipes that include this combination. These are Pro/Fats and Veggies meals. Whole-milk ricotta has trace amounts of carbohydrates, but it is a small imbalance.

Cottage cheese is on the Pro/Fats list, but you said no whole-milk products. Is there something I am missing?

You are absolutely correct. Nonfat cottage cheese is the only cottage cheese allowed and it should only be listed in the Carbos group. This was an error from the earlier books.

I am a vegetarian. I get my protein from tofu and fish. How should I treat tofu cheese?

Tofu cheese should be treated as a Pro/Fat. It does contain some carbohydrates, but we make exceptions for vegetarians.

I bought some shredded cheese and the ingredients say part skim milk. Does that make it Funky? It also has at the end of the ingredients list potato starch to prevent caking. Is this okay?

All cheese is made with milk. The carbs are eliminated in the process. As for the starch, the more processed your food gets, the more additives you wind up with. I doubt that the imbalance from eating this food would be very great, but if you have time, it's certainly better to shred your own cheese.

I have a question about cream cheese. How do I combine this with other foods? Level One or Level Two?

Regular cream cheese is a Pro/Fat. There are nonfat cream cheeses, but many of them are filled with starches and chemicals to make up for the missing fat. Technically, nonfat cream cheese is a Carbo, but check the ingredients list for yucky stuff.

I have been buying sliced farmer's cheese, which is a form of yogurt cheese. Is this okay for Somersizing (Level One)?

The rules are the same as the rules for yogurt. If it's nonfat farmer's cheese, it would be a Carbo. If it's low-fat or whole-milk farmer's cheese, it would be a Funky Food, as it contains both Carbos and Pro/Fats.

I know you said we could have fat-free cottage cheese on whole-wheat bread, but can we also have fat-free mozzarella cheese? Or any other fat-free cheese with whole-wheat bread?

Yes, technically you can have any kind of fat-free cheese with a Carbos meal, such as whole-wheat bread. However, please check the label. Many times the fat that is removed from cheese is replaced with all kinds of fillers, so watch those labels!

I live in Canada and I can't buy fat-free cheese. I can buy low-fat cheese with different amounts of milk fat. Can you tell me how much milk fat is in the fat-free cheese the book says I can have?

Fat-free cheese has 0 percent milk fat. One percent would actually be considered low-fat.

I love having grilled-cheese sandwiches. Is there a way I can eat them on Level One? Can I eat grilled cheese if I use nonfat cheese and whole-wheat bread?

You could do your grilled cheese with nonfat cheese. However, most nonfat cheeses do not melt very well. Have real cheese and fry eggplant slices as your "bread."

If cheeses are considered to be proteins, why can't nonfat cheeses and yogurts also be considered in this category? Why are they thought to be only carbohydrates?

Any kind of milk—nonfat, low-fat, or whole—has protein and carbohydrates. Since we don't combine fat and carbohydrates, we put low-fat and whole milk in the Funky Food category. Even though nonfat milk also has protein, we treat it as a Carbo. Yogurt falls into the exact same category as milk. Nonfat is a Carbo, low-fat and whole-milk yogurt are Funky Foods. Cheese is different because in the process of making cheese, cream, and butter, all of the carbohydrates are separated from the original milk and only the proteins and fats remain. These foods are therefore grouped as Pro/Fats. Now to answer your question. Look on the label. If nonfat cheese has carbohydrates, you should treat it as a Carbo (just beware of starchy fillers that are sometimes used to replace fats). You may not group it as a Pro/Fat because we don't want to eat carbohydrates with proteins and fats. Same goes for nonfat yogurt. It has carbohydrates and we don't want to eat carbohydrates with proteins or fats because carbohydrates cause our bodies to secrete insulin. Remember, insulin must be present for food to be stored as fat. We can eat proteins, fats, and low-starch vegetables freely because they do not cause an insulin response. Whole-grain carbohydrates and nonfat dairy products cause a moderate release of insulin and, therefore, are eaten separately.

Is Parmesan cheese allowed on top of my whole-wheat spaghetti?

In Level Two you can add a little fat, like Parmesan and olive oil, to your whole-wheat pasta.

Is there a limit to how much cheese I can eat in a day?

No, but don't forget to eat plenty of vegetables.

May I eat regular cottage cheese with a Pro/Fat meal? Is nonfat cottage cheese a carb?

Nonfat cottage cheese is a Carbo. Low-fat and whole-milk cottage cheese are technically Funky Foods, as they contain both fat and carbs. However, if you're doing well on the plan, you may incorporate some whole-milk cottage cheese with your Pro/Fats meals and see if it disrupts your weight loss.

Where do pimientos fit in? Can I have pimiento cheese?

Pimientos are peppers that have been pickled. They are considered Veggies. Pimiento cheese is fine.

Will eating oranges and cheese be enough nutrition for my body without drinking whole milk or drinking orange juice?

Absolutely! Whole oranges are much better for you than orange juice because they have all the added fiber. Cheese has all the same qualities as milk, without the carbohydrates.

I have heard you say that you can eat American cheese when Somersizing. I thought American cheese was a Funky Food since it has milk and fat in it. Could you clarify this?

American cheese has trace amounts of carbohydrates, but I have included it in the Pro/Fats group. When I was creating the program, I found there were places where it seemed appropriate to bend the rules slightly. This minor imbalance will not likely throw anyone off course.

You have said that some foods are okay if they have "trace" amounts of carbs and/or sugars. How much would you consider a trace? For example, I'm concerned about using spray cheese on my celery. It has 2 grams of carbs and 1 gram of sugar, but it's cheese, so is it allowed? Should I use 2 grams of carbs as a cut-off point . . . or should there always be 0 carbs in order to eat it with a Pro/Fats meal?

I cannot advocate spray cheese. It may say "cheese" somewhere on the label, but spray cheese is a distant cousin of real cheese. It is probably called "cheese food." When Somersizing, we always try to stick to real foods. I don't know how big the serving size is, but it sounds like a lot of sugar for a little squirt of cheese. There are many soft cheeses like goat cheese and Brie that would spread on celery without the addition of all those fake foods.

CHOCOLATE, CAROB

Can I have chocolate?

On Level Two you may enjoy dark chocolate in moderation. It must be at least 60 percent cocoa. I like Valhrôna, but there are many others. You may enjoy a variety of SomerSweet chocolates as an Almost Level One treat in moderation. They are available at SuzanneSomers.com.

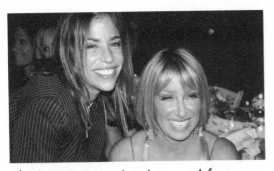

Leslie, my step-daughter and business partner.

Can I purchase 60 percent chocolate from a grocery store? Can I use it for snacking as well as baking purposes?

My grocery store, Whole Foods in Los Angeles, carries 60 percent chocolate. Valrhôna is the brand. You may use it for snacking and baking on Level Two. Somer-Sweet Chocolate is also acceptable and is made with no refined sugar.

Can I sweeten unsweetened chocolate? Is it allowed on Level One?

Unsweetened chocolate is still a Funky Food because it has caffeine, which can spike insulin all on its own. It contains a small amount of carbohydrate. Overall, it is only a minor imbalance; if you are steadily losing weight on Level One, you can try incorporating this treat every now and then.

The Chocolate Almond Torte recipe calls for 8 ounces of dark chocolate. I used baking chocolate and it tasted a little bitter. Should I have used sweetened chocolate? How can you tell if it has at least 60 percent cocoa?

Dark chocolate has some sugar in it. Baking chocolate is unsweetened. This recipe was done before I had SomerSweet. Now I would use unsweetened chocolate and SomerSweet or SomerSweet Chocolate.

What's the final word on carob?

Carob is similar to chocolate in that it has fats and carbohydrates. Sorry, it's Funky.

COFFEE, TEA, DRINKS, COCOA

Can I have a cup of decaf with cream between two Pro/Fats meals?

Yes.

Can I have hot cocoa made out of Hershey's pure cocoa with artificial sweetener and skim milk? Would it be counted as a Carbo?

Technically, cocoa is a Funky Food and should be eliminated on Level One. Cocoa has caffeine, which can spike insulin levels. But if you're going to have hot chocolate, the recipe you devised would create the least amount of imbalance, and yes, it would be considered a carbohydrate. Look for my Somersize Hot Cocoa, too.

Can I have iced tea?

Yes, but it should be decaffeinated.

Can I have some club soda with just a splash of 100 percent fruit juice to give it some flavor?

A splash of fruit juice equals a splash of insulin. This combo is only acceptable with

Fruit meals. Otherwise, try a splash of lemon or lime juice.

Can Perrier take the place of my water intake, or can it just be used as an acceptable drink alternative in addition to eight to ten glasses of water per day?

Perrier counts toward your eight to ten glasses.

Everybody always says to drink eight to ten glasses of water a day. Only problem is they never state what size glass we should be drinking.

This would be referring to drinking an eight-ounce glass of water.

How long after eating can you drink water?

Try to wait until you're at least halfway through your meal to drink anything. The majority of your drinking should occur between meals—two hours after your last meal.

I am hooked on crème brûlée flavored decaf coffee. They are coffee grinds, not the flavored coffee with syrup.

Assuming these are coffees flavored with extracts, you may enjoy them on Level One.

I drink a hot beverage called Caro (the ingredients are soluble solids of roasted malt barley, barley, chicory, and rye). I have it hot with skim milk, which I know you treat as a Carbo. So is it okay to drink? I was put on to it as a healthy coffee substitute, and if allowed, I presume I should have it with cream after a Pro/Fats meal?

I can't tell from the ingredients list if these are whole grains or refined grains. If they are whole grains, you can have Caro with skim milk as a Carbo. You cannot combine cream with it for a Pro/Fat because you would be combining Pro/Fats with Carbos.

I drink decaf in the morning with nonfat milk. Do I have to wait three hours before having a Pro/Fats meal?

Technically the answer is yes; however, a splash of milk will probably not take three hours to leave your system. Use your weight loss as a guide. If you are steadily losing weight on Level One, try waiting less time and see if your body reacts negatively. I doubt you'll have a problem.

I found a sugar-free and caffeine-free and fat-free cocoa powder in the health food store. Is it okay?

Wondercocoa is a great product. It still has carbs, so technically it's Almost Level One, but it's a better choice than regular cocoa.

I know that for coffee after a Pro/Fats meal, I should use cream, and for coffee after a Carbos meal, I should use fat-free milk. But what about coffee between meals (i.e., mid-morning coffee break)?

If you are switching from Pro/Fats to Carbos, or vice versa, you need to wait three hours. The same rule applies for milk or cream in your coffee. For example, if you had a Carbos breakfast, wait three hours and then have decaf coffee with cream to prepare for a Pro/Fats lunch.

I need my caffeine in the morning. How long do I have to wait for my insulin to drop back to a normal range after one cup of coffee?

If you absolutely must have a cup of coffee, wait a couple of hours before your next meal. Just know that caffeine boosts your adrenaline, which drops your serotonin levels. Low serotonin levels make us crave comfort foods, which are usually carbs and sugars. Try decaf!

I was curious about ordering coffee drinks from places such as Starbucks. Besides getting a decaf coffee, would it be safe to order a drink that is decaffeinated and sugar free that uses fat-free milk? Or do you have any other suggestions for good drinks? Are there any rules about when to drink it? For example, do I have to drink it a certain amount of time after one meal or before a meal or does it matter?

A decaf, sugar-free, fat-free drink is fine. I love decaf herbal tea and decaf nonfat iced cappuccinos! When you drink coffee with nonfat milk, that is a Carbo and should be considered the same as a member of the Carbo food group. If you drink decaf coffee with cream, that is a Pro/Fat and should be treated like a Pro/Fat food.

If I am drinking Somersize drinks or other decaf iced teas, does that count toward my water intake?

Yes, you may count this as water.

Is flavored tea, especially fruit, a free food as long as it is decaffeinated?

Flavored teas, as long as they are decaf and have no added sugar, are fine. Enjoy!

Is green tea allowed?

Yes, as long as it's decaffeinated.

Is it okay to have the sugar-free lemonade drinks like Country Time and Crystal Light?

Yes, and try my Somersize Drink Mixes, made with SomerSweet.

Is it safe to have lattes in the afternoon three hours after a Pro/Fats or Carbos meal if it is decaf, no sugar, and skim milk?

Yes, it is a Carbo because of the skim milk.

Where can I find decaf cappuccino? Is it considered a Carbo or Pro/Fat?

A cappuccino is made from espresso and steamed milk and/or frothy, foamed milk. To make it Somersized, it would be a Carbo made with decaf espresso and nonfat milk. I get mine at Starbucks, but you should be able to find one at any local coffee house.

Will drinking caffeinated coffee slow down my weight loss?

Quite possibly, yes. Caffeine causes a spike in your insulin level, and as you know, insulin is the deciding factor on whether your food is used for energy or stored as fat. Weaning yourself off caffeine is difficult for the first couple of weeks. I know, I used to be *addicted* to the stuff! I had headaches for the first few days, but now I don't even crave it anymore. Try treating yourself to a quality decaf coffee to help you get through the process. If you must incorporate caffeine on Level One, it's best to drink it alone.

That way, when your insulin rises, you won't have a meal in your stomach in jeopardy of being stored as fat.

You said coconuts are a Funky Food. What about the water inside the coconut and the coconut milk you get out of shredded coconut?

The water/milk you speak of is also high in sugar, and therefore a Funky Food.

MILK, CREAM, HALF-AND-HALF, EGGS, YOGURT, BUTTER, SPRAYS

Are Egg Beaters allowed with carbs? As an example, in muffins, pancakes, and such or served with whole-wheat toast?

Egg Beaters are 99 percent egg whites and 1 percent fillers. I am not an Egg Beaters fan. Real eggs are one of nature's most perfect foods. They are an excellent source of protein and the egg yolk has all the essential omega-3 fatty acids. If you want to include Egg Beaters, they would be considered a Pro/Fat. I know you are hoping for more ways to expand your Carbos meals, but I don't want to give you more options for Carbos meals. You will be much healthier and much thinner if you choose the Pro/Fats meals.

Are heavy cream and light cream both considered Pro/Fats?

Most likely, yes, but check the ingredients for hidden sugars.

Can I have whipped cream with a Pro/Fats meal?

Absolutely, if it is made without sugar.

Can I have yogurt?

Yogurt with Grape-Nuts is a nice snack or breakfast; however, the yogurt must be plain or vanilla nonfat, with no sugar, and no added thickening agents containing any type of starch.

Can I use "I Can't Believe It's Not Butter" spray on my whole-wheat bread? If not, is there another fat-free spray I can use?

I don't recommend these fat-free sprays because they are made from fake foods. You'll be amazed at how much better you'll feel when you eliminate all these processed foods from your life. As for Somersizing, this spray will cause a modest imbalance on Level One with your toast. Technically it's not allowed, but use your body as a guide. If you are steadily losing, you can include it as long as your progress continues. Me? I'll have my bread warm with a slice of tomato, or with some nonfat cottage cheese. On Level Two I'll use some real butter or some SomerSweet Jam.

Can I use cooking sprays such as Pam?

Pam is simply vegetable oil in a spray can. You may use it freely as a Pro/Fat.

Can you give me information about where to find Pavel's yogurt?

The yogurt is sold pretty much only in California at Whole Foods, with the exception of parts of Arizona and New Mexico. In northern California, they sell the yogurt at Safeway. There is no mail order because it is too small a quantity and it also shakes up the yogurt. They are currently working on selling it in Dallas and Chicago.

Can you use the nonfat milk in a can, like Carnation, for your Carbos meal?

If the only ingredient is nonfat milk, yes, it's a Carbo. If it's a Carnation Drink filled with sugar and such, then the answer is no.

Egg whites are Pro/Fats, but because they don't contain any fat, can't I eat them with the Carbos?

Technically the answer is no. Egg whites are still a protein and should only be eaten with Pro/Fats and Veggies. For a lengthy explanation on this topic go to the Discussion Forum on my website under Somersize, "Messages from Suzanne."

I cannot seem to lose weight. I am using heavy cream in diet root beer and on strawberries. So, I actually am using a lot of heavy cream. Could this be the problem? I thought heavy cream in big quantities is okay.

It is possible that you are overdoing it, especially if you are unknowingly creating imbalances. Make sure you are following all the guidelines. If you still are not losing, cut back on the cream. Remember you should only mix fats (cream) with berries if you are losing well as it causes a slight imbalance. You can have the two, just not together.

I have been using Molly McButter for years as a substitute for butter and would like to know if it fits into your program. If so, would you consider it a Carbo? Molly McButter is great on veggies.

Substitutes for butter are generally filled with fake foods, so I would suggest that you put the substitutes aside and use real butter.

I have been using Promise fat-free margarine, which has no trans fatty acids. Is this all right for Somersizing?

I do not like margarine, but at least this one does not have trans fatty acids. You may use margarine, but real butter is a better choice.

I have just started Somersizing and would like to know about lactose-free skim milk and how I can keep it in my diet. Should I only use it with Carbos or because it is lactose-free can I also use it with Pro/Fats?

You would need to consider this as a Carbo. Treat it just like regular skim milk.

I noticed that on the label of half-and-half it lists milk and cream as ingredients (thus we would assume carbos in the milk); however, on the label it also states 0 Carbos. Which is it? Can I use half-and-half and be safe not to spike insulin? Cream in the grocery store without sugar is hard to find and it is so thick.

Technically half-and-half is a combination of cream and milk. Since milk has carbohydrates and cream has fat they should not be eaten together. However, if you can only find cream with added sugars, certainly half-and-half would be a better choice. If you are steadily losing weight, you should be able to incorporate a small amount of it without a problem. I would not substitute large amounts of half-and-half for cream because then those carbs may start adding up. Hunt for pure cream. It is curious that no carbohydrates were listed on the nutritional panel of the half-and-half. It is probably because the serving size was very small, and they rounded to the nearest whole number.

I used to put a banana in my morning smoothie for a thicker consistency. I also put in nonfat vanilla yogurt for a little flavor and consistency. I can live without the banana, but can I still use some yogurt in the smoothie? Also, I like to start the day with a large glass of water, especially after I go jogging. Should I drink water before or after my smoothie?

You cannot combine nonfat yogurt (Carbo) with Fruit on Level One. You could make a decaf coffee and nonfat yogurt smoothie with some ice cubes. If you want a Fruit smoothie, it must be all fruit. If you want a nonfat yogurt smoothie, it must be all Carbos. As far as water, you need to replenish your body after a run, so drink it before your smoothie.

If I make a spinach dip with nonfat sour cream, could that be a Carbos/Veggies meal and be served with whole-wheat bread?

Yes, and it sounds great. Try it with pita bread triangles.

Is nonfat frozen yogurt in the same category as regular yogurt?

Nonfat frozen yogurt is filled with sugar and definitely a no-no for Somersizing. There are some nonfat frozen yogurts that are also sugar free. Technically you can have this because it is made from nonfat dairy products and artificial sweetener. Please use good judgment when you choose to include processed products. It's great to have a treat like this every now and then on Level One, but don't overdo it! Even on Level Two, you are much better off having real ice cream (made from milk, cream, eggs, and sugar) rather than nonfat frozen yogurt, which is filled with sugar and starch or artificial sweeteners to make up for the missing fat.

Is nonfat milk the same as skim milk? Is skim milk a Funky Food?

Nonfat milk is the same as skim milk. It may also be called fat free. It is not a Funky Food, but it is considered a Carbo and should only be used with Carbos.

Is nonfat plain yogurt allowed, even though in the nutritional panel is says there are more or less 16 grams of sugar?

As I always say, check the ingredients list, not the nutritional panel. If there are no added sugars, it is fine. The reason you see sugars in the nutritional panel is because nonfat milk has carbohydrates, which convert to sugar upon digestion. That is why nonfat yogurt is grouped as a Carbo.

Is sour cream allowed on Level One?

Yes, full fat sour cream is a Pro/Fat. Nonfat sour cream is a Carbo.

One of the ingredients in skim milk is sugar. Is that still okay?

Your skim milk should not list sugar in the ingredient list. If it does, I would look for another brand. It may, however, list "Sugars" on the nutritional panel. This is because milk has carbohydrates and natural sugars. That is why we list nonfat milk with the Carbos. It is perfectly fine to eat food in the approved Carbos list even if you see sugars appearing on the nutritional panel.

Should I use margarine?

Even though margarine is listed as a Pro/Fat, you may want to avoid it because of the trans fatty acids. Also try to avoid any food that has a significant amount of hydrogenated oil listed on the package. Adding hydrogen to fat makes it a cheap filler for the producer. Unfortunately it raises your LDL cholesterol (bad) and lowers your HDL cholesterol (the good one that helps get rid of the bad). It's a personal choice, but at least you're informed.

What about low-fat dairy products?

Low-fat milk is not included in this program because it contains fat and carbohydrates. Low-fat cheese contains less fat and usually no carbohydrates. But full-fat cheese tastes so much better and is perfectly okay on Level One.

What do you suggest for people who are lactose intolerant?

Obviously, you need to eliminate the dairy items that cause a problem for you. You may substitute nonfat soy or nonfat rice milk in the Carbos group. Otherwise, enjoy all the wonderful meats, vegetables, fruits, and whole grains.

What is the least harmful way to eat nonfat yogurt with fruit at the bottom?

The least harmful way is not to eat it at all. Fruit should be eaten by itself. If you want to have yogurt, you should have the plain nonfat yogurt. The least amount of imbalance from yogurt with fruit would be to have nonfat yogurt with fresh berries. Yogurt with fruit at the bottom is filled with sugar. It's definitely a no-no.

When drinking decaf green tea or decaf herbal tea, are the rules the same as they are with decaf coffee concerning either heavy cream or nonfat milk? Can either cream or milk be used with each of them depending on the kind of meal they are going with (heavy cream with Pro/Fats, skim milk with Carbos meal)?

The rules remain the same for decaf tea as for coffee. Use skim milk as a Carbo and

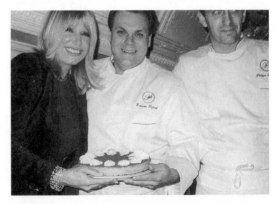

François Payard presenting me a Somersized cappuccino cheesecake in New York.

cream as a Pro/Fat. The same guidelines apply for switching between food groups. Wait three hours when switching between food groups.

Where does buttermilk fit into Somersizing?

Buttermilk is a Funky Food because it has fat and carbohydrates, just like whole milk or low-fat milk. I do use a bit of buttermilk powder in my Somersize Ranch Dressing mix, and it does the trick without the carbs.

DESSERTS, ICE CREAM

At what point can I introduce some Level Two desserts? I have not reached my goal weight, but am really feeling deprived of some sort of sweets.

If you are steadily losing weight on Level One and would love some type of a sweet, check out some of my delicious dessert recipes. You could certainly have some of my sugarless cheesecake or a decaf coffee granita on Level One. My dessert mixes, like Somersize Crème Brûlée and Somersize Chocolate Mousse, are made with Somer-Sweet and may be enjoyed in moderation as an Almost Level One treat. Also, keep a box of SomerSweet Chocolates in the house. SomerSweet allows you to eat sweets without disrupting your weight loss at all. Just don't overdo it! There are great recipes in my dessert cookbook, *Somersize Desserts,* featuring SomerSweet.

Do you have a recipe for cookies that I could make for Level Two that would incorporate acceptable ingredients according to your plan?

Cookies, by their nature, are not easily Somersized. They almost always contain Pro/Fats and Carbos, which, as you know, is not a good combo. I have several cake recipes that have this combination, but with the cakes I can greatly reduce the amount of flour, which lessens the problem. With cookies you must use quite a bit of flour, so they create a larger imbalance. If you just have to have a cookie, use whole-grain flour and try SomerSweet instead of sugar, but you'll have to experiment. Sugar and brown sugar are essential to a good soft cookie.

How long should you wait to have your desserts after a Pro/Fats meal or a Carbos meal?

If you are having a dessert made with mostly Pro/Fats, like sugarless cheesecake, you may eat it right after a Pro/Fats meal. If you are having SomerSweet Chocolate, the best time to eat that is all by itself, in the middle of the afternoon. If you are having a fruit-based dessert, like fruit sorbet, you should wait two hours after your last meal. Of course, all of these guidelines loosen up as you enter Level Two, or get close to entering Level Two.

I know I can have sugar-free ice cream (with the fat in). But is it a Carbo or a Pro/Fat?

Ice cream of this type is a Pro/Fat. I have awesome SomerSweet Ice Cream Mixes and Somersize Triple Hot Fudge and Hot Caramel. Yum!

I recently made the Decadent White Chocolate Cake and found the ganache very thin. Since there are only two ingredients in the ganache, what could be the problem?

The ganache will be thin before it hardens. Letting it cool will help. Place your cake on a cooling rack with something underneath to catch the extra ganache. Pour the ganache over the cake, letting the remainder drip down the sides. Then transfer the cake to a plate and refrigerate until the ganache sets, like the exterior of a chocolate candy. Also, make sure the white chocolate you're using is a high-quality chocolate. Most white chocolates today are made from oil and sugar. If you can find a chocolate made from cocoa butter, that would be best. Also, you may try using a little less cream.

Can a person eat too much of the sugarless cheesecake? I tend to eat a piece every day as a treat. I know it is all protein, but I want to make sure it won't hinder my weight loss.

One slice a day is fine. Just because my sugarless cheesecake is all Pro/Fats, that's not an excuse to eat a whole one in one sitting! One piece a day is very reasonable.

I'm confused. You say we can have no-sugar-added, full-fat ice cream, but they always have milk or cream. I thought only fat-free milk was okay, and then as a Carbo?

Remember that cream is a Pro/Fat. When I say full-fat ice cream, I mean one that is made with cream, not milk. I have never been able to find a store-bought ice cream with no sugar that is made from all acceptable Pro/Fats. Sometimes you find ones that are sugar-free and made with a combination of milk and cream. The milk would create a

modest imbalance. The problem is that most sugar-free ice creams are also fat-free. Those are filled with starches and fillers to make up for the missing sugar and fat. I know you want Somersize ice cream! That is why I created recipes for my own ice cream made from cream, eggs, and vanilla beans, and now we have SomerSweet Ice Cream Mixes. Invest in an ice cream maker and try this fabulous Level One ice cream. It's so rich, you'll only want a little bowl.

Is sugarless ice cream and no sugar added the same?

The FDA has different categories for food products. To call a product "sugar free," it must contain less than .5 grams of sugars (that means sugar or sweeteners) per serving. To call a product "no sugar added" means that absolutely no sugar or sweetener was added as an ingredient. The nutritional panel may list sugar, because of natural sugars (like those that occur in milk).

The only kind of cream I can find is either table cream or light cream, and it also has one carbo per serving. Do you have advice, or is one carbo normal and okay?

Check the ingredients list. All should fit into the Pro/Fats group.

What about the popsicle rule? What kind is it that we have to have?

You want to look for all-fruit-juice-sweetened ice pops. You can have sugar-free ice pops, but watch out for artificial sweeteners.

What brand of sherbet would you recommend? The ones I have checked in my local grocery stores are all made with sugar as the second or third ingredient.

You actually want to look for sorbet that is sweetened only with fruit juice. Remember that concentrated fruit juice is still quite high in sugar, and therefore should only be eaten in moderation on Level One. I have a few recipes for sorbet and granita in *Somersize Desserts*.

What kind of chocolate should I be using to make your chocolate desserts? I know it should be 60 percent, but is that semisweet or unsweetened?

Chocolate with at least 60 percent cocoa is somewhere between unsweetened and semisweet. High-quality chocolate usually lists the percentage of cocoa it contains. Semisweet chocolate has too much sugar in it for Somersizing. Some dark chocolate is 60 percent cocoa or more, but you can't know for sure unless the percentage is listed. Look for this good-quality chocolate in fine food shops or through catalogs. If you can't find chocolate with the percentage on it, use bittersweet or dark chocolate. These recipes were created before I had SomerSweet. Now I would use unsweetened chocolate and SomerSweet or SomerSweet Chocolate.

FLOUR

Are egg rolls or wonton wrappers allowed? They say wheat flour.

If you can find the type that says whole

wheat, then they are fine. For Level Two, these wheat flour wrappers are fine.

Are you allowed to have enriched wheat flour?

It must say whole wheat to be acceptable. Enriched wheat flour is just white flour. Look for enriched whole-wheat flour, or whole-wheat flour.

Can I make fried chicken if I use whole-wheat flour?

This is fine for Level Two, but on Level One we do not combine starches with fats. I fry foods with no flour at all and they taste delicious. You still get the flavor, just not the floury crust. Or try my Somersize Shake It and Bake It Chicken (p. 234).

How about King Arthur's white whole-wheat flour?

I recommend it. This flour is made from hard white wheat. The product states that it is made from 100 percent of the wheat germ and bran, so it would be the same as whole-wheat flour.

It is difficult to find whole-wheat phyllo dough. What should I use instead?

If you are having a hard time finding whole-wheat phyllo, use the regular kind in Level Two.

Is unbleached wheat/whole-wheat flour okay to use?

This is probably a combination of unbleached wheat flour (which is white flour) and whole-wheat flour. Only the latter is okay, so I would avoid this combination.

Is white unbleached organic flour a Funky Food?

Sorry, it's still white flour. Look for whole-grain flour, like whole-wheat flour.

What is the substitute for flour when making white sauce?

I make white sauce with cream, butter, and Parmesan cheese. You may not use starch with cream sauces because you may not combine fat with starch.

FRUIT

Are dried fruits allowed?

Only sparingly because the sugar content has been concentrated during the drying process. You will see results more quickly if you avoid dried fruits.

Are plantains allowed, and if so, are they a Fruit or a Veggie?

Plantains are a type of banana, so they are full of sugar and, therefore, a Funky Food.

Are raisins considered a fruit?

Raisins, as you know, are dried grapes. Any dried fruit has an intense concentration of natural sugar. It is best to hold off on all dried fruit in Level One. Or, if you are doing well on Level One and losing steadily, try incorporating dried fruit in moderation and see how your body reacts.

Are there fruits I should avoid?

Even though bananas are high in potassium, they are also very high in starch. That is why they are a Funky Food. With all the other fruits you can eat, you won't miss them. Berries are very high in fiber, so they cause only a slight imbalance when eaten with other foods. As an Almost Level One treat, you may enjoy berries with whipped cream after a Pro/Fats meal. On Level Two, I sometimes use all-fruit-juice-sweetened berry jam on my whole-grain toast in the morning.

Avocados are listed as a Funky Food. Are they allowed in Level Two?

Absolutely. Avocados are one of those foods that I hate to have on the Funky Foods list. They are filled with healthy fats and are only listed on the Funky Foods because they also have some carbohydrates. You may eat them freely on Level Two, and I am sure you will not have a problem.

Can strawberries be eaten at any time?

Berries are grouped with the Fruits. When you are just beginning to Somersize you should include berries with all the other fruits and follow the guidelines for when you may have them. However, berries are very high in fiber and cause less of an insulin surge than other fruits. If you are doing well on Level One and are steadily losing weight, you may loosen the reins on berries and treat them as a free food. Enjoy them with whipped cream after a Pro/Fats meal. Or swirl them into nonfat yogurt for a Carbos

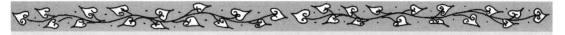

Dear Suzanne,

For years I had been going to the gym and starving myself in order to stay skinny. I worked out for two hours every day, had a cup of coffee for breakfast, and then ate a huge dinner. I was always hungry and thin but not healthy. This strenuous lifestyle burned me out, and I just gave up. The next couple of years I ate everything and didn't exercise. I went from a size 3/4 to busting out of a size 10.

I walked into a Jenny Craig office and learned about their program. I knew immediately that it wasn't for me because it was quite costly and you had to purchase their food. I was so embarrassed with how I looked, I was afraid that someone I knew would see me leaving the building. Then, one afternoon when I was waiting for my son to get out of school, a friend told me she was reading one of your books and that your program sounding interesting. So the next day I went and picked one up for myself.

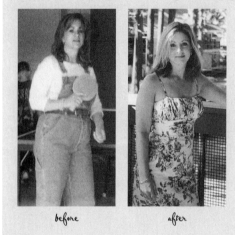

befone   after

The results are staggering: I'm 5 feet 2 inches, and in May 1999, I weighed 142 pounds. Today, I weigh 107, and I'm back into my size 3/4 pants and into an exercise routine that doesn't wipe me out.

The recipes in all three of your books are great. I've made the Buffalo Wings and Blue Cheese for my family, and they didn't even know they were Somersizing. I have also been coaching my mother and aunt through the program. They've lost a total of 115 pounds.

I feel great. I weigh the same as I did years ago, but the difference is, now I am healthy. Thanks for all your help, Suzanne.

Sincerely,
Teri Passanisi

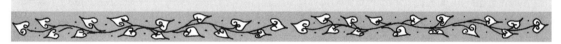

breakfast or afternoon snack. (Sweeten the whipped cream or yogurt with a little vanilla and SomerSweet.)

Can we eat canned fruit if we drain the juice and wash the fruit before eating it?

You may eat canned fruit that does not have added sugar or corn syrup. I don't think washing it will get rid of the soaked-in sugar. You'd be better off eating frozen fruit.

How much fruit can I eat? Is there a limit?

I don't give you any limits on how much fruit you should eat, but remember, fruit is a natural sugar. If you are eating a lot of fruit and find you are not losing weight, I would try cutting back to see if that helps. I usually eat fruit in the morning and occasionally as a snack in the afternoon.

I realize bananas are a Funky Food, but on Level Two, can you have mashed bananas on wheat toast for breakfast? I would guess the imbalance to be the same as fruit-sweetened jam. Please advise.

Because of their high starch content, bananas would create a somewhat greater imbalance than a bit of fruit-sweetened jam. However, as you are on Level Two, give it a try and see how it affects you. If it's creating too great an imbalance, go back to Level One until your body has readjusted.

Is it okay to eat sugarless applesauce with ascorbic acid?

Yes, treat it as Fruit.

JUICE

Can I have juice?

By the time you make juice from fruit you have taken out most of the nutrition and are left with fruit sugar. Technically, if you are drinking juice alone, you may have it in the same way you eat fruit alone. However, many juices are very high in natural fruit sugar and I recommend you drink them sparingly. The whole fruit also contains fiber, which helps to reduce the effects of insulin. But sometimes on Level One it's great to enjoy an ice pop made from fruit and fruit juice only. Beware of eating too many products with concentrated fruit juice because it will make your insulin spike.

Can juice be used in smoothies for Level One?

Yes, as long as it does not have any added sugar.

I cannot find sugarless orange juice. Any recommendations for the making of smoothies? I love the fruit fix for breakfast.

When you say you cannot find sugarless orange juice, are you checking the ingredients or the nutritional panel? It has natural sugar that will show on the nutritional panel. However, as long as there is no form of sugar added in the ingredients, it is okay. Usually it will say 100 percent pure orange juice on the carton.

I know I can have tomato juice, but is it a Carbo or Pro/Fat?

Tomato juice would be considered a vegetable, so you may have it with either.

I know V-8 juice is a Funky Food, but would it cause too much of an imbalance if I used a small can to make meatballs?

I don't think you'll have a problem. If you want to be a purist, you could substitute tomato juice and add onion powder, garlic powder, celery seed, salt, pepper, and Tabasco sauce.

MEATS, FISH, CHICKEN

Can I eat any meat I want?

Yes, just make sure it is not cured with sugar. (Pork is most often the culprit.) Watch out for cold cuts and be sure to read the ingredients list.

Can I use regular turkey sausage for your stuffing recipe?

Yes. Feel free to improvise on any of my recipes as long as you stay within the same food groups.

Can we have oysters?

Oysters have trace amounts of carbohydrates, but it should not be enough to inhibit your progress on Level One. Beware of fried oysters, though, because they are usually coated in flour.

Can I eat sugar-cured meats?

Generally, try to avoid sugar-coated hams, because they can be quite high in sugar. Many sausages and bacon have small amounts of sugar, and I have found that it has not been a problem to include them on Level One. Use your own body as a guide.

If I can't use lamb, what meat can be substituted?

Beef, chicken, pork, or whatever you like.

I'm finding dextrose listed in the ingredients in many meat products. Isn't this a form of sugar and not allowed?

Sometimes packaged cold cuts have dextrose and other sweeteners. It's best to get fresh cold cuts from a deli, because it's healthier. However, I doubt the small amount of dextrose in meat will affect your weight loss.

In your pork recipes, can I substitute beef for the pork?

Absolutely. Feel free to make substitutions that suit your liking and your budget.

Is beef jerky allowed?

Beef jerky is usually made with some kind of sugar, but some are dried and seasoned without any sugar or sweeteners. As always, check the ingredients list. If there are no Funky Foods on the ingredients list, you may have it.

Is it okay to eat store-bought buffalo wings with blue cheese dressing and celery?

Check the ingredients list; as long as there is no sugar and flour, they are fine. I fry my own wings, then toss them in hot sauce and dip in my homemade blue cheese dressing.

Is liverwurst or braunschweiger allowed?

No. Liverwurst and braunschweiger are both made from liver, which is a Funky Food because it has protein, fat, and carbohydrate. You may enjoy liver on Level Two without a problem.

Is sushi okay to eat on Level One? I commonly have the California roll . . . but there is a vegetarian roll with just cucumber, white rice, and seaweed. Is this okay? How about the wasabi (horseradish paste) and light soy sauce? Do you have any suggestions for alternatives to Japanese food if these are not allowed?

As you know, white rice is a Funky Food, since it spikes your insulin level, so it is not allowed on Level One. The cucumber, seaweed, wasabi, and soy sauce are all fine. You may want to try sashimi, which is sushi without the rice. Or you could also have a Carbos meal of buckwheat noodles with steamed vegetables and soy sauce. Or have chicken or steak grilled with oil and soy sauce with some vegetables. Steer clear of teriyaki sauce, as it's full of sugar.

Is canned chicken okay? Also, how do you feel about canned tuna? How much mayo should I add to these salads?

As long as there are no added sugars or starches in canned chicken it is okay. It's certainly not as healthy as fresh, but it's okay for Somersizing. Every now and then I enjoy a can of tuna fish mixed with mayonnaise and celery. You can use as much mayo as you want as long as you are eating all Pro/Fats and Veggies.

I've had a hard time finding bacon or sausage that isn't sugar-cured or doesn't contain sugar or

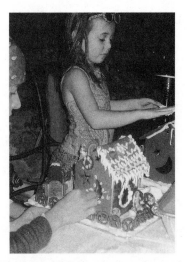

Leslie the artist teaching the kids how to make gingerbread houses.

some type of corn syrup solids. Can you suggest a few obtainable brands? I travel a lot, and hotel breakfast buffets have fluffy scrambled eggs and fried bacon. I suspect that the eggs have milk added and the bacon might contain sugar. Any suggestions?

The trace amounts of sugar in bacon and sausage shouldn't affect your weight loss. The small amount of milk possibly added to the scrambled eggs would create a very minor imbalance, so they should be fine.

HEALTH-RELATED QUESTIONS

Could breast-feeding be the cause for not losing any weight while Somersizing?

Absolutely! Your hormones go through a big change when you are breast-feeding. This happened to my daughter-in-law, Caroline. Dr. Schwarzbein explained that sometimes the hormone progesterone becomes elevated when we are breast-feeding. This elevation can keep us from losing weight. It's like Mother Nature's way of making sure we hang on to some body fat so we can keep producing healthy milk for the baby. Keep on your Somersizing path so as not to make the problem any worse. Breast-feeding is so great for your baby. Keep it up. As your baby starts to eat solids, the weight will begin to melt away.

Diabetics are supposed to eat Carbos evenly throughout the day to keep a level sugar level. How about a Somersize plan for us?

As with all medical questions, you must check with your doctor. I highly recommend you read Dr. Schwarzbein's book, *The Schwarzbein Principle.* She is a brilliant endocrinologist who has helped many diabetics turn their health around.

How can I counteract acid in my system?

There is a wonderful book called *Alkalize or Die,* by Dr. Theodore A. Baroody. It explains how we are facing a crisis of illness and disease linked to overacidity in our bodies. We want our bodies to be alkaline, not acidic. Many factors lead to this dangerous acid condition—polluted air, chemically filled food and water supply, and high stress levels. One of the easiest ways to get your body alkaline is to eat asparagus. I have it several times a week. Pick up a copy of the book to get all the information.

I recently cooked a celery root purée, which made us extraordinarily gassy. Is this a normal reaction to celery root? Is it like cooked cabbage? Or is there a way to prepare it so that it produces less gas?

Celery root, also known as celeriac, comes from the umbrel family. This family of aromatic plants includes celery, parsley, carrots, and fennel. I have never heard of celery root giving one gas, but certainly if it makes you uncomfortable, avoid it. A tip to keep beans from giving you gas is to add a slice of ginger while you're cooking them. Maybe you should try this with your celery root.

I'm afraid that beef, bacon, cheese, and other fats on the Somersize plan will promote cancer. Do you have any feelings on the subject?

I recommend you read Dr. Schwarzbein's book, *The Schwarzbein Principle.* After I wrote *Eat Great, Lose Weight,* I knew that fat would not make you fat, but I was still worried about health concerns. After I met with this doctor, she changed my feelings about fat. Read for yourself. The information is compelling.

Is it normal for a person following the program 100 percent to feel dizzy or lightheaded?

No, it is not normal to feel dizzy. Check with your doctor. You should feel energized and great. Make sure you are balancing your meals and not just eating all Pro/Fats. Are you eating Carbos for breakfast? Are you including plenty of fresh vegetables? Are you eating enough food? Balance is the key.

Is it true that a large waistline is usually caused by an improper insulin level in the system?

People with raised insulin levels have more glucose than their cells can store. If the cells are filled with this sugar and cannot take any more, the glucose will be sent to the fat cells, where it is converted to fat and reserved for later use. Insulin is like the gatekeeper; it decides if the glucose gets burned as fuel or stored as fat. If the fuel cells are full, the first place glucose looks for a home is in the fat cells around the midsection. For men, it's the love handles and beer belly. For women, it's the reproductive areas like the tummy, hips, butt, and thighs. Once you deny your body fuel in the form of sugar and carbohydrates, your body turns to its stored fuel as an energy source. That's when "The Melt" begins. Your body goes from being a carbo-burning machine into a fat-burning machine.

Is Somersizing safe during pregnancy?

As always, check with your doctor. I have had so many letters from pregnant women who say Somersizing is an excellent program during pregnancy. It is low in sugar and high in foods that include protein and calcium. During pregnancy I would recommend that you stick to Level Two and enjoy real foods, vegetables, proteins, and fats, whole-grain carbohydrates, and fruit. My daughter-in-law, Caroline, Somersized her way through both pregnancies and can't praise it enough.

Is too much protein hard on the liver?

Many people say high-protein diets are hard on the liver. Dr. Schwarzbein does not agree.

My gallbladder was removed in 1995 and I've had nothing but problems. I understand that eating too much protein is not good for my system. How can this program help me?

If you shouldn't eat a lot of protein, then you would have to Somersize without eating a lot of protein. It's possible, but Somersizing is high in protein by design, so perhaps this is not the program for you. Please ask your doctor.

Some say that no matter what program you're following, if you eat more calories than you use during the day, they will be stored as fat. Is this true?

The hormone insulin must be present for food to be stored as fat. This is scientifically undisputed. Insulin is the fat-storing hormone. If you are eating foods that do not cause an insulin response, then they cannot be stored as fat. You can sit down and eat a Somersized meal, like a steak with broccoli and salad, and as long as there are no hidden sugars, this meal will not be stored as fat because these foods do not cause an insulin response. *But,* if you follow up that meal with just a bite or two of cake, you have blown the whole thing! Now the entire meal may be stored as fat because the insulin released from the sugar in the cake may trap the steak dinner as well, and send the entire meal to the fat reserves. You must be diligent!

Somersizing gets my monthly cycle out of whack. Why?

If your monthly cycle is out of whack, you should check with your doctor. There are several factors that could be affecting your cycle.

What can you suggest for people who suffer from hypothyroidism and have gained weight? Will your program help them?

I'm not a doctor, so I can't give medical advice. We have heard from many people like you who have lost weight by Somersizing. Please check with your doctor to see if this program is safe for you.

Will the program work for me if I am postmenopausal?

People of all ages have had success Somersizing. However, your own personal hormonal state can greatly affect your ability to lose weight. Try it and see if it works for you. Many menopausal and postmenopausal women have done well Somersizing. If you are not losing weight, I recommend that you see an endocrinologist and have your hormone levels checked.

SOMERSIZING FOR THE FAMILY

Is it safe for children to follow this food plan?

If your child is overweight, you should check with your doctor. The letters I have received from parents indicate this is the easiest way their children have ever lost weight. Plus, it eliminates sugar, which keeps their moods more even. For children who don't need to lose weight, Level Two with proteins, fats, whole grains, and fruit provides a very balanced, healthy way of eating.

My kids are really picky. Do you have any suggestions to switch them over to this way of eating?

Start slowly. If they are used to eating pizza and pasta, they may not learn to love beef and broccoli overnight. Kids will follow your habits. Remember, you introduced them to the foods they consider staples. There are simple things you can begin with. Get them off the soda pop and convert them to drinks made with SomerSweet. Replace your sugary condiments with Somersize Ketchup and Somersize Barbecue Sauce. Delete the sugary desserts and serve them

Somersize Hot Fudge Sundaes or Somersize Chocolate Mousse. As for their meals, most kids are thrilled with Somersize foods. Begin by replacing their white bread with wheat bread. Introduce them to brown rice instead of white rice. This book is filled with kid-friendly options like Somersize Chicken Nuggets, even Mini-Pepperoni Pizzas and Somersize Macaroni and Cheese. Most kids welcome this food because it's delicious and loaded with flavor.

I'm a working mom and I have to be able to make meals quickly for my family. I'm so used to making pasta. Any suggestions?

Invest in some tools like a slow cooker and a pressure cooker. They'll change your life! With a slow cooker, you throw your meal together in the morning and arrive home to a beautiful dinner. With a pressure cooker you can have delicious meals in minutes. Vegetables take a minute or two and there are many one-pot recipes in this book designed for people who don't have a lot of time. Also, continue to check my website for shortcuts to delicious meals, like Somersize Taco Seasoning Mix for fast and easy tacos and taco salads.

I don't have time to make two meals, one for me and one for my family. How can I avoid this and stay on the program?

If your family does not want to Somersize, you can easily adapt your meals to please both of you. Make yourself chicken with a vegetable and a sauce and add a side of rice or pasta for the non-Somersizers in the house. Make a great spaghetti sauce and serve it to yourself over zucchini noodles and over white pasta for the family. Everyone's happy.

It's a tradition in my family to have pancakes or waffles every Sunday morning. We love your Somersize Pancake and Waffle Mix, but isn't it a no-no to oil the waffle maker with Carbos?

Somersize Pancake and Waffle Mix is Level One (except Wild Blueberry, which is Level Two). All are made with whole grains and SomerSweet. When you make waffles with the Somersize Waffle Maker, the grids are nonstick, so you don't need to add butter or oil. Adding a bit of fat would make this Almost Level One, fine for once a week. Just don't add bacon or sausage to this meal.

Is this program safe for teens?

As always, check with your doctor. I know many teenagers who have had great results.

MISCELLANEOUS

About half an hour after I have a Pro/Fats meal I am hungry again. Am I doing something wrong?

Eat more! Have larger portions. Eat until you feel satisfied. Keep hard-boiled eggs in the fridge to help fill you up after a meal.

Can I eat hummus with a bagel?

Yes, fat-free hummus on a whole-grain bagel is fine.

Can I have Chinese food? I know I can't have the rice, but what can I have?

Eating in a Chinese restaurant is very difficult because they use sugary sauces as a base in most of their preparations. Some Chinese restaurants are offering brown rice and steamed vegetables, or you could order stir-fried vegetables with chicken, meat, or fish and ask them to cook it in oil and soy sauce only.

Can I have grits?

Grits are made from corn and are, therefore, a Funky Food.

Can I have pickles?

Sure, as long as they are dill pickles and not sweet pickles. As with all foods, check the ingredients to make sure there is no added sugar.

Do I have to be concerned if a product has a small amount of sugar in it, like bottled salad dressing or bread or meat?

When you first start the program you should be very strict about eliminating all sugars, even the small amounts to which you refer. Then use your weight loss as a measuring stick. If you are steadily losing weight, try incorporating these minor imbalances and see if they affect your weight loss.

Do you have a suggestion for storing Parmesan chips?

I would suggest you store the Parmesan chips in an airtight container and refrigerate them.

Do you have any suggestions as to what I can add to a Carbos meal to keep me from being so hungry shortly after I have finished eating? This doesn't happen with a Pro/Fats meal.

Carbos are a form of sugar and can get your body craving more and more. Even the good carbohydrates on my program can have this effect. That is why I recommend you eat more Pro/Fats meals than Carbos meals. Even with my good carbohydrates, your body does not feel as satisfied. The best way to get rid of hunger pains is to eat Pro/Fats. A piece of cheese really does the trick for me.

Does Somersizing work if I am on birth control pills?

Any medication that you are taking could have an effect on your hormonal balance; and as you know, Somersizing is all about balancing your hormones. However, I have not heard of anyone having a problem Somersizing while taking birth control pills.

Does the fact that I don't have a lot of weight to lose mean that it might take a little longer for me?

It really varies for everyone. Some lose it very quickly regardless of how much they need to lose. For others, it takes a little longer to get started.

How do you know when to move from Level One to Level Two?

When you like the way you look and have reached your goal weight, you move to Level Two to maintain your weight.

How does lowering your carb intake affect a nursing mother?

Check with your doctor. Here's my opinion: Your body needs protein, fat, and calcium to produce healthy milk for your baby. Carbohydrates are used for energy. Your body can break down your own energy by converting your fat reserves into energy. Cutting back on carbohydrates will only help you lose weight. That's an effect most of us are looking for! If you find you are getting too thin, you could risk losing your milk supply. In that case, you'll want to move to Level Two to maintain your weight and keep your milk supply.

How long should it take me to lose twenty pounds?

It took me two months before I started seeing any weight loss. Everybody is different. Some people see results in the first week and for other people, like me, it takes a little longer. Be patient; it will work.

How much exercise do you recommend daily?

Although you don't have to exercise to lose weight when you Somersize, I highly recommend exercise three times a week for at least twenty minutes. It doesn't have to be strenuous, just something that gets your heart moving. As I always say, be *fit,* not fanatic! The benefits of regular exercise are so great—not just for weight loss, but to live a longer, healthier life. I also recommend weight training to prevent osteoporosis.

How much should I be eating? Do I have to count calories or fat?

Do not count fat grams, carbs, or calories or weigh anything. Follow the Level One guidelines and eat what you want until comfortably full. Try to eat a wide variety of foods each day.

I am a little nervous about starting Level Two when the time comes. I am concerned that when I start creating imbalances, the cravings will return. Is this a possibility?

When you start Level Two, it's wise to start out slowly. You're absolutely right—if you jump into imbalances that your body can't handle, the cravings will return, and you'll find yourself in a downward spiral that will have you craving more and more sugar. The good news is, now that you've attained your goal weight, the sugar has been cleansed from your cells, allowing you to create some minor imbalances without throwing your body into a tizzy. So start slowly, pay attention to your body, and enjoy the treats (in moderation!) that Level Two brings. You've earned it!

I am a vegetarian. How will your eating plan work for me?

I have many vegetarians who love my plan. They simply eliminate the foods they don't eat and follow the rest as it is outlined. I also allow soy products on Level One to be added for vegetarians, even though they are a Funky Food. Your level of comfort will depend on how strict you are as a vegetarian. If you eat poultry, seafood, and dairy prod-

ucts, you will still have plenty of choices on my program. If you are a strict vegetarian, I would say you already have enough dietary restrictions and do not need to add any more. Overall, just about everyone can benefit by reducing sugar in their diet.

I am trying to begin Somersizing, but my sugar lust is bringing me down and it seems I can't get started. Can you give me any advice to overcome it, or is cold turkey the only possibility?

Unfortunately, only you can decide to do this. You have to really make the commitment to do this and to follow the program diligently. You have to decide when you are ready mentally to make that commitment. You have to totally cut out the sugar to make it work. Also know that the sugar cravings really only last a couple of weeks. Plus SomerSweet is available and we can have "legal" desserts when we want something sweet. Also, try Crave Control to help with the cravings.

I had lost 3.5 pounds the first week and then suddenly I gained 1.5 pounds in one day! I weighed 127 pounds on Saturday and on Sunday I weighed 128.5. What happened?

You've just learned why it is best to weigh yourself once a week. It is totally natural that our weight fluctuates from one day to the next. So many things can affect it, including the time of the month. You were probably just retaining some water that day. This happens to everyone. It is only temporary, so don't worry.

I have a good breakfast but at lunch I can't

prepare these nice lunches from your book. So what kind of sandwiches can I make?

How about making extra for dinner and having leftovers for lunch? Make a big pot of soup ahead of time that can be reheated. As far as sandwiches, if it's with whole-grain bread, remember it needs to be Carbos and Veggies, so you could have a veggie sandwich with lettuce, tomato, pickles, onions, sprouts, cucumber, and mustard. You can also make whole-wheat tortilla roll-ups by mixing my Somersize Dip Mix with nonfat ricotta cheese and using it as a spread. Then layer with tomatoes, herbs, onion, or any veggies you like. Roll it up and you have a Somersize Wrap. You could also have egg salad, tuna salad, chicken salad, BLT, sliced turkey with mayo but on all of these, instead of bread roll them up in lettuce leaves like tacos.

I have been laid off work and can't afford most of the ingredients you suggest for Somersizing. Can you recommend things that are less expensive?

I've received several letters saying that my food is too expensive. You don't have to eat lamb chops, duck, and filet mignon. Simply choose less expensive cuts of meat like ground turkey, chicken, and hamburger, and check out the recipes in this book—you will find many recipes that don't cost a lot to make.

I have been on your diet for two weeks and am caffeine free. I am eating more cheese than I have for quite a while. I am constipated all the time. Do you have any tips? I eat a fruit smoothie and this just does not seem to be enough.

It takes a while for your body to adjust to not having caffeine. Make sure you're eating plenty of vegetables with your Pro/Fats meals, as veggies contain lots of natural fiber to keep your system running smoothly. Fruit is also full of fiber, so a fruit smoothie is a great idea. Consider adding a whole-grain cereal in the morning, such as Grape-Nuts or All-Bran. (All-Bran does list a small amount of sugar in the ingredients, but it's so minor, it shouldn't be a problem.) You could also try my Somersize Supplements to help your digestive system run more smoothly.

I have followed your program to the letter and have not lost as much weight as I had hoped.

You need to look over what you are eating and make sure you are not straying from Level One guidelines. If you are following Level One to the letter, be patient. I swear it will happen. It took me two months and then "The Melt" began.

I haven't lost any pounds, but I'm down two dress sizes! What am I doing wrong?

You've lost two dress sizes and you think you're doing something wrong? You're doing great! Many Somersizers notice that they lose inches before they lose pounds. The old adage "Muscle weighs more than fat" is actually true!

I know I do not need to count fat grams, but is there a point at which you can eat too much fat in one day and not lose weight?

It is very difficult to overeat fat, unless you ignore the signs from your body. When you

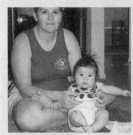

before

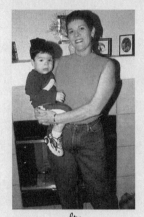

after

Dear Suzanne,

I had used your program previously when I wanted to shed 15 pounds and it worked beautifully. However, when I became pregnant, I unfortunately fell back into bad habits. I succumbed to my cravings instead of eating more healthfully, rationalizing that I would easily drop the weight because I was going to be breast-feeding. (Wrong!) After months of gorging on drive-thru burritos and hot buttered popcorn, I had ballooned up to over 200 pounds.

One year after my son was born, I was still 50 pounds overweight and wearing maternity clothes, miserable and disgusted with myself. Changing my eating habits seemed to be too much of a struggle. Finally, when I realized I couldn't continue living this way, a little voice of reason reverberated, "Somersize! Somersize!" I restarted the program and lost 15 pounds the first month. I regained my energy and started feeling better about myself. Even though I experienced some tough plateaus, I kept with the program because it made me feel great and I kept losing weight—a total of 40 pounds thus far. I am confident I will achieve my ultimate goal. Anyway, I weigh 6 pounds less than I did when I found out that I was pregnant. Guess that first trimester weight is no match for Somersizing after all!

Considering the fantastic meals I am able to prepare for my family, we never feel deprived. I can't say enough to thank you for bringing this marvelous program into our lives. We are healthier and happier for it.

Sincerely,
Janet Mikealson-Lenox

eat fat your brain releases an enzyme that signals your body you are full; that is why these full-fat meals are so satisfying. Don't overdo it. You need to use common sense. Balance your meals with plenty of vegetables and include fruit as snacks.

I used to follow Dr. Atkins' plan and recently switched to Somersizing. Do you believe in ketones in the urine as an indicator of fat burning?

Although Dr. Atkins has wonderful information, our programs have many differences. You do not need to count your carbs and you do not need to pee on a stick. Simply enjoy the freedom and ease of Somersizing and I'm sure you'll have great results.

I was wondering if Somersizing would be good for me even though I do not need to lose weight. I do get low blood sugar. I'm thin, but after I eat even a little bit, I'll have a very poochy belly. I also have some digestion problems.

Yes, this would be a great way to eat even if you do not need to lose weight. I am sure you are aware we cannot make any medical claims. However, many Somersizers have told us that eating this way has helped their digestion.

I weigh 450 pounds. I'm 5 feet 9 inches, so I'm a really fat person. I can eat three Whoppers, large fries, a large Coke, and a large milkshake at one sitting, so you know I'm a big eater. Although I don't think I eat as much on your diet, is it really true that portion sizes don't matter, even if you are a big, big eater?

We always say in Somersizing that you can eat as much as you want, but most people need less food to get full. However, the fact that you'll be eating foods that won't cause your insulin levels to spike is going to create a great improvement for you.

Since your diet is based on fats and proteins, is my body fat percentage going to increase dramatically?

Eating dietary fat will not make you gain weight, as long as you do not combine it with carbohydrates. This is the basic premise of Somersize. You can actually lose weight and body fat by following the Somersize guidelines to achieve your ideal body composition. Remember, sugar is the real enemy.

If I use your stuffing mix to stuff the veggies, do I need to mix it with egg before filling them (as your other stuffing recipes call for)?

You don't have to, but it helps bind the stuffing to hold it together.

I'm not a breakfast eater. Is it important to have breakfast?

If you skip breakfast, your body has gone sometimes over twelve hours without any food. By the time you eat lunch, your body may hang on to every morsel for fear it might not get food again. The best way to increase your metabolism is to eat. Try to have a little something for breakfast.

Is couscous allowed on Level One?

Yes, it's a Carbo.

Is hominy allowed on Level One, and would it be a Vegetable or a Carbo?

Hominy is a type of corn, a Funky Food.

Is it better for me to eat my Carbos in the morning, or doesn't it matter?

The earlier in the day the better, because you are more likely to burn it off as fuel. Remember, carbohydrates equal sugar equals energy. You don't want your last meal of the day to be fuel, because most likely you are going to go to bed shortly after. If fuel is not burned off, it has the potential to be stored as fat even if it is a whole grain or fruit.

Is it okay if two out of three meals are Carbos meals? If so, will I still lose weight?

You will lose weight more quickly if you limit your Carbos to breakfast only. When you cut back on the carbs, you force your body to use your fat reserves as an energy source. That's when "The Melt" begins.

Is it okay to use pork rinds to coat chicken and fry it?

Pork rinds and chicken are both Pro/Fats, so it is allowed.

Is it possible to just start Somersizing at Level Two and get results?

It depends on your body and your metabolism, as well as how much healing your metabolism has to do. You will see results much faster on Level One.

Is wheat germ allowed?

Yes, wheat germ belongs in the Carbos group. Sprinkle it on your whole-grain cereal.

My husband is Japanese and we love sushi—especially California rolls. I know I can't eat the rice with it, but what about the seaweed? Is this classified as a vegetable? And is imitation crabmeat a protein? I like to eat the crabmeat, the seaweed, and mayonnaise together and eliminate the rice. Is this okay?

Seaweed is fine—it's a Veggie. Mayo, of course, is a Pro/Fat. Imitation crab is full of starches and sugar, so it is considered a Funky Food.

Now that I'm Somersizing, if a special event comes up or if I have a bad day, will it screw everything up?

As far as a special event messing you up, number one, make sure it's worth it and not a regular occurrence. Do the best you can and try to keep cheats at a minimum. Just because one thing throws you off for the day, don't throw in the towel for the rest of the day. After it's over, get back to strict Level One right away. Drinking extra water helps too. Most important, if it's a special event, enjoy it, don't worry about it, and get right back on track the next day.

Some of your recipes are quite in depth. Do you have any tips or advice for someone with a busy work schedule?

This book is for you. Most of the recipes take less than thirty minutes to prepare. I'm very busy, too. I have to eat frequently on the road and in restaurants. The key to cooking at home is keeping meat, fish, or poultry in the freezer to thaw for a quick meal, and plenty of fresh vegetables that can be steamed.

The book doesn't limit the number of Carbos I can have in the morning. Is that possible?

Yes, as long as you follow the Somersize combinations; however, use your common sense. Most people find that they lose weight faster if they limit their carbohydrates.

We are having a problem learning your program and knowing how to plan meals. We are plain people and don't eat gourmet meals, which most of yours seem to be. Any suggestions?

This book has some real basics. You do not have to eat gourmet meals to Somersize. I enjoy fancy foods, but most of the time I eat very simply. Look at the food lists. For breakfast you can have eggs. Cook them however you want. If you don't want to make a feta cheese omelette, use cheddar cheese or American cheese. If you don't want to make pepper steak for dinner, eat hamburger patties! The beauty of this program is that you can eat however you want. I try to give you recipe ideas to make your meals more flavorful, but adjust the ingredients to your taste! Just follow the simple guidelines and enjoy all the benefits.

What are the differences between your plan and Dr. Atkins' plan?

Dr. Atkins' plan limits your carbohydrates, so people tend to cut back on a lot of fruits and vegetables. In my plan, I give you a list of acceptable vegetables that are all low in starch so you may eat as much as you want. As for fruit, I ask that you not combine them with any other foods. I have a lot of respect for Dr. Atkins. He's done some amazing research. What I like about Somersizing is that you get the same kind of results, but you are allowed a more balanced array of foods.

When I was doing my grocery shopping, I tried to be very careful about what I bought. I checked labels, and I noticed that many products have some sugar in them (1 to 2 grams) and they also have carbohydrates listed.

The best way to determine what you can and cannot eat is to check the reference guide in the back of the book. Here you will find the allowed foods by food group.

You can even copy it and take it with you to the grocery store. It's really very simple. Stick to the foods and combinations for Level One and avoid all Funky Foods. It is important that you check ingredients lists and not nutritional panels on food products. Some foods have natural sugars and Carbos (such as tomatoes). As long as the ingredients show no added sugars and all the ingredients fit properly into the Somersize food groups, you are fine. Looking at the nutritional panel sometimes just makes it more confusing.

When reading labels, what is a good rule of thumb for determining the carbohydrate levels since everything contains carbs? For example: under 25 grams?

We do not have a set number of carbohydrates that are permitted in a day. That is one of the nice things about this program. You don't have to count anything. It is best to ignore the nutritional panel. Always check the ingredients list instead to make sure the ingredients fit properly within the Somersize food groups. When having Pro/Fats, always make sure there are no Carbos added to the ingredients. You don't have to worry about the natural carbs.

Your recipes say serves two, four, or six. Since I will be fixing the food for one only, can I freeze the rest for another time?

Feel free to freeze the leftovers or cut the recipes down to your desired servings. Also, many Somersizers like having extra meals prepared for lunch the next day.

PASTA, NOODLES, RICE, BEANS

Can I use brown rice pasta?

Yes, because it is made from the whole grain.

Can you recommend a brand of whole-wheat pasta as well as a place to buy it?

I like De Cecco brand. They carry it at my grocery store and in Italian delis. Now we have Somersize Pasta! It's available at SuzanneSomers.com.

Can you tell me if brown rice cakes are acceptable as long as the only ingredients are brown rice and salt?

Yes, they are a Carbo. But don't overdo it.

I have been unsuccessful in finding whole-wheat wontons and whole-wheat lasagna noodles or spinach lasagna noodles. Each brand I have checked includes some white flour with spinach flour or the store does not carry whole wheat at all. I was wondering if you could recommend a place where I might be able to locate and purchase these items.

Try your local health food store. If they don't carry these items, ask if they can special order them for you.

I have found a terrific-tasting pasta made by Eden Foods, Inc., but I'm not sure it's legal. The ingredients are: organic durum wheat, red bell pepper, paprika, saffron, garlic, cloves, and pepper.

Durum is the hard interior of a kernel of wheat. Durum flour, therefore, is not a whole-grain flour. Any pasta you use must say "whole wheat," so I'm afraid this one is not, as you say, legal.

I was recently at a Thai restaurant and ordered steamed shrimp with vegtables and bean threads. Are the bean threads, which look like clear noodles, allowed?

Sorry, but the bean threads are very high in carbohydrates, so they are not allowed.

Is basmati rice allowed?

Brown basmati rice is fine. White basmati rice is a Funky Food.

Is it okay to eat wild rice on Level One?

Wild rice is a Carbo and may be eaten on Level One with Carbos and Veggies. When you graduate to Level Two, wild rice can be eaten with your Pro/Fats, in moderation. It is a much better choice than white rice, or even brown rice.

Can you explain whether durum wheat semolina, durum wheat pasta, and semolina pasta are okay?

This has been a confusing issue, even for me. Here's the final say on pasta. Semolina pasta and durum wheat pasta are not okay. Durum wheat semolina is not okay. It must say "whole wheat" or whole grain. I think there is some confusion because in a previous Reference Guide I listed "pasta made from whole grains," then listed the different types of grains, including durum wheat.

Any of the grains listed must be in their whole-grain form, so durum wheat would need to be durum whole wheat. Actually, durum wheat should come off the list, because it is technically the hard interior of the wheat kernel, and, therefore, cannot come in a whole-grain form. Use your gut—if it looks too white and too good to be true, it probably is.

PLATEAUS

Do you have any suggestions on what I can do to jump-start my weight loss once I have hit a plateau?

The only thing I can recommend is that you stick with the program. We all hit plateaus, and going off the program is just going to make it worse. Know that you're on the right track, and keep it up!

POTATOES

Are yams okay for Level Two?

Yams are pretty high in starch, similar to white potatoes, and should be treated as such. Anything is okay in Level Two, but only in moderation. As for yams, reserve them for your treat if you really like them. You will diminish the effect of any high-starch food by eating it with plenty of fiber, like a big green salad.

My husband loves steak and potatoes. Is this allowed? If not, what can you suggest to serve with steak?

Potatoes are a Funky Food because they are high in starch. These kinds of foods turn directly into sugar in our bodies upon digestion. I would suggest you try the Celery Root Purée on page 228. There also is a recipe in *Eat Great, Lose Weight* on page 98. It is a great substitute for mashed potatoes. I would also include a vegetable with this.

When cooking a roast for family and there are potatoes cooked with it, can we still eat the meat?

You are probably okay if you pull out the potatoes and just eat the meat.

PROTEIN BARS AND SHAKES

Are there any high-protein bars that are okay for Somersizing?

I've had so many questions about this. I finally made my own. Somersize Protein Bars are delicious and perfectly designed for my program.

Besides fruit smoothies, are there any other "shake" recipes?

In my last book, *Eat, Cheat, and Melt the Fat Away,* you'll find two new coffee-flavored smoothies. Yum! Plus, I now have Somersize Protein Shakes.

Recently I discovered protein bars—on the ingredients list there are no added sugars but the bars do contain 2 grams of sugar. All of the bars contain cocoa and I was wondering if they would be okay for Level One. They also make a protein drink. I know you recommend getting protein from real foods but it is hard for me to eat three meals a day since I am in college. Would this protein drink be allowed even though it contains soy protein?

If the ingredients are all proteins and fats, with no carbohydrates or sugars, then they are okay for Level One. If unsweetened cocoa is the only Funky Food listed, then they are Almost Level One. Cocoa still has caffeine in it, so it remains on the Funky Food list, even though it only creates a very minor imbalance. You can probably eat these bars in moderation on Level One. Try Somersize Protein Bars and Shakes, then you'll know they are okay.

PUDDING, JELL-O

Can I have sugar-free Jell-O and/or sugar-free puddings?

Sugar-free Jell-O is okay, but you should be aware that it contains aspartame. When you need a dessert fix, it is great with whipped cream, but I would eat it sparingly. The sugar-free Jell-O can be eaten after a Pro/Fats meal or a Carbos meal. Sugar-free pudding is made with cornstarch and should be considered a Funky Food, so save it for a special treat. Try my Jiggly Fruit Gels recipe on pages 308–311 in this book.

Can I have tapioca pudding if I use cream instead of milk and Equal instead of sugar? I'm still on Level One.

Tapioca is very high in starch, and therefore a Funky Food.

Is gelatin a protein or a carb?

Plain gelatin is a Free Food, so you can have it with anything. You may also enjoy sugar-free gelatin in moderation.

SALAD DRESSINGS, DIPS, MUSTARD, KETCHUP

Can I eat ranch dressing on Level One?

Ranch dressing is made with buttermilk, which is a Funky Food. In my Creamy Salad Dressing Mixes I have a ranch dressing that is made with buttermilk powder, which is fine.

Can I have mayonnaise and oil?

You can't have oil and mayo with carbs, but you can have them with protein, which is chicken, meat, or fish. For instance, a chicken salad with mayo would be perfect.

Can I have salad dressing?

Yes! The great thing about Somersizing is that you can have the oil and the fats. Watch out for bottled salad dressings. Beware of commercially prepared dressings that have sugar or some type of starch or thickener in them. Of course, these are all dressings you would use when having Pro/Fats and Veggies. If you are having a Carbos and Veggies meal, your dressing can have no fat. Try my line of Somersize Salad Dressing Mixes.

Can I use ketchup on Level One?

Now we have bottled Somersize Ketchup, or check out the recipe on page 245. Regular ketchup is usually sweetened with some form of sugar. It is important in the early stages of Somersizing to eliminate all sugars so you get rid of all cravings. I have a whole line of Somersize condiments made with SomerSweet.

Can you recommend store-bought salad dressings?

I don't use bottled salad dressings because I don't like the preservatives they add. There are several Italian types that are great, and Paul Newman's and Girard's are both good. It's hard to find blue cheese or Thousand Island without sugar. My Somersize Secret Sauce tastes just like Thousand Island.

I know you have a recipe for mayonnaise, but can we use store-bought mayonnaise even though it has some sugar in it?

Yes. In my second book, *Get Skinny*, I made store-bought mayo okay because I realized it only has trace amounts of sugar. I like Best Foods.

Most store-bought salad dressings have both fats and carbs. I usually eat salads with my Pro/Fats meals, and I am wondering how few carbs is few enough to qualify for a Pro/Fats meal. I'm sticking to ones with two or fewer grams of carbs per serving.

Please remember to check the ingredients list as opposed to the nutritional panel. There are some natural carbohydrates that will show up and that is fine as long as there are no carbohydrates added. Make it easy on yourself. Stop looking at the nutritional panel. Just check ingredients and make sure all the ingredients fit in with the Somersize food groups in the proper combination.

Should I stay away from a brand of salad dressing or anything else if it lists sugar as the last item in the ingredients and says there are 0 grams of sugar in the nutritional panel?

In my early Somersizing days I would have said not to include anything that has sugar in the ingredients list. I even had Best Foods mayonnaise on the no-no list because it has sugar listed in the ingredients. I have since learned that the amount of sugar in my beloved Best Foods is so slight that it does not even show up on the nutritional panel. Best Foods is back on the acceptable list and I would say your salad dressing is probably fine, too. If you are doing well and steadily losing weight, you can incorporate it without a problem. Just be sure not to include these questionable treats around every corner, or they will start to catch up with you.

What is fat-free dressing considered? Or should it even be eaten?

You need to check the ingredients. My sense is that you are having a hard time categorizing fat-free dressing because you cannot pronounce any of the ingredients! Acceptable fat-free dressings are made from vinegar, lemon juice, herbs, nonfat yogurt, or nonfat sour cream, and would be considered Carbos. Check my recipes for some cleaner versions, rather than the nasty bottles in the grocery store.

When having an Oriental chicken salad and making my dressing from scratch, can I use balsamic vinegar?

I recently found out that balsamic vinegar does have some natural sugars, but I've been using it for so long that I didn't eliminate it. Just don't overdo it. If you're interested, check out my recipe for Chinese Chicken Salad on page 188 in *Get Skinny*.

You list mustard in the Carbos section. Does this mean we can only have mustard with Carbos meals?

I used to avoid mustard with Pro/Fats because I thought it had trace amounts of carbohydrates. Since then I have changed my tune and now allow it with Pro/Fats, Carbos, and Veggies. It's a Free Food.

SHOPPING

Do you have any suggestions on where to find nonfat, whole-wheat tortilla shells?

I find nonfat whole-wheat tortillas at my grocery store in Los Angeles, Whole Foods. Try a health-food store.

Where can I purchase whole-wheat pastry flour to make your delicious popovers?

Try your local health-food store. If they don't carry it, ask if they can order it. I get mine in Los Angeles from Whole Foods.

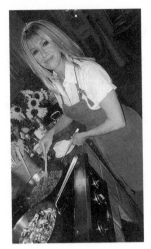

Cooking again.

PRETZELS, NUTS, CRACKERS, SNACKS, SEEDS

Are nuts okay to eat?

Nuts are a Funky Food. When you get to Level Two, you can enjoy them in moderation.

Are sesame seeds allowed?

Sesame seeds have carbohydrates and fat, so technically they are a Funky Food. They only create a slight imbalance. If you are doing well on Level One, you probably will not have a problem if you decide to include a few with your Pro/Fats and Veggie meals, or with your Carbos meals. Tahini is a purée of sesame seeds and should be treated similarly.

Are Triscuits legal to have as a snack? The ingredients are whole wheat, partially hydrogenated soybean oil, and salt.

Because Triscuits contain both whole wheat and oil, they combine Carbos and Pro/Fats, which is not allowed on Level One. But remember, hydrogenated fats are harmful to your health.

Are water chestnuts and bamboo shoots Funky Foods, or can I use them in stir-fry?

They are fine for a stir-fry. They have been added to the vegetable list in my books.

Can flaxseed be eaten? Can it be used for an oil replacement in bread?

Flaxseed has similar qualities to other nuts and seeds . . . they contain fats and carbohydrates. These foods have many health benefits, but on Level One we like to keep fats and carbohydrates separate. Of all the imbalances, these combo foods create only a minor imbalance. If you are doing well on Level One, you may incorporate flaxseed without a problem. On Level Two it is perfectly fine. Flaxseed would be delicious in bread and would create only the slightest imbalance.

Can you suggest a cracker I can eat?

I don't eat crackers, but just look at the ingredients list. Many are made with added oils so they are not okay. I think RyKrisp is okay. Myself, I'd rather have a piece of cheese or celery sticks dipped in blue cheese dressing.

Can you suggest some snacks that do not have to be refrigerated as cheese does?

There are individually wrapped cheeses that are okay out of the refrigerator for quite some time. Hard-boiled eggs are okay for a couple of hours without refrigeration. If you're snacking on an empty stomach, fruit is great. Veggies, again, are an excellent snack option. If you're looking for a Carbos snack, try whole-wheat pretzels with no fat.

How much time should elapse before I have a snack?

Snacks follow the same guidelines as meals. If you have a Pro/Fats breakfast, you may have a Pro/Fats snack at any time afterward. If you have a Pro/Fats meal and want a Carbos snack, you must wait three hours. The reverse is true if you have a Carbos meal and want a Pro/Fats snack; you must wait three hours.

I am having a difficult time trying to pack a lunch and snacks for my husband. Any suggestions?

Some good snacks would be fruit, veggies and dip, or cheese. For lunch, he could take grilled chicken breast, leftover meatloaf or roast beef, sliced meat wrapped in cheese, a bowl of chicken or tuna salad with tomatoes, lettuce, cucumbers, and other veggies. He can even go to a burger joint and have a couple of hamburgers or cheeseburgers . . . without the bun. He can have a taco salad without the tortillas, beans, or guacamole. See "Brown Baggin' It" on page 115.

Spelt pretzels have .5 gram of fat for eighteen pretzels. Would that be too much to include on Level One?

The trace amount of fat should not affect your weight loss. It's a very minor imbalance.

I found something in the health store called taro root chips. They are fried and seem to resemble potato chips. Are they allowed?

Taro is a very starchy root that is grown in Hawaii. Unfortunately, the high starch content makes it a Funky Food that is not allowed on Level One.

If I eat a small snack or treat (on Level Two), do I still have to wait three hours before eating a different type of meal? If I eat a couple squares of dark chocolate, do I wait three hours to eat a Pro/Fats dinner? Or if I have ice cream (Level Two), do I have to wait three hours after a Pro/Fats dinner?

On Level Two, we loosen the reins a bit, so you can ease up on the amount of time between switching to a different type of meal. Just know that you're creating a minor imbalance by changing from one type to another without waiting the full three hours, and keep it in check.

Is popcorn allowed with a Carbos meal?

Popcorn is a Funky Food, which is why it's not allowed on Level One. If you'd like to have it on Level Two as a treat, it's best to eat it alone.

What about sunflower seeds?

Sunflower seeds belong in the same category as nuts and seeds. They have carbohydrates and fats, so technically they are a Funky Food. They only create a slight imbalance. If you are doing well on Level One, you probably will not have a problem if you decide to include a few as a snack.

What can I snack on between a Carbos meal and a Pro/Fats meal so I don't get such an empty bloated stomach?

Two to three hours after your Carbos meal, you could snack on a hard-boiled egg, a piece of cheese, or maybe some fruit. Of course, veggies and dip are always a great snack!

SOUPS, SAUCES

Am I allowed miso soup with seaweed?

Yes, it usually has a touch of tofu, but it's a very small amount.

Can canned soups be eaten on the Somersize plan?

Canned soups can be eaten if all of the ingredients fall into either the Pro/Fats and Veggies category or the Carbos and Veggies category. It's rare to find a canned soup that falls strictly into one of those categories, so, again, check those labels!

Can I eat Campbell's tomato soup (canned)? I would add cream to the soup instead of water and would have a chunk of cheese. I would make this a Pro/Fats and Veggies meal.

Sorry, but not allowed. When in doubt, always check your ingredients. In this case you will see it contains corn syrup and wheat flour, which would make it funky.

Can I have canned or jarred gravy if it says it is 98 percent fat free?

As always, check the ingredients, but I

doubt it. Gravy almost always contains white flour or cornstarch, both of which are Funky Foods. In this case, there have probably been even more starches added to make up for the fat being removed.

Can you eat sour cream with your proteins and fats?

Yes, sour cream is a Pro/Fat.

Can you recommend a good fat-free pasta sauce to use with carbo meals?

Yes, Somersize Pasta Sauce! Also, check out the fat-free pasta sauce recipes in my books—they are quick, easy, and delicious.

I have a great tomato soup recipe but it calls for a quarter teaspoon of honey. Is this enough to worry about? Supposedly it's to counter the acid from the twelve fresh tomatoes.

Try a bit of SomerSweet instead. I use a touch in my tomato sauce to balance the acid.

My mother recently made a pot of homemade chicken soup. She makes her soup with fresh-cut potatoes. Is it okay to eat the soup if I pick out the potatoes, or does it still affect the carbs in the soup?

The best cooks know that adding potato to your broth makes it nice and rich. Unfortunately, the starch that cooks into the soup from the potatoes is technically going to spike your insulin. If you were to follow the Level One guidelines to the letter, you could not eat the soup. However, as we always say, experiment with your own body and see if eating this soup affects your weight loss. If you are steadily losing weight, you may be able to incorporate this soup, in moderation, without a problem.

Are cream soups, like Campbell's cream of chicken or cream of mushroom soup, allowed?

If you ever have a question, just look at the ingredients list. Cream, chicken, and mushrooms are all allowed on the Pro/Fats and Veggies list; however, I believe these soups have cornstarch in them, so these soups would be okay for Level Two, not Level One.

SOY

Can I use soy sauce?

Yes, soy sauce is a free food that may be used on Pro/Fats, Carbos, and Veggies.

I buy soy milk that has 3 percent fat. Is that okay, or does it have to have no fat? I really don't want to drink cow's milk.

Technically, no, but use your body as a guide and see if it disrupts your progress.

I was wondering about a soybean called edamame. Are these allowed while Somersizing?

Edamame are wonderful snacks, full of nutrition, protein, and healthy fats. Unfortunately, they also contain more carbohydrates than the low-starch vegetables in our Veggies group. Therefore, technically, you must save them for Almost Level One. However, they cause only a small imbalance so if you are losing steadily on Level One you could try to incorporate them and see if your body reacts.

If I followed your program but had a soy latte or two a day, would that be counterproductive?

If you want a soy latte, switch and have a decaf soy latte. If you just have to have your caffeine, you won't see results as quickly. You're still reducing the effects of insulin by Somersizing, so it's better than not doing anything. Pro/Fats and Veggies meals are far more satisfying than Carbos meals. That is why I recommend you eat Carbos only for breakfast and stick to Pro/Fats and Veggies for lunch and dinner.

Is soy flour permissible for frying foods?

Soy flour is still starch, and on Level One we do not mix starches with fats (oil). Try frying your foods without any flour. It still has a great flavor, and I don't miss the floury crust. You could try the soy flour for frying in Level Two. Or try my yummy Somersize Bake and Fry Mix (p. 235).

What about soymilk and other soy products, like soy nuts?

Nonfat soymilk is included in the Carbos group because it has carbs without fat. Regular soymilk, tofu, and soy nuts are considered Funky Foods because they contain protein, fat, and carbs. If you are a strict vegetarian and you need additional protein sources, I make an exception with tofu and soy products because the carbohydrate content is not terribly high. In addition, on Level Two, these are some of the first foods I encourage you to put back into your eating plan because soy has such important nutrients.

How much sodium are you allowed to have per day?

The Somersize program does not have limits for sodium. If you are concerned about your sodium intake, please see your doctor.

I know you say olives are a Funky Food because they contain Pro/Fats and Carbos, but the jar of olives I have right in front of me says zero carbohydrates. Can I eat them?

Go for it. There seems to be some variance depending on the olives.

I love sesame oil and pumpkin oil on my salads. Is this allowed? I know not to eat the seeds, but is the oil okay?

You've got it right. You can't have the seeds, but the oils are fine to use. Enjoy!

I thought peanuts were a Funky Food, so why is peanut oil used in some recipes?

Peanuts are funky because they contain a combination of carbs, fats, and proteins. In the process of making peanut oil the carbs are removed so you no longer have the bad combination of carbs and fats.

Are flavored extracts okay?

Flavored extracts are fine to use as long as they do not have added sugars, like corn syrup. Since you use a minimal amount the alcohol in it should not be a problem.

Is it okay to use cinnamon?

Absolutely! Spices and herbs are Free Foods.

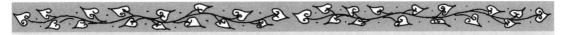

Dear Suzanne:

I have had a weight problem all my life. I'm sixty-four years old now and I've been up and down like a yo-yo since my teens. Let's face it, I just love the taste of food. Every time I would lose weight, I would be so proud of myself, but then I would go back to my old habits and gain it all back again. I am only 4 feet 11 inches, and so I had a hard time fitting into clothes. I would get out of breath when I climbed stairs and walked very far. I was constantly getting colds and had a very bad time with reflux and heartburn.

Then a friend told me about *Get Skinny on Fabulous Food*. I read the book and swore this would be the last diet I would try in my life. The first couple of weeks were a little hard, giving up all those sug-

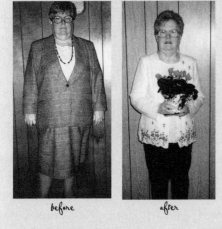

before   after

ary treats, but I stuck to it and wow, the weight started coming off. I took it slow and only lost one or two pounds a week, but being able to eat all the fat and healthy snacks made it all worthwhile. I reached my goal weight in about a year. I had a 55-pound loss and I've been able to keep the weight off for almost two years now.

Eating this way completely cured my heartburn and reflux problem. I haven't had to take any antacids since I started Somersizing. No more colds either. I feel great, and I went from a size 18/20 to a 10/12. My husband is so proud of me, and I can't tell you how happy I am.

Sincerely,
Joan Coleman

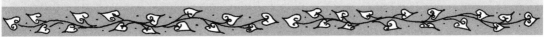

What can I use for oil or oiling a baking pan for homemade breads?

Technically you should not use any fat with your Carbos, but if you need a thin layer of oil, I would use a nonstick spray oil like Pam, so that you use the minimum amount.

Why can I use olive oil and I can't have olives?

You can have olive oil because it is a pure fat, but olives contain fat and carbohydrates.

You use sea salt in your cooking video. Is sea salt better than regular table salt?

Yes, yes, yes! Please give it a try, it has a wonderful flavor!

You've mentioned that malted barley is an acceptable ingredient in Grape-Nuts cereal. What about using malted barley extract as a sugar substitute for making homemade bread?

The difference between malted barley and malted barley extract is that in the extract, the carbohydrates from the barley have already been converted into sugar. Malted barley extract is very high in sugar and therefore a Funky Food.

SUGAR, SWEETENERS

Are sweeteners like brown rice syrup and barley malt acceptable? If so, what are they considered?

These sweeteners have a lower glycemic index than sugar, but they do have some naturals sugars. Use sparingly if you must.

Can fructose be used in Somersizing?

I used to have fructose on the Funky Food list, because I thought it would spike your insulin, but since then we have found that certain types of fructose will only cause moderate rises in blood sugar. Use pure crystalline fructose in moderation only. If you use too much, you could have a problem. SomerSweet contains a small amount of fructose, but because SomerSweet is concentrated, you only get a trace amount.

I am confused about the sugars we are looking for on the ingredients label. Aren't there several different names for sugar, such as sucrose? Can you tell me what some of them are?

Here are some of the other names for sugar: sucrose, refined sugar, high fructose corn syrup, dextrose, glucose, honey, maltose, concentrated fruit juice, confectioners' (powdered) sugar, barley malt syrup.

How much sugar is allowed in canned food (canned peas, spaghetti sauce, green beans, and so on) at Level One?

Added sugars are not allowed on Level One. Always check the ingredients list for added sugars and avoid products that have them. Some items have natural sugars that will show up on the nutritional panel. That is okay as long as there are none in the ingredients.

Is Splenda okay to use?

Splenda will not spike insulin. It goes in the same category as saccharin and aspartame, artificial sweeteners that can be used in moderation when you really want something sweet. I prefer SomerSweet because it's blended with natural, sweet fiber and tastes great.

What is your opinion about a sweetener called stevia?

I have a whole writeup on it in *Get Skinny*. It's an all-natural sweetener; that part I like. It also has a bitter aftertaste; that part I don't like. And I find it difficult to cook with. SomerSweet doesn't leave a bitter aftertaste and cooks and bakes like a dream.

TOFU

Can I have tofu?

Tofu has protein, fat, and carbs, so it is a Funky Food, technically. However, there are many people who use it in Pro/Fats meals with oil, cheese, and veggies or in Carbos meals with Veggies and they have no problem. It is a very minor imbalance. If you are doing well on Level One, you should not have a problem adding tofu.

VEGGIES, VEGGIE BURGERS

Are green beans considered carbs or not? I believe that they are listed one way in one book, and the other in another book.

Green beans are considered a Veggie.

Can you tell me which kinds of squash are allowed? I know winter squashes (butternut and acorn) are Funky Foods. How about spaghetti squash?

Spaghetti squash is low in starch, which means it's on the Veggies list. Look for my recipe in *Get Skinny*.

Do you know of a specific veggie burger that is allowed?

We have not found a specific veggie burger for Level One. Most are made with a combination of carbs and fats. They are suitable for Level Two.

I don't eat any vegetables, not even salad. I've tried them but I just do not like them. Is there any way I can still do this diet?

When you're eating your Pro/Fats meals, it is important to include vegetables, because that's where you're getting your fiber. Also, vegetables provide a small amount of carbohydrates, which is necessary to keep your body balanced. Clearly, we would not recommend just eating meat, cheese, and eggs every day. That's not a healthy, balanced diet. If you absolutely refuse to eat any vegetables, please make sure you are dividing your meals between Pro/Fats and Carbos, and eat fruit in the morning and for snacks.

I have always thought that a tomato is a fruit, but you have recipes that include tomatoes and tomato products. Do you consider it a vegetable?

Tomatoes are technically fruits, but they are lower in sugar than most fruits, so I include them as a vegetable for Somersizing.

Is celery root a Carbo or a Veggie?

Celery root is a Veggie because it is low in starch.

Is gem squash legal? It's dark green, round, and bright yellow inside.

Sorry, but this is like pumpkin and considered a Funky Food.

Is it okay to have spaghetti squash with meat sauce on it?

Absolutely. Yum.

Is sauerkraut allowed?

Yes, it's a Veggie.

Is the vegetable rutabaga allowed?

Rutabaga is fairly high in starch and should be included in the Funky Foods. However, it's not as bad as a potato, so if you are doing well on Level One, you could incorporate a little without a problem.

Is veggie chili allowed?

Vegetable chili is usually made from tomatoes, fresh vegetables, and beans. All of these foods fit into the Carbos and Veggies group. Here's the catch: if you are eating Carbos, then you may not include any fats on Level One. Most Veggie chili is made by sautéing the veggies in oil. This will create a minor imbalance with a Carbos meal. (It is fine for Level Two.) Therefore, if you want to sauté your vegetables in oil, make your Veggie chili a Pro/Fats meal and add cheese and sour cream. For this Pro/Fats option you would not add any beans (or brown rice) to your chili. If you want the beans and brown rice, eliminate any fats (like oil, cheese, or sour cream) and make it a Carbos and Veggie meal.

Is yucca root okay to use? Is it a Carbo or a Veggie?

Yucca is a starchy root that is a Funky Food.

Is chayote okay?

I believe chayote has too much starch to be included on the Veggies list. If you're looking for a potato substitute, try celery root.

What is pattypan squash and where would I be able to buy it?

Pattypan squash is in the summer squash family. It's green, round, and flattish with a scalloped edge. It looks a bit like a UFO! You should be able to find it in the produce section of most grocery stores.

What type of food are chickpeas considered?

Chickpeas are the same as garbanzo beans and are considered a Carbo. You can eat them in combination with Veggies.

Which are Carbos and which are considered Veggies: wax beans, water chestnuts, snow peas?

All of these are Veggies.

Why can't we have pumpkin or any other orange squashes?

Sorry, these foods are too high in starch. We eliminate starchy foods so that your body is forced to burn your fat reserves as a fuel source, rather than burning the sugars and carbohydrates we eat for fuel.

VITAMINS, SUPPLEMENTS, PAINKILLERS, HORMONES, DRUGS

By avoiding or limiting Funky Foods, are you depriving yourself of any vitamins and minerals that aren't supplemented in the rest of the diet?

Somersizing has a wide variety of foods from every food group. If you eat from all the food groups, you will get all the vitamins and minerals you need.

Can psyllium fiber, like Metamucil, be used on Level One?

Fibers like Metamucil are fine as long as they do not contain sugar. Try to find the sugar-free Metamucil. Better yet, get your fiber from real foods, like whole grains, plenty of fresh vegetables, and fruit.

Do you have any information on weight-loss products such as Chitosan and carb blockers? Also do you have any information regarding the

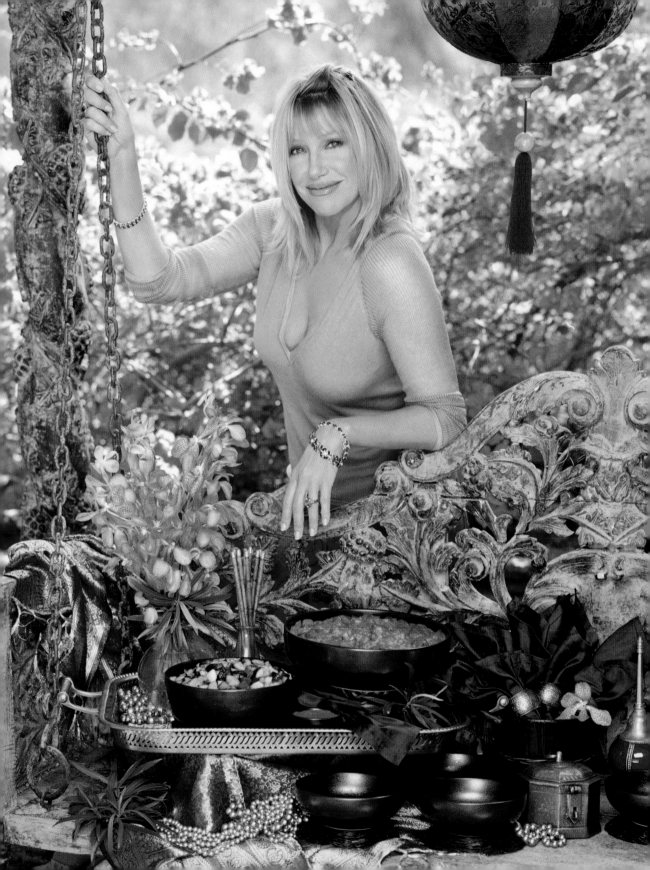

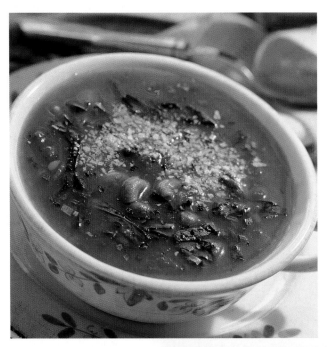

Previous page:
Cumin-Scented Zucchini and
In a Hurry Beef Curry

Fast and Easy Minestrone

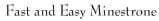

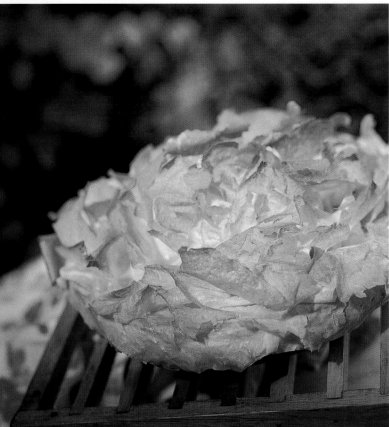

Chicken Pot Pie

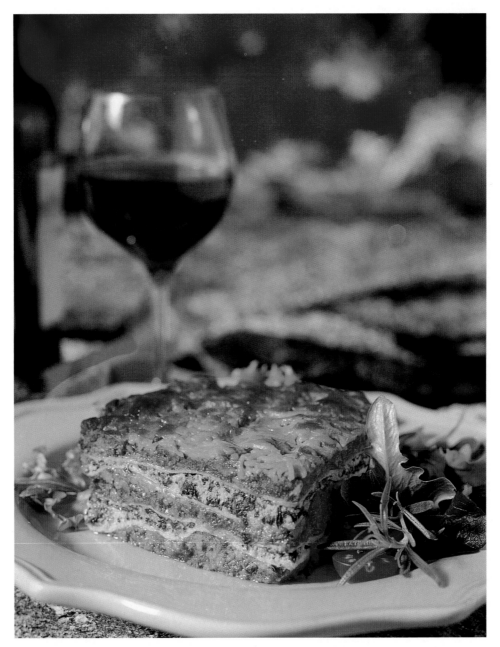

You must try this Somersize Lasagna!

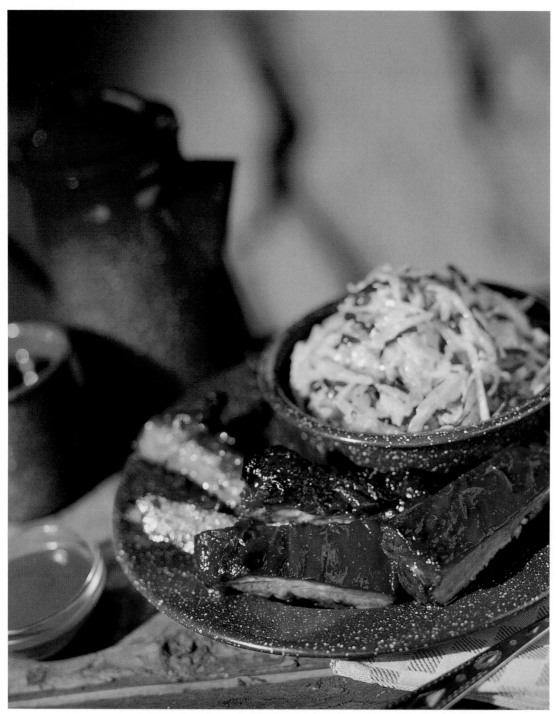

Baby-Back Barbecue Ribs and Crunchy Coleslaw

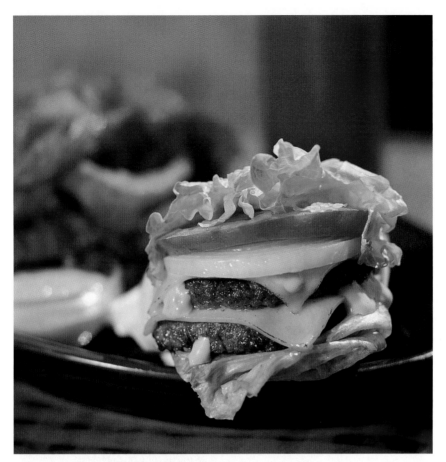

Somersize
Double Double
Cheeseburger

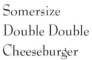

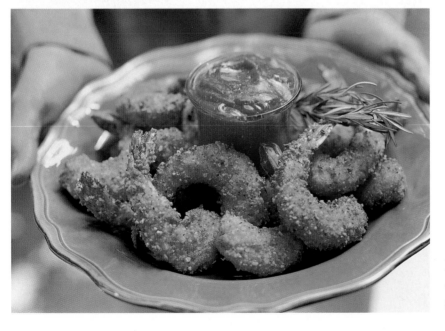

Fried Shrimp
with Spicy
Cocktail Sauce

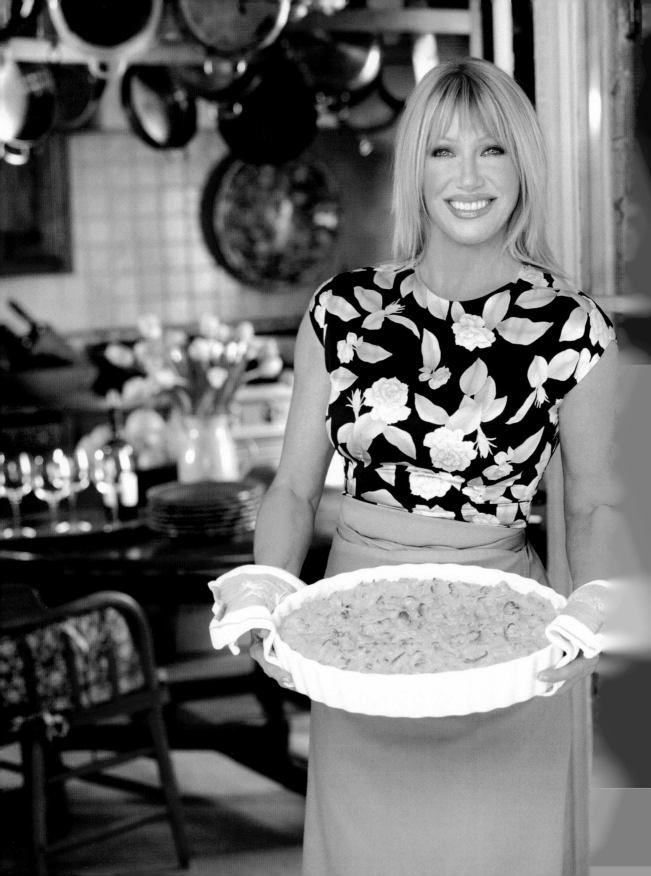

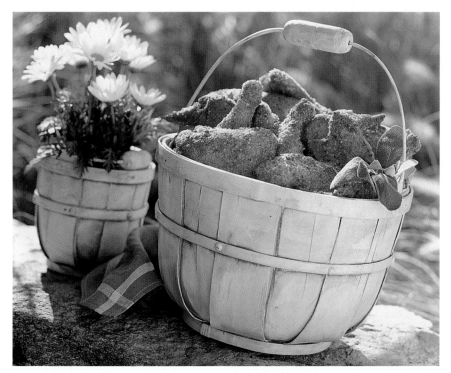

Somersize
Shake It and
Bake It Chicken

Opposite: It's such a pleasure
to present Somersize
Macaroni and Cheese to
hungry family and friends.

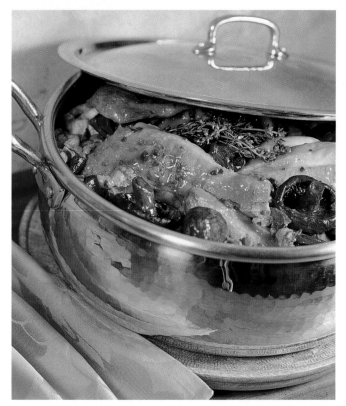

Coq au Vin

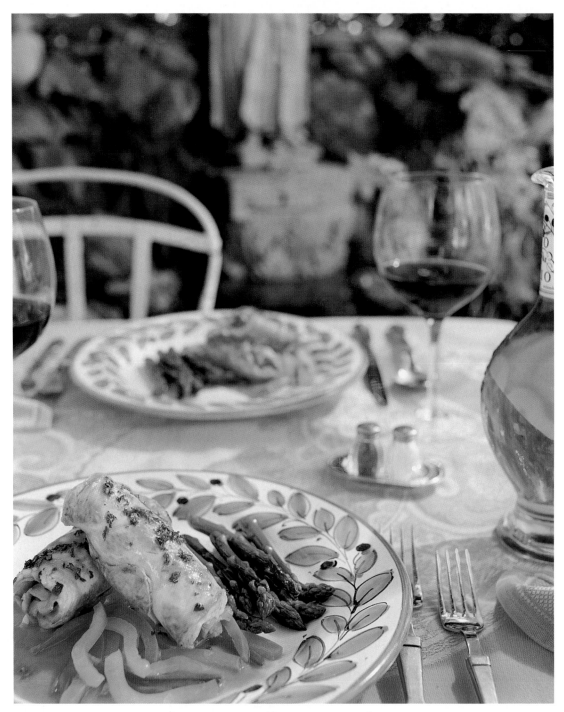

Saltimbocca in a Tarragon Butter Sauce

use of stimulants like xandrine that contain ephedra and ma huang?

I'm not familiar with these products. Any product that contains stimulants will mess with your metabolism. Don't look for weight loss in a diet pill. You will only subject yourself to a lifetime of roller-coaster dieting. Heal your metabolism the natural way by eating real foods, the Somersize way.

Every time I see an article on the diet or see a TV program it always mentions that the diet is well balanced but lacks calcium. I find I eat a lot of cheese and have cream in my coffee, but obviously, with no enriched white flour or milk in cereal, this is a concern. Should I be taking some sort of calcium supplement? If so, how much? Also are there any other nutrients the diet is lacking that should be supplemented?

Calcium is essential to protect us from osteoporosis. There are many calcium-rich foods in the Pro/Fats, Veggies, and Carbos. Cheese, cream, sour cream all have calcium. Broccoli and kale are excellent sources of calcium. And all the nonfat dairy products in the Carbos group, like milk, yogurt, cottage cheese, and ricotta cheese, have loads of calcium. Still, it never hurts to add a calcium supplement. There are no specific nutrients that this program is lacking, but it depends on how you choose your meals. Balanced eating is up to you. I eat a very balanced diet, but I still take a variety of supplements.

I am on Depo-Provera. Will that hinder my weight loss?

Hormonal imbalance is a major reason for weight gain. The type of hormones and the amount of hormones can affect your weight. I choose natural hormones. Ask your doctor about natural hormones. I also recommend you see an endocrinologist to get your hormones balanced during menopause.

I am on the drug tamoxifen. Can that be slowing down my weight loss?

It is quite possible. Tamoxifen interferes with your hormones; when there is hormonal imbalance, there can be weight gain.

I just began HRT (hormone replacement therapy) with Premphase and I'm worried about the warned weight gain. Have any of your readers been on HRT and been able to avoid the weight gain by Somersizing?

The hormone replacement therapy does not cause weight gain. Weight gain results when your hormones are imbalanced. Somersizing is a great way to help keep your hormones balanced. However, if you are going through menopause, some women experience severe loss of hormones that cannot be balanced by diet alone. Please ask your doctor about natural hormone replacement, rather than synthetic. Synthetic hormones only take away the symptoms of menopause, such as hot flashes, irritability, loss of libido, and so on. Natural hormones actually replace the lost hormones, which keeps you happier, healthier, and thinner! You do not need to resign yourself to being the shape of a pear just because you are going through menopause! Replace your lost hormones with natural hormones and keep on Somersizing.

I know that some of the over-the-counter ibuprofen tablets I take (Advil) are coated with a sweet candylike coating. Will this have a negative effect on my Somersize results?

The minimal amount of candylike coating on Advil should not have an effect on your results.

I need to drink a whey protein drink in the morning (has no sugar). If I combine this with soymilk, will that be okay? If not, can you make some suggestions? With this protein drink can I still have a carb breakfast, or is it like eating a protein breakfast so I must stick with protein?

Whey protein is fine as a Pro/Fat. Soymilk is a Funky Food.

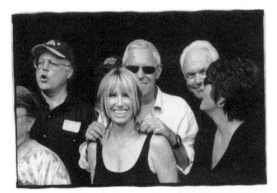

Me and Al, my pal, at a family picnic.

I take one tablespoon of flaxseed oil in the evening. I have not lost any weight and have been on the program for three weeks. Do you think the flaxseed oil is keeping me from losing weight?

Flaxseed oil is an excellent supplement. I don't think the flaxseed oil is the problem. Just be patient. It takes longer for some than others.

Over-the-counter painkillers such as Excedrin Migraine contain caffeine. How does that affect my hormone balance and does it cause my insulin level to rise?

Over-the-counter medications can affect your weight loss. You'll have to check with your doctor to find pain medications without caffeine. Depending on how many you take, yes, the caffeine can cause an insulin response.

Is it okay to put brewer's yeast, fibro flax, bee pollen, and MSM in my fruit smoothie in the morning? I feel like my weight loss is being inhibited, but I am trying to eat those things because they are a cancer preventative.

Usually we don't add anything to fruit. Have you tried sprinkling these things on whole-grain cereal or oatmeal? If you are steadily losing weight I would not worry about this addition, but if your weight loss is slowed, try taking these things in pill form during a Carbos meal.

FOURTEEN

The Somersize Revolution: Products and Foods to Help You Lose Weight

The easiest way to stay on any weight-loss plan is to make it convenient to make fast meals. The recipes in this book will help you make meals quickly and easily, but sometimes we need even more help than that. I have been developing a line of packaged Somersize foods, appliances, protein bars, shakes, and supplements that will make it even easier to stay on the program.

This great variety of packaged Somersize foods will help you make meals in minutes. Somersize Whole-Wheat Pastas, Somersize Pasta Sauces, Somersize Dip Mixes, Somersize Salad Dressings and Condiments, Somersize Crème Brûlée, even Somersize Ice Cream Sundaes . . . that's just a sampling of what's out there and there's so much more to come. The drink mixes come in Decaf Iced Tea, Passion Fruit Decaf Iced Tea, Peach Mango, and Lemon Lime. You just add water and stir. And since they are made with SomerSweet, you

may enjoy them freely. Please keep checking SuzanneSomers.com to see what new food products we are offering—you are going to be delighted with all the choices available to you!

There are days when we don't have time to prepare a full meal, even with the help of my Somersized food products. Sometimes we need a quick snack or meal and just don't have time to fit it in. That's when we usually blow it and grab a candy bar, or protein bar (which is just as bad because most are filled with sugars and carbohydrates). I have resisted advocating protein bars of any kind because I have been trying to teach all my Somersizers to eat real food, but I know that time pressures sometimes make it impossible to do so now. I have my own Somersize Protein Bars and Somersize Protein Shakes that are not filled with a bunch of junk. Somersize Protein Shakes and Protein Bars are made from the finest ingredients, and they provide important omega-3 and omega-6 fatty acids and sources of protein. Plus, they are sweetened with SomerSweet, and you won't believe how great they taste! You no longer need to ask which protein bar or protein shake is "legal" for Somersizing . . . now we have our own!

We are also developing small kitchen appliances with coordinating food items to make Somersizing a breeze. If you really want to make this program fast and easy, we are providing you with the tools to do so. How about a Somersize Bread Maker with Somersize Bread Mix and SomerSweet Jam? How about a Somersize Waffle Maker with Pancake and Waffle Mix and even Maple Syrup? How about a Somersize Ice Cream Maker with SomerSweet Triple Hot Fudge and Caramel Sauce? Fast, easy, delicious and totally Somersized! How about SomerSweet Ketchup, Barbecue Sauce, Secret Sauce, and Tartar Sauce? How about a Somersize Fast and Easy Cooker so you can make one-pot Somersize Meals in minutes! Or a Somersize Slow Cooker so you can start your dinner in the morning and have

it waiting for you when you get home? These are time savers!

With the recipes I've included in this book and my others, the prepackaged foods you can get on SuzanneSomers.com, and the appliances I offer, you have so many ways to Somersize. For example, I also have recipes for Somersize Ketchup, Somersize Barbecue Sauce, and Somersize Tartar Sauce made with SomerSweet; but if you don't have time to make them, you can buy a whole line of condiments on my website. I have numerous recipes for pasta sauces . . . or you can buy my Somersize sauces. Same with the whole-grain breads . . . you'll find recipes for breads in my books, or you can buy my Somersize Bread Mixes. Just add it to the bread machine, set the timer, and you're done. Somersize meals in minutes are a reality with this exciting new line of foods and appliances. There's really no excuse not to Somersize now, so let's get going!

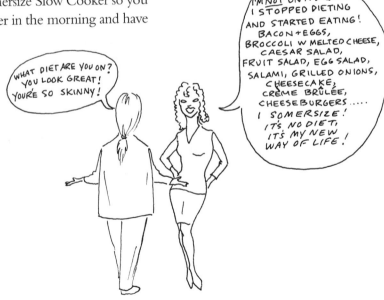

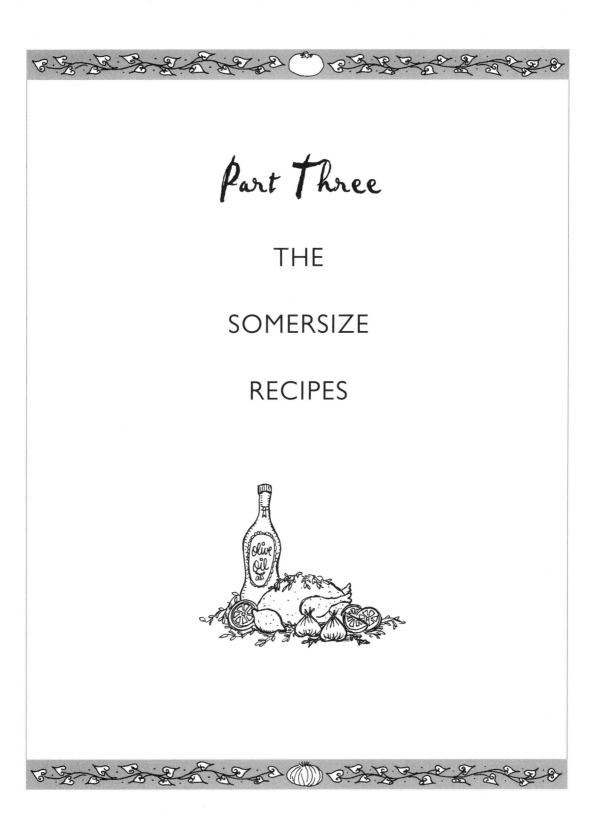

Part Three

THE

SOMERSIZE

RECIPES

Breakfast

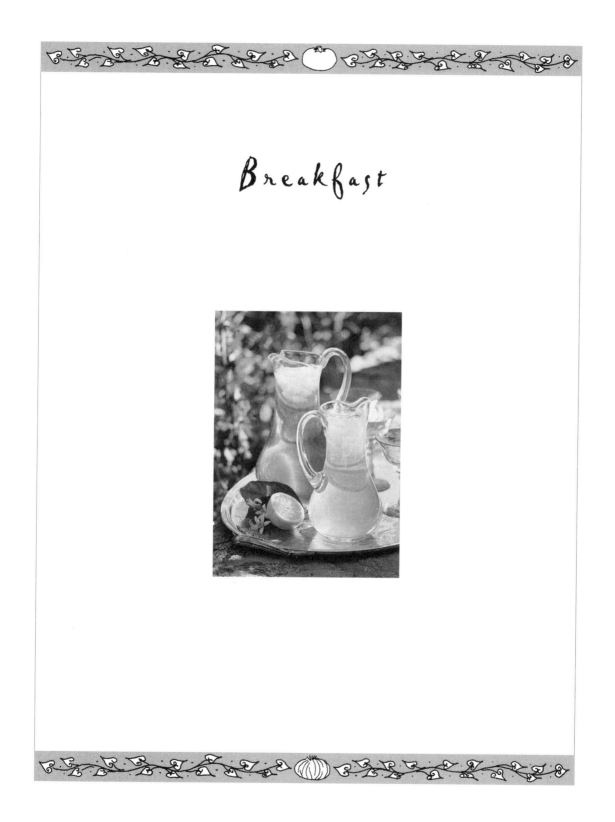

Cream Cheese Pancakes

PRO/FATS—LEVEL ONE

SERVES 4 TO 6

This is a recipe submitted to me by Kamelia Calvert for the Somersize recipe contest on my website, SuzanneSomers.com. This is an awesome choice for breakfast. They taste like the lightest little soufflé pancakes. My granddaughters love them. Absolutely delicious. If you like thinner pancakes, let the batter rest for 20 minutes before serving. And the SomerSweet cinnamon syrup is to die for. You can also use Somersize Maple Syrup.

1 (8-ounce) package cream cheese
4 eggs, separated
½ teaspoon SomerSweet
½ teaspoon cinnamon
Butter, for the griddle

SYRUP
2 teaspoons SomerSweet
½ stick butter, melted
½ teaspoon cinnamon

In a medium bowl, mix together cream cheese, egg yolks, SomerSweet, and cinnamon until well blended.

In another bowl, beat egg whites with an electric mixer until stiff peaks form. Fold egg whites into cream cheese mixture.

Heat a griddle to medium heat. Dollop about ⅓ cup of the batter onto the buttered griddle.

Cook until golden brown, about 2 to 3 minutes. Flip and cook other side to a golden brown, adding butter to griddle as needed.

To make SomerSweet Syrup:

Mix SomerSweet with melted butter until dissolved. Stir in cinnamon and pour over pancakes.

Green Eggs and Ham Sandwiches
PRO/FATS AND VEGGIES—LEVEL ONE

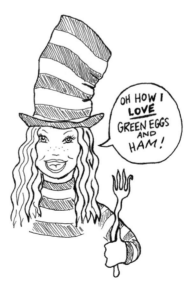

MAKES 2 SANDWICHES

This is one of my favorite recipes in the whole book. Finally, a Level One sandwich! The Spinach "Bread" is like a dense, delicious egg-and-spinach frittata. It's sliced into pieces, then layered with bacon and cheese. Get it? Green Eggs and Ham!

PREP TIME: 2 MINUTES
COOKING TIME: 8 MINUTES

8 slices bacon, or 4 slices of your favorite ham
4 slices Swiss cheese

4 slices Spinach "Bread" (p. 182)

Cook bacon in a large skillet until crisp. Drain bacon on paper towels. Add Spinach "Bread" slices to the bacon fat in the skillet and cook for 1 minute. Turn "bread" over and lay 1 slice of cheese on top of each. Put 4 slices of bacon on 2 of the slices. Top bacon with the remaining 2 slices of spinach bread with cheese. Cook for 2 to 3 minutes, or until cheese starts to melt. Cut each sandwich in half diagonally and serve.

Spinach "Bread"

MAKES 4 SLICES

This is a must-try recipe! I consider it one of the cornerstone recipes of this book. I have given you two ways to make this bread—in a glass baking dish or tripling the recipe and baking it in a loaf pan. It takes longer to cook in the loaf pan, but you end up with a whole loaf of bread that you can slice and freeze. Then you have Spinach "Bread" for a whole variety of sandwiches. Try my Green Eggs and Ham Sandwiches (p. 181), or invent some of your own.

PREP TIME: 2 MINUTES
COOKING TIME: 15 MINUTES

Butter for greasing baking dish
1 (10-ounce) package frozen chopped
   spinach, thawed and drained
4 large eggs, beaten

¼ teaspoon crushed garlic
Salt and freshly ground black pepper

Preheat oven to 400 degrees. Butter an 8 × 8-inch glass baking dish.

Mix together spinach, eggs, and garlic. Season with salt and pepper. Pour into prepared pan. Bake for 15 minutes, or until mixture has set. Allow to cool slightly. Cut into 4 squares. Use a spatula to remove squares from pan. Refrigerate or freeze until ready to use.

Variation

To make a whole loaf of this bread, triple the ingredients and pour into a well-buttered loaf pan. Place loaf pan on a baking sheet and bake for 1 hour and 15 minutes at 350 degrees. A whole loaf will yield 12 slices. Use what you need; wrap well and freeze extra slices or loaves.

Southwestern Eggs-in-a-Pan Casserole

PRO/FATS AND VEGGIES—LEVEL ONE

SERVES 6

This spicy egg dish uses a Mexican sausage called chorizo. If you can't find chorizo, you may use any sausage you like.

PREP TIME: 5 MINUTES
COOKING TIME: 27 MINUTES

1 pound chorizo sausage, casing removed
   and meat crumbled
1 large onion, chopped
6 ounces mushrooms, sliced, about 1 cup
1 package Somersize Salsa Dip Mix, or
   1 cup drained fresh salsa

1 cup sour cream
6 large eggs
1 cup shredded cheddar cheese
Salt and freshly ground black pepper
3 tablespoons cilantro, chopped

Brown sausage in a large skillet, about 5 minutes. Add onion and cook for 5 more minutes. Add mushrooms. Cook for an additional 5 minutes.

Blend dip mix (or drained salsa) and sour cream together. Add to sausage mixture.

Bring mixture to a simmer, then crack 6 eggs on top. Cover pan and cook on low heat for 8 minutes. Add shredded cheese, replace cover, and cook for 4 minutes more. Season with salt and pepper. Sprinkle with cilantro and serve.

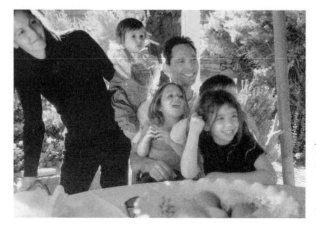

Breakfast in Palm Springs. All the kids love Uncle Marc.

Easy Eggs Florentine

PRO/FATS AND VEGGIES—LEVEL ONE

SERVES 6

They're like cupcakes, but they're made with ham, spinach, cheese, and eggs. Adults and kids love 'em! For a more elegant presentation, dress them up for brunch with my Easy Blender Béarnaise Sauce (p. 185).

PREP TIME: 5 MINUTES
COOKING TIME: 15 MINUTES

Unsalted butter for greasing 12-cup muffin tin
12 thin ham slices, about 8 ounces
1 (10-ounce) package frozen chopped spinach, thawed and drained

Salt and freshly ground black pepper
12 eggs
¾ cup finely shredded cheddar cheese

Preheat oven to 375 degrees.

Butter a 12-cup muffin tin. Place a slice of ham into each muffin cup and press to form a cup. Divide spinach equally among cups, about 1 tablespoon each. Lightly season spinach with salt and pepper. Crack an egg into each cup, being careful not to break the yolk.

Bake for 10 minutes. Top each egg with 1 tablespoon grated cheese. Return to oven for an additional 5 minutes, or until the cheese has melted.

Using a heatproof spatula, carefully remove the Florentine cups from the muffin tin. Serve immediately.

Easy Blender Béarnaise Sauce

PRO/FATS—LEVEL ONE

MAKES ABOUT 1 CUP

This is a delightful lemony sauce to serve over my Eggs Florentine (p. 184). Here's a tip: if you over-cook the sauce, it will separate. If that happens, pour the sauce back into a clean blender and add a tablespoon of mayonnaise and a teaspoon of ice-cold water. Blend until sauce becomes smooth again.

PREP TIME: 5 MINUTES
COOKING TIME: 8 MINUTES

4 egg yolks
2 tablespoons mayonnaise
2 tablespoons lemon juice
1/8 teaspoon Tabasco hot sauce (optional)

1/8 teaspoon salt
1 cup (2 sticks) unsalted butter, cut into
   1/2-inch pieces
1 1/2 teaspoons tarragon

Heat a small saucepan of water until it boils. Turn heat down to simmer.

Place egg yolks, mayonnaise, lemon juice, Tabasco, and salt in a blender. Blend for 10 seconds.

Place butter in another small saucepan. Melt butter over medium heat. Add tarragon. Turn heat to high and cook until butter is bubbling.

Start the blender. With the blender running, slowly add hot butter in a steady stream.

Turn off the blender and pour mixture into a small stainless-steel bowl. Set bowl over the saucepan of simmering water. Cook, stirring constantly, until sauce thickens, about 2 minutes. Serve immediately.

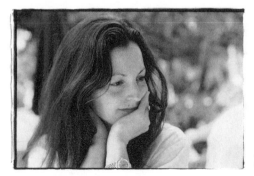

Beautiful Caroline.

Sausage and Egg Breakfast Enchiladas

PRO/FATS AND VEGGIES—LEVEL ONE

MAKES 4

In this recipe I use the Egg Crêpes as tortillas to make enchiladas.

PREP TIME: 4 MINUTES
COOKING TIME: 25 MINUTES

Unsalted butter for greasing baking dish
1 package Somersize Salsa Dip Mix, or
   1 (8-ounce) can enchilada sauce
1 cup heavy cream
1/2 cup sour cream, plus additional for
   garnish
3 tablespoons tomato paste

8 ounces breakfast sausage, cooked and
   crumbled
4 Egg Crêpes (p. 188)
1 cup plus 1/2 cup shredded jack or cheddar
   cheese
4 scallions, sliced thin

   Preheat oven to 350 degrees. Butter an 8 × 8-inch baking dish.

   Mix dip mix (or enchilada sauce), cream, sour cream, and tomato paste together in a medium bowl. Spoon 1/2 cup of sauce into bottom of prepared pan. Set aside.

   Put a quarter of the sausage down the center of each crêpe. Top each crêpe with 1/4 cup cheese. Divide half the scallions among the 4 crêpes. Roll up crêpes and place side by side in prepared pan. Spoon remaining sauce over enchiladas, then top with remaining cheese and scallions. Bake uncovered until cheese is bubbly and beginning to brown, about 25 minutes. Garnish with sour cream and scallions before serving.

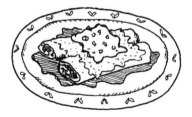

Breakfast Burritos

PRO/FATS AND VEGGIES—LEVEL ONE

MAKES 4

Another great invention with Egg Crêpes. These tasty burritos can be made ahead of time and reheated in the microwave for about a minute. You can also wrap them individually, freeze, and reheat them whenever you want a quick breakfast.

PREP TIME: 2 MINUTES
COOKING TIME: 9 MINUTES

12 slices bacon
4 Egg Crêpes (p. 188)
Salt and freshly ground black pepper
1/2 cup shredded jack cheese

1/2 cup shredded cheddar cheese
1/4 cup sliced scallions
Salsa and sour cream, for garnish

Cook bacon in a large skillet over medium-high heat until crisp. Drain on paper towels and set aside. Drain all but 1 tablespoon of the bacon fat from the skillet.

Lay crêpes out on a clean work surface. Season to taste with salt and pepper. Divide bacon, cheeses, and scallions equally among the 4 crêpes. Fold bottom third of crêpe up and over the filling. Fold over the 2 sides, leaving one end open. Cook burritos in reserved bacon fat over medium-low heat until golden, about 2 minutes. Turn and cook for an additional 2 minutes. Serve with salsa and sour cream.

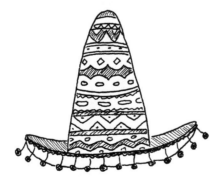

Egg Crêpes
PRO/FATS AND VEGGIES—LEVEL ONE

SERVES 4

These are Alan's mother's egg crêpes, from Eat, Cheat, and Melt the Fat Away. *They've become a Somersize staple, and since they're used in some of my new recipes, I'm including the recipe in this book too!*

6 eggs
Salt and freshly ground black pepper

Butter

In a mixing bowl, lightly beat the eggs. Season with salt and pepper. Heat a crêpe or omelette pan over medium to medium high heat and lightly coat the bottom and sides with butter.

Using a ladle, put enough egg in the pan to make a thin coating. When it sets,

lift up with a spatula, being careful not to tear the crêpe, and turn. Cook one more minute and then slide the crêpe out of the pan and onto a dish. Continue making egg crêpes in this way until you have used all the batter. Stack the crêpes as you would pancakes.

Irish Oatmeal Pancakes with Raspberry Sauce
CARBOS—ALMOST LEVEL ONE

MAKES 12 PANCAKES

These pancakes are so satisfying. Rather than flour, they are made with McCann's Irish Oatmeal, which is cooked, then formed into pancakes and fried on the griddle with a touch of oil (that's what makes it Almost Level One). They have an incredible flavor and texture. The Raspberry Syrup is simply made from fresh raspberries, SomerSweet, and nonfat yogurt. You may also use Somersize Maple Syrup.

1½ cups cooked McCann's Irish Oatmeal
or 1½ cups quick-cooking oatmeal
(uncooked)
1 cup nonfat yogurt
½ cup nonfat milk
1 egg white

1 teaspoon baking soda
½ teaspoon salt
1 teaspoon vanilla
1 tablespoon SomerSweet
Oil for greasing pan

Place oatmeal, nonfat yogurt, nonfat milk, egg white, baking soda, salt, vanilla, and SomerSweet into a mixing bowl. Stir until well blended. Allow to stand for 5 minutes.

Heat a nonstick skillet over medium heat. Add enough oil to lightly coat bottom of pan. Add a scant ¼ cup of batter to pan for each pancake. Cook for 2 to 3 minutes per side, or until golden-brown. Serve with Raspberry Sauce or Somersize Maple Syrup.

For Level Two
Add 1 slightly beaten egg white for lovely, light oatmeal pancakes.

Raspberry Sauce

FRUIT—ALMOST LEVEL ONE

MAKES 1½ CUPS

6 ounces fresh raspberries
1 cup water

¼ cup nonfat yogurt
1 tablespoon plus 2 teaspoons SomerSweet

Bring raspberries and water to a boil in a small saucepan over medium-high heat. Turn heat to low and simmer for 15 minutes. Place mixture in a sieve set over a bowl.

Allow mixture to drain, pressing lightly on pulp to extract all juices. Add nonfat yogurt and SomerSweet. Stir until SomerSweet has dissolved. Serve over Oatmeal Pancakes.

Cinnamon Bread

CARBOS—LEVEL ONE

MAKES 1 LOAF

Enjoy this delicious bread toasted for breakfast or even an afternoon treat. It tastes like dessert, especially with my Sweet Orange Cream Cheese Spread (p. 191). I use King Arthur whole-wheat flour for best results. Look for it in most markets. Also, before you start, make sure your bread machine is a two-pound-loaf capacity. Make sure you measure accurately! You must use dry measuring cups for dry ingredients and calibrated glass measuring cups for liquid ingredients. Most people know this, but if you don't, it makes a big difference! Also, you will need an instant-read thermometer for this recipe. It's a handy kitchen tool if you don't already have one. Cinnamon Bread is also available as a Somersize Bread Mix.

PREP TIME: 8 MINUTES
BREAD MAKER/PROOFING AND BAKING TIME: 2 1/2 HOURS

4 cups whole-wheat flour
3 tablespoons SomerSweet
3 tablespoons cinnamon
1 teaspoon salt
1/3 cup nonfat dry milk
1 cup nonfat plain yogurt
2 cups nonfat milk

2 teaspoons vanilla extract
2 1/4 teaspoons bread machine yeast, or
   1 (1/4-ounce) packet active dry yeast

EQUIPMENT
Bread maker

Mix together flour, SomerSweet, cinnamon, and salt.

In a medium saucepan, stir together nonfat dry milk, nonfat plain yogurt, nonfat milk, and vanilla. Cook over low heat, stirring, until liquid reaches a temperature of 120 degrees on an instant-read thermometer. Pour liquid into bread maker. Add all dry ingredients except the yeast to the bread maker. Make a 1/2-inch well in top of dry ingredients. Sprinkle yeast into well.

Set bread maker to whole-wheat cycle. Cool and remove loaf according to your bread maker's instructions.

If well wrapped, this bread can be frozen for 1 week.

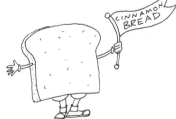

Sweet Orange Cream Cheese Spread

CARBOS—LEVEL ONE

MAKES 1 1/2 CUPS

The orange in this spread goes wonderfully with my Cinnamon Bread (p. 190). Make sure you look for fat-free cream cheese that does not contain a bunch of unpronounceable ingredients. Kraft Philadelphia brand is a good one.

PREP TIME: 3 MINUTES

1 (12-ounce) package fat-free cream
   cheese, softened
1 tablespoon SomerSweet

1/2 teaspoon orange extract
1/2 teaspoon vanilla extract
2 teaspoons grated orange zest

Combine all ingredients in a small bowl. Blend until SomerSweet is completely dissolved. Refrigerate in an airtight container for up to 1 week.

Watermelon Icy

FRUIT—LEVEL ONE

SERVES 4

I just love fruit smoothies. This one may be the most refreshing of all! Fresh watermelon, lime juice, and ice . . . that's it. It's actually a Mexican tradition. Try it in the height of watermelon season. If your melon is not quite sweet enough, add a touch of SomerSweet. For an extra-frosty drink, freeze the chunks of watermelon before you blend it. That way you don't have to add any ice and it concentrates the taste.

PREP TIME: 10 MINUTES

1½ pounds ripe watermelon, rind and
    seeds removed, cut into chunks (about
    ¼ of a watermelon)
1 teaspoon SomerSweet (optional)

Juice of 2 limes
6 ice cubes
Lime slices, for garnish

Place watermelon, SomerSweet, lime juice, and ice in a blender. Purée until smooth. If mixture is too thick, add a touch of very cold water until the smoothie blends well. Adjust taste by adding a little more SomerSweet or lime juice. Serve in tall, frosty glasses garnished with a slice of lime.

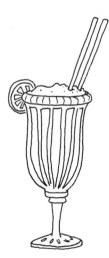

The Somersize Recipes

Appetizers and Snacks

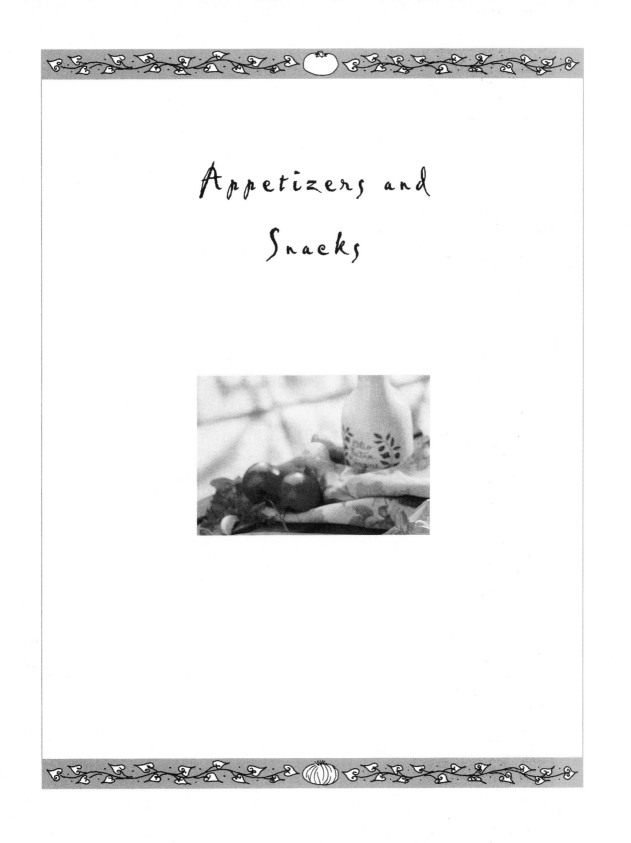

Fried Shrimp

SERVES 6

These delicious shrimp taste just like they've been breaded and fried, but there's no breading! They are dipped in my Somersize Bake and Fry Mix, which makes them crispy and golden brown. It takes only ten minutes to make this great appetizer or entrée. I buy the frozen raw shrimp already peeled and deveined, so my prep time is minimal.

PREP TIME: 2 MINUTES
COOKING TIME: 8 MINUTES

1 pound medium shrimp, peeled and
    deveined
3 large eggs
2 cups Somersize Bake and Fry Mix
    (p. 235)

Peanut oil for frying
1 recipe Spicy Cocktail Sauce (p. 195)

EQUIPMENT
Deep fryer

Using paper towels, blot shrimp dry. Set aside.

Beat the eggs in a medium bowl. Place Bake and Fry Mix in a separate medium bowl. Dip shrimp first into egg, then into Bake and Fry Mix. Heat oil in a deep fryer or a large deep pot to 375 degrees. Fry shrimp until golden, about 2 minutes, depending how hot your oil is. Shrimp are done when they are golden brown on the outside and a whitish pink on the inside. Drain on a baking sheet lined with paper towels. Serve with Spicy Cocktail Sauce.

Spicy Cocktail Sauce

PRO/FATS—LEVEL ONE

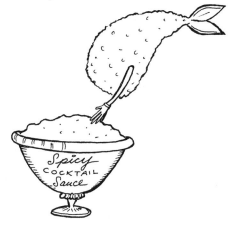

MAKES 2¼ CUPS

This is a zesty cocktail sauce made with my Somersize Ketchup. It has a great kick, but if it's too spicy for you, back off on the cayenne pepper and the horseradish. Or you can simply buy Somersize Cocktail Sauce.

PREP TIME: 2 MINUTES

2 cups Somersize Ketchup (p. 245)
1 tablespoon lemon juice
3 tablespoons prepared horseradish

1½ teaspoons Worcestershire sauce
1 teaspoon cayenne pepper
Salt and freshly ground black pepper

Mix all ingredients together. Refrigerate in an airtight container for up to 10 days.

Artichoke and Onion Dip

PRO/FATS AND VEGGIES—LEVEL ONE

MAKES 2 1/2 CUPS

Artichokes are one of my favorite vegetables. They are so versatile. Here I use artichoke bottoms or crowns and my Somersize Onion Dip Mix to create a truly divine dip for artichokes and crudités or a spread for a chicken breast. The flavor is great if you use fresh artichokes, but the fast and easy version calls for canned artichoke bottoms or crowns. This is also wonderful served warm. See the variation below.

PREP TIME: 5 MINUTES

1 package Somersize Onion Dip Mix
1 cup sour cream
1 (8-ounce) package cream cheese, softened
1 (14-ounce) can artichoke bottoms or crowns, drained

1/2 cup grated Parmesan cheese
1 teaspoon lemon juice
Salt and freshly ground black pepper

Place all ingredients in a food processor. Process until smooth, scraping the sides of the bowl with a spatula if necessary. Season with salt and pepper. Refrigerate until ready to use.

Note
This may also be served warm. Simply place purée in an oven-proof dish and bake for 15 minutes at 350 degrees.

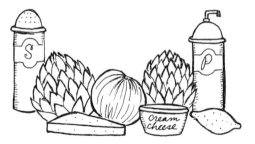

Cucumber Dill Dip

PRO/FATS AND VEGGIES—LEVEL ONE

MAKES 3 CUPS

In Indian cuisine, a yogurt-based side dish is often served with a spicy entrée to cool the heat. This light and refreshing Cucumber Dill Dip is the perfect companion to my In a Hurry Beef Curry (p. 270). When serving this with Pro/Fats, you use full-fat sour cream. For the Carbos version, you use a combination of nonfat yogurt and nonfat sour cream. This is also a great dip for crudités.

PREP TIME: 3 MINUTES

4 medium cucumbers, peeled, seeded, and
   cut into 1-inch pieces
$2/3$ cup chopped onions
1 bunch fresh dill, stems removed

$2\frac{1}{4}$ cups full-fat sour cream
1 tablespoon plus 1 teaspoon lemon juice
2 teaspoons salt
$\frac{1}{4}$ teaspoon black pepper

Place cucumbers, onions, dill, sour cream, lemon juice, salt, and pepper in the bowl of a food processor. Pulse until mixture is the consistency of salsa. Chill for 1 hour.

Variation
To serve with a Level One Carbos meal, substitute 1 cup nonfat yogurt and $1\frac{1}{4}$ cups nonfat sour cream for the full-fat sour cream.

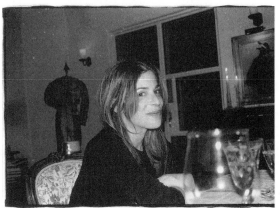

Darling Leslie.

Appetizers and Snacks

White Bean Rosemary Spread

CARBOS AND VEGGIES—LEVEL ONE

MAKES 2 CUPS

This recipe is great as a dip or sandwich spread. I love it on a toasted whole-wheat bagel or toasted whole-wheat pita triangles. You can even make your own tortilla chips by cutting wheat tortillas into wedges and baking on a cookie sheet in a 400-degree oven for 10 to 12 minutes.

PREP TIME: 4 MINUTES

2 (15-ounce) cans small white beans,
   rinsed and drained
1 teaspoon chopped fresh rosemary or
   ½ teaspoon dried
1 teaspoon chopped fresh thyme or
   ½ teaspoon dried

¼ teaspoon salt
¼ teaspoon black pepper
Pinch of cayenne pepper
2 tablespoons lemon juice
3 tablespoons nonfat yogurt
¼ cup minced red onions

Place beans in the work bowl of a food processor, along with the rosemary, thyme, salt, black pepper, cayenne pepper, lemon juice, and yogurt. Process until smooth, about 2 minutes. Stir in the red onions. Adjust seasonings. Refrigerate in an airtight container for up to 4 days.

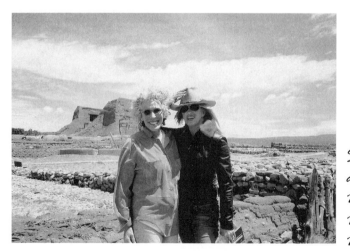

Susie and me at the Pecos National Monument in New Mexico.

Ginger Chicken Wontons

PRO/FATS AND VEGGIES—LEVEL ONE

MAKES 40

My daughter-in-law, Caroline, always makes great Asian food. To make these Somersized, Caroline just used the flavorful filling of the wonton, to keep it Level One. For Level Two you can wrap them in whole-wheat wonton wrappers, which can be found in the refrigerator section of your local supermarket. Try them with Chinese-Style Hot Mustard Dipping Sauce or Gingered Soy Sauce.

PREP TIME: 15 MINUTES
COOKING TIME: 10 MINUTES

1 pound ground chicken
1 large egg
1 teaspoon ground ginger
3 cloves garlic, minced
¼ cup finely chopped scallions
¼ teaspoon allspice
⅛ teaspoon cinnamon
¼ teaspoon cayenne pepper
1 teaspoon salt

1 teaspoon black pepper
Peanut oil for deep frying
1 recipe Chinese-Style Hot Mustard
   Dipping Sauce (p. 200)
1 recipe Gingered Soy Sauce (p. 201)

EQUIPMENT
Deep fryer

In a large mixing bowl, combine ground chicken, egg, ginger, garlic, scallions, allspice, cinnamon, cayenne pepper, salt, and black pepper. Mix well until all ingredients are evenly distributed.

Heat oil to 375 degrees in a deep fryer or a large deep pot. Carefully place a heaping teaspoon of chicken mixture into hot oil. Cook in batches of 8 to 10 at a time, until golden brown. Remove from oil and drain on paper towels. Serve with Chinese-Style Hot Mustard Dipping Sauce or Gingered Soy Sauce.

For Level Two

For Level Two you will need a package of wonton wrappers (whole-wheat if you can find them). Place 1 teaspoon of chicken mixture into the center of a square wonton wrapper. Lightly dampen the edges with water. Fold one corner over to the opposite corner to from a triangle. Press edges to encase filling. Deep fry as above until golden brown.

Chinese-Style Hot Mustard Dipping Sauce

PRO/FATS—LEVEL ONE

✦

MAKES ¹/₂ CUP

*This one of the **dipping sauces** for Ginger Chicken Wontons (p. 199). It's also great to spice up a hamburger or hot dog.*

PREP TIME: 2 MINUTES

¹/₄ cup Dijon mustard
¹/₄ cup sour cream
2 teaspoons Worcestershire sauce
2 teaspoons SomerSweet

1 teaspoon Tabasco sauce
2 teaspoons soy sauce
Salt and freshly ground black pepper

Combine mustard, sour cream, Worcestershire, SomerSweet, Tabasco, and soy sauce in a mixing bowl. Mix until smooth.

Season with salt and pepper. Add more Tabasco to taste if desired. Refrigerate in an airtight container for up to 5 days.

Gingered Soy Sauce

LEVEL ONE

MAKES 1 CUP (ENOUGH FOR 2 FILLETS)

This is the other dipping sauce for the Ginger Chicken Wontons (p. 199). It's also a wonderful marinade for chicken, fish, or beef. Check out the recipe for Ginger Scallion Grilled Mahi-Mahi (p. 283) using this marinade.

PREP TIME: 3 MINUTES

1 cup soy sauce
2 teaspoons freshly grated ginger

3 cloves garlic, minced
2 scallions, finely chopped

Combine all ingredients and set aside to let flavors meld. Store in an airtight container in the refrigerator.

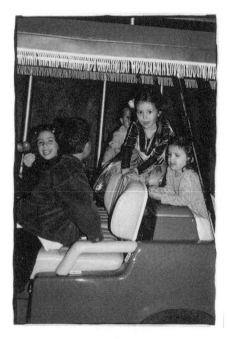

All the grandkids love to pile into Alan's golf cart.

Pinwheels

MAKES 24

These pinwheels are made with whole-wheat tortillas, fat-free cream cheese, and vegetables. They make great appetizers or sandwich rolls. It only takes about seven minutes to make, but you can make it even faster by blending my packaged Somersize Onion Dip Mix with nonfat cream cheese.

PREP TIME: 7 MINUTES

1 (8-ounce) package nonfat cream cheese, at room temperature
$\frac{1}{4}$ cup very thinly sliced scallions, plus diagonally cut scallions for garnish
$\frac{1}{4}$ teaspoon salt
$\frac{1}{4}$ teaspoon black pepper
2 whole-wheat tortillas
1 red bell pepper, thinly sliced
1 English cucumber, peeled and sliced thin
2 red leaf lettuce leaves

In a small bowl, mix together cream cheese, scallions, salt, and pepper until well combined.

Lay a tortilla on a clean work surface. Spread half of the cream-cheese mixture evenly over the tortilla. Then layer with half the red pepper slices, cucumber slices, and 1 lettuce leaf. Roll up like a jelly roll. Repeat with the other tortilla, cream cheese, and vegetables.

Slice tortilla rolls about $\frac{1}{2}$ inch thick. Garnish with a scallion slice.

Soups

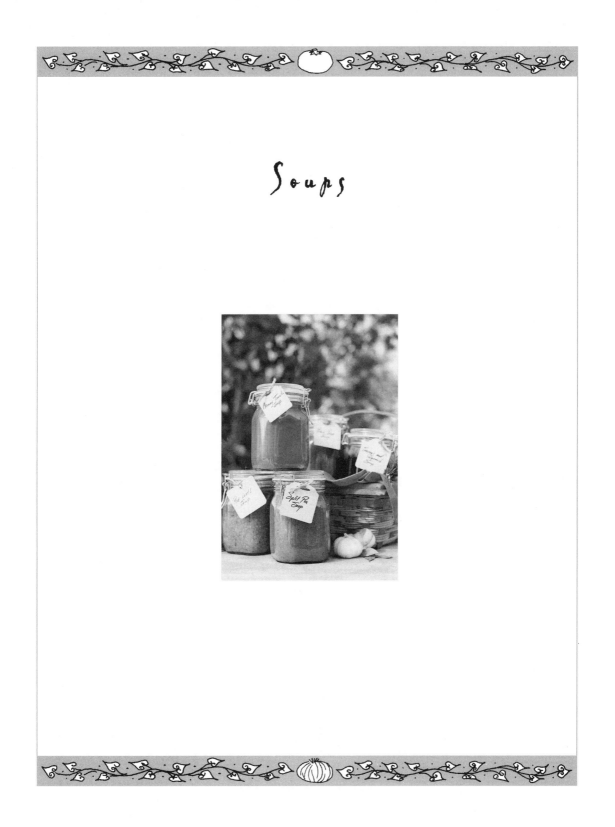

Red Lentil Cumin Soup

CARBOS AND VEGGIES—ALMOST LEVEL ONE

SERVES 6

Red lentils cook faster than brown lentils because they are softer and do not have a seed coat. They are sometimes called Egyptian lentils. Look for them in your grocery store. This is an Almost Level One recipe because I use fat-free chicken broth with the Carbos. I think it tastes best this way, but if you want to make this a true Level One soup, use vegetable broth instead.

PREP TIME: 5 MINUTES
COOKING TIME: 30 MINUTES

5 cups fat-free chicken broth
1 cup chopped onions
$\frac{1}{4}$ teaspoon crushed ginger
$\frac{1}{4}$ teaspoon crushed garlic
1 teaspoon cumin

1 (14-ounce) can crushed tomatoes
3 cups (1 pound) red lentils, rinsed
Salt and freshly ground black pepper
4 whole scallions, sliced

In a large pot, bring $\frac{1}{2}$ cup chicken broth to a boil. Add onions, reduce heat, and simmer until onions are soft and most of the liquid has evaporated. Add ginger, garlic, cumin, and tomatoes. Stir to combine. Let simmer over low heat for 2 minutes.

Add lentils and the rest of the chicken broth. Bring to a boil, reduce heat, and simmer for 20 to 25 minutes. Season with salt and pepper. Garnish with scallions.

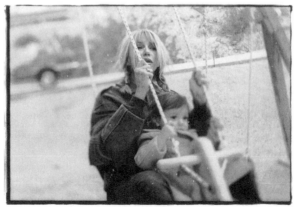

Me and my sweet granddaughter on the swing "horsey."

The Somersize Recipes

Chicken Sausage and Spinach Soup

PRO/FATS AND VEGGIES—LEVEL ONE

SERVES 6

I love soups that make a whole meal. This is hearty and satisfying with bites of sausage and wilted spinach leaves. You can shorten the cooking time by slicing up cooked sausage.

PREP TIME: 5 MINUTES
COOKING TIME: 20 MINUTES

1 pound sweet Italian chicken or turkey
 sausage
1½ tablespoons unsalted butter
1½ tablespoons olive oil
1 (49-ounce) can chicken broth, about
 6 cups

1 (10-ounce) package frozen whole-leaf
 spinach
Salt and freshly ground black pepper
Shredded Parmesan cheese, for garnish

Remove sausage meat from casing and form into 1-inch balls. If using cooked sausage, cut into quarter-inch slices.

Heat butter and oil in a large heavy pot over medium-high heat. Brown sausage in butter and oil, about 7 minutes. Add chicken stock to pot. Bring to a boil, reduce heat, and simmer until sausage is cooked through, about 12 minutes.

Add spinach and simmer for 1 minute. Season with salt and pepper. Serve with Parmesan cheese.

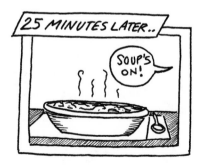

Cauliflower and Red Bell Pepper Soup

PRO/FATS AND VEGGIES—LEVEL ONE

SERVES 4 TO 6

This two-colored soup is twice as delicious. I love to alternate spoonfuls from each side . . . a little cauliflower, a little red pepper, back to the cauliflower . . .

PREP TIME: 20 MINUTES
COOKING TIME: 18 MINUTES

1 (1-pound) bag frozen cauliflower florets, thawed (or fresh, if desired)
½ cup water
Pinch of salt
½ cup shredded Swiss cheese
4 tablespoons butter
4 cups chicken stock
⅓ cup plus ½ cup heavy cream

Salt and freshly ground black pepper
1 (12-ounce) jar roasted red bell peppers, drained
½ cup chopped onions

EQUIPMENT
Microwave

Put cauliflower in a microwave-safe bowl with the water and a pinch of salt. Cover with plastic wrap and microwave on high for 9 minutes. Drain. Place cauliflower in work bowl of a food processor with Swiss cheese, 2 tablespoons butter, and 2 cups chicken stock. Process until smooth. Add ⅓ cup of cream and pulse until incorporated. Season with salt and pepper. Pour into microwave-safe bowl and cover with plastic wrap. Set aside.

Place peppers in a microwave-safe bowl with 2 cups chicken broth and chopped onions. Cover with plastic wrap and microwave on high for 5 minutes. Place peppers, onions, and stock in bowl of a food processor. Process until smooth. Add ½ cup heavy cream and remaining 2 tablespoons butter. Pulse to blend. Pour into microwave-safe bowl and cover with plastic wrap.

To serve, heat soups in microwave until hot, about 2 minutes each. Using two 1-cup measuring cups, each filled three-quarters with soup, pour both soups into soup bowl simultaneously. Swirl soups together with a toothpick. Serve hot.

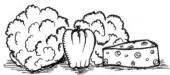

Eight-Minute Creamy Tomato Soup

PRO/FATS AND VEGGIES—LEVEL ONE

MAKES ABOUT 5 CUPS

Have you got eight minutes? That's all you need to make this delicious soup.

PREP TIME: 1 MINUTE
COOKING TIME: 7 MINUTES

2 tablespoons unsalted butter
½ cup chopped onions
1 (28-ounce) can diced tomatoes

1 cup chicken stock
1 cup heavy cream
Sour cream, for garnish (optional)

Melt butter in a 3-quart heavy-bottomed saucepan. Add onions and sauté for 2 minutes. Add tomatoes, chicken stock, and cream to onions. Bring to a boil, reduce heat, and simmer 5 minutes.

Pour into a blender or food processor. Blend until smooth. Pour into soup bowls, garnish with sour cream, and serve.

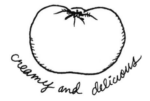

creamy and delicious

Tex Mex Black Bean Soup

CARBOS AND VEGGIES — ALMOST LEVEL ONE

SERVES 4

I love this spicy soup. Black beans really fill you up. Serve this beside a simple green salad with a squeeze of lemon. Again, this soup tastes best when made with chicken broth, but that combo makes it Almost Level One. For a true Level One soup, make it with vegetable broth.

PREP TIME: 2 MINUTES
COOKING TIME: 11 MINUTES

2 (14-ounce) cans fat-free chicken or
   vegetable broth
1 cup chopped onions
3 (15-ounce) cans fat-free black beans,
   drained
1 tablespoon plus 2 teaspoons cumin
1 teaspoon Tabasco sauce

$\frac{1}{4}$ teaspoon cayenne pepper
$\frac{1}{4}$ cup fat-free sour cream
Salt and freshly ground black pepper
3 tablespoons chopped cilantro
2 tablespoons lime juice
Salsa, for garnish

In a medium saucepan over medium-high heat, bring 1 cup broth to a boil. Add onions and cook in broth for 6 minutes. Add beans, remaining broth, cumin, Tabasco, and cayenne. Simmer for 5 minutes. Transfer mixture to a food processor.

Process for 30 seconds. Add sour cream and pulse until mixed. Season with salt and black pepper. Add cilantro and lime juice. Stir well. Serve immediately with a dollop of fresh salsa.

Split Pea Soup

SERVES 8

Cooking this split pea soup in the pressure cooker makes it really fast. It tastes great on a cold afternoon or evening. For Level One, make this soup with vegetable broth. For better flavor, use chicken broth and enjoy it as Almost Level One.

PREP TIME: 2 MINUTES
COOKING TIME: 12 MINUTES

2 cups chopped onions
1 pound dried split peas, rinsed
8 cups (2 quarts) fat-free chicken or
    vegetable broth
2 tablespoons fresh dill
2 bay leaves

Salt and freshly ground black pepper
Nonfat sour cream or yogurt, for garnish

EQUIPMENT
Pressure cooker

Place onions, split peas, broth, dill, and bay leaves in the pan of a pressure cooker. Lock lid into place. Bring to pressure over high heat. Lower heat and cook for 12 minutes.

Release pressure slowly. Remove and discard bay leaves. Season with salt and pepper. Garnish with nonfat sour cream or yogurt before serving.

Alternate Stovetop Method

Soak split peas according to package directions. In a large saucepan, bring 1 cup of the broth to a boil. Add the onions, lower heat, and simmer until the onions are soft, about 5 minutes. Add the rest of the broth, split peas, dill, and bay leaves to the saucepan. Bring to a boil, reduce heat, and simmer, covered, for 1½ hours or until split peas are tender. Remove bay leaves. Season with salt and pepper and garnish with nonfat sour cream or yogurt before serving.

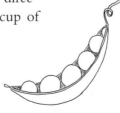

Fast and Easy Minestrone

CARBOS AND VEGGIES—ALMOST LEVEL ONE

SERVES 6

I'm always looking for delicious ways to eat kale. Kale is a super green vegetable that is loaded with vitamins and minerals. This soup is chock-full of great beans and veggies. I make this soup in big batches and freeze it for those nights when I get home late and want a home-cooked meal. When made the super-yummy way with chicken broth, it's Almost Level One. When made with vegetable broth, it's Level One.

PREP TIME: 2 MINUTES
COOKING TIME: 22 MINUTES

1 medium onion, chopped
3 (14-ounce) cans chicken broth
4 cloves garlic, finely chopped
1 (28-ounce) can diced tomatoes
1 (15.5-ounce) can garbanzo beans, rinsed and drained
1 (15.5-ounce) can red kidney beans, rinsed and drained
2 cups chopped fresh kale, Swiss chard, or baby spinach leaves
1/2 cup dried Somersize Spinach Macaroni (or any whole-grain pasta)
1 teaspoon Italian seasoning mix
1/4 teaspoon dried rosemary
1/4 teaspoon red pepper flakes
Salt and freshly ground black pepper

In a large saucepan, cook onions in 3/4 cup chicken broth over medium-high heat until onions are translucent, about 5 minutes. Add another 1/2 cup broth and garlic. Cook 5 minutes more. Stir in tomatoes, the rest of the broth, garbanzo and kidney beans, kale, pasta, Italian seasoning, rosemary, and red pepper flakes. Bring to a boil. Reduce heat. Cover and simmer 10 to 12 minutes, or until pasta is tender. Season with salt and pepper before serving.

Salads

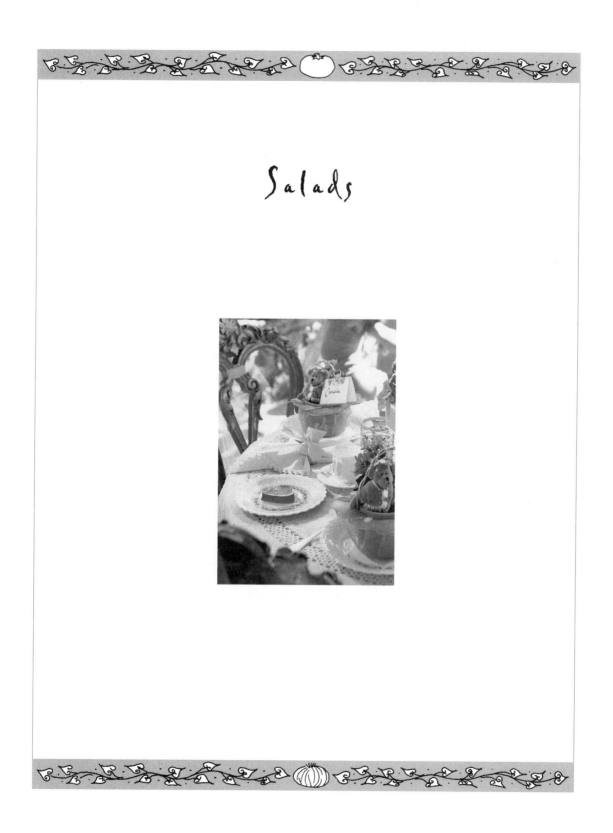

Shrimp Scampi and Gorgonzola Cheese Salad

PRO/FATS—LEVEL ONE

❖

MAKES 2 MAIN-COURSE SERVINGS, OR 4 APPETIZER SERVINGS

This recipe is almost too fast and too easy! It makes an elegant starter for a dinner party or is a wonderful light dinner all by itself.

PREP TIME: 2 MINUTES
COOKING TIME: 5 MINUTES

3 tablespoons olive oil
5 cloves garlic, chopped
1 pound large shrimp, peeled and deveined
$\frac{1}{4}$ cup fresh lemon juice (about 2 lemons)
Salt and freshly ground black pepper
2 tablespoons unsalted butter

$\frac{1}{4}$ cup fresh parsley, chopped
$\frac{1}{2}$ pound mixed baby greens
$\frac{1}{4}$ cup crumbled gorgonzola, or other blue cheese
Lemon wedges, for garnish

Place oil and garlic in a large sauté pan. Turn heat to low. Cook garlic for 2 minutes, stirring occasionally. Do not let garlic brown. Turn heat to high and add shrimp to pan. Add 2 tablespoons lemon juice, scraping any bits from the bottom of the pan. Season with salt and pepper. Cook for 2 minutes. Remove shrimp from pan and set aside.

Deglaze pan with remaining lemon juice. Add butter to pan and stir until melted. Taste sauce and season with salt and pepper. Return shrimp to pan. Add parsley and toss in mixture to coat shrimp. Remove from heat. Place greens on plates. Spoon shrimp and sauce over greens. Sprinkle with gorgonzola and serve. Garnish with lemon wedges.

Warm Steak and Arugula Salad with Parmesan Shavings

PRO/FATS AND VEGGIES—LEVEL ONE

SERVES 4

This is my kind of salad: hearty, satisfying, and beautiful. For a wonderful flavor combination use my Lemon Olive Oil (p. 279) in place of the extra-virgin oil.

PREP TIME: 4 MINUTES
COOKING TIME: 10 MINUTES

3 tablespoons plus 1 tablespoon extra-
    virgin olive oil
1 tablespoon balsamic vinegar
Salt and freshly ground black pepper

4 ounces arugula
1 pint cherry tomatoes, cut in half
1 pound beef tip steak
Parmesan shavings

Whisk 3 tablespoons olive oil in a bowl with balsamic vinegar. Season with salt and pepper. Add arugula and tomatoes and toss to coat. Place on a large serving platter or 4 dinner plates.

Pat steak dry with paper towels. Season liberally with salt and pepper. Heat a large sauté pan on medium-high heat. Add 1 tablespoon olive oil, then the steak. Sauté steak until browned, about 5 minutes on each side. Place steak on a cutting board. Allow to rest for 3 minutes before slicing thin. Arrange hot steak slices over arugula. Top with Parmesan shavings before serving.

Buffalo Mozzarella and Cherry Tomato Salad

PRO/FATS AND VEGGIES—LEVEL ONE

MAKES 4 SERVINGS

Alan and I eat buffalo mozzarella and tomatoes at least three times a week. When it's the height of tomato season you can get wonderful tomatoes from local growers. Once you've tasted a tomato like that, it's impossible to enjoy the pink store-bought version. I find that if you are shopping at a regular grocery store, your best option is cherry tomatoes. Here's my salad made with the sweet little ones.

PREP TIME: 3 MINUTES

12 ounces cherry tomatoes
8 ounces buffalo mozzarella
1 ounce fresh basil leaves (1 bunch)

1½ tablespoons extra-virgin olive oil
Salt and freshly ground black pepper

Cut tomatoes in half and place in a salad bowl. Cut mozzarella into chunks roughly the size of the cherry tomato halves. Add mozzarella to salad bowl. Chop basil leaves into fine strips and add to the tomatoes and mozzarella. Drizzle olive oil over the top, then season with salt and lots of coarsely ground pepper. Toss and serve.

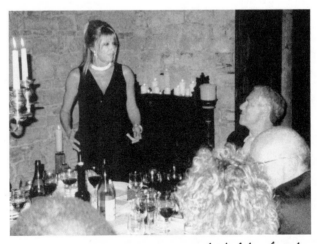

*Me giving a toast to my wonderful husband,
Alan, on his birthday.*

Tomato and Cucumber Salad with Feta Vinaigrette

PRO/FATS AND VEGGIES—LEVEL ONE

MAKES 6 SERVINGS

I love feta cheese. The salt in the cheese combined with the tomatoes and cucumbers is perfect. Serve this all on its own, or with grilled baby lamb chops or chicken breast for a delightful summer meal.

PREP TIME: 3 MINUTES

1 tablespoon balsamic vinegar
¼ cup extra-virgin olive oil
¼ teaspoon salt
¼ teaspoon coarsely ground black pepper

6 ounces crumbled feta cheese
4 medium Roma tomatoes, sliced
1 small English cucumber, sliced

Place balsamic vinegar in a small bowl. Whisk in olive oil a little at a time. Keep whisking until all olive oil has been added and vinaigrette is creamy. Whisk in salt and pepper. Stir in feta cheese. Cover and refrigerate until ready to use.

To serve, place slices of tomato and cucumber on individual salad plates. Drizzle vinaigrette over tomato and cucumber. Spoon some of the feta on top.

For Level Two
Add ½ cup of Kalamata or oil-cured olives.

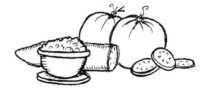

Rock Shrimp with Citrus-Serrano Vinaigrette

PRO/FATS AND VEGGIES—LEVEL ONE

SERVES 4 AS AN APPETIZER, 2 FOR LUNCH

This is a Caroline creation made with delicious rock shrimp, crunchy jícama, and a tart-and-spicy citrus dressing. Rock shrimp are small shrimp that have a wonderful flavor reminiscent of lobster. If you can find them, they are a real treat. (Of course, you may substitute any shrimp.)

1 red onion, sliced into thin rings
1 pound cooked rock shrimp
1 jícama, peeled and sliced into thin strips
1 recipe Citrus-Serrano Vinaigrette
   (p. 217)

1 head of torn butter lettuce
1 pint cherry tomatoes

Place the red onion rings, cooked shrimp, and jícama into a stainless-steel or nonreactive (nonmetallic) bowl and pour the Citrus-Serrano Vinaigrette over the top. Gently toss to combine. Let mixture stand to allow flavors to develop (30 minutes is best, but it still tastes great with less marinating).

Place the torn butter lettuce leaves and cherry tomatoes into a salad bowl. Pour the shrimp mixture over the lettuce and toss to combine. Serve immediately.

Note
Rock shrimp usually come raw and peeled. They cook very quickly. Simply place in salted boiling water until they turn pink. Remove immediately and drain.

Citrus-Serrano Vinaigrette

PRO/FATS AND VEGGIES—LEVEL ONE

MAKES ABOUT ²/₃ CUP

Fresh lemon, fresh lime, serrano chilies, mint, and olive oil . . . a great flavor combination! If you can't find serrano chilies, use a jalapeño instead. This really gives your salad a kick.

PREP TIME: 5 MINUTES

1 serrano chili
2 tablespoons lemon juice
2 tablespoons lime juice
3 tablespoons chopped fresh or freeze-
   dried mint leaves

2 cloves garlic, chopped
Salt and freshly ground black pepper
½ cup extra-virgin olive oil

Slice the serrano in half lengthwise and remove seeds. Finely chop the serrano, or process in a mini–food processor until minced.

Whisk together lemon juice, lime juice, serrano, mint, garlic, salt, and pepper in a small bowl. Slowly add olive oil in a steady stream, whisking until the oil is emulsified.

Taste for seasoning and adjust salt and pepper as necessary.

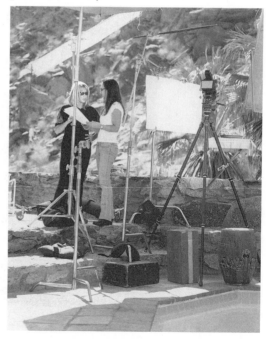

Caroline and me at work.

Fennel, Red Onion, and Hearts of Palm Salad

PRO/FATS AND VEGGIES—LEVEL ONE

SERVES 4

I am a huge fennel fan. What I love about this salad is that you can make it ahead of time, and it will stay crunchy for several hours. Try this with my Pink Goddess Salad Dressing or any of the vinaigrettes from my previous books.

PREP TIME: 6 MINUTES

2 large bulbs fennel
1 medium Vidalia, Maui, or other sweet
  onion, sliced thin
1 (14-ounce) can hearts of palm, drained

¼ cup packed fresh basil leaves
Salt and freshly ground black pepper
⅔ cup Pink Goddess Salad Dressing
  (p. 219)

Trim stalks from fennel. Slice fennel thin. Place in a large salad bowl with the onion. Carefully cut hearts of palm into quarter-inch slices and add to fennel and onion. Chop basil leaves coarsely and add to bowl.

Season with salt and pepper. Add Pink Goddess Salad Dressing to salad and toss gently, taking care not to break hearts of palm. Refrigerate for 1 hour before serving.

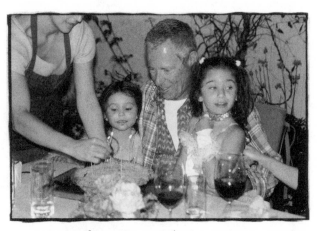

Alan flanked by his gals.

Pink Goddess Salad Dressing

PRO/FATS—LEVEL ONE

❖

MAKES 1¼ CUPS

You've tried my Green Goddess—now we have Pink Goddess! Raspberry vinegar makes it pink, or for Level Two you add fresh raspberries for a truly spectacular color. Serve this lively dressing with my Fennel, Red Onion, and Hearts of Palm Salad (p. 218) or on any salad that makes you feel like a goddess.

PREP TIME: 2 MINUTES

½ cup red raspberry vinegar
⅓ cup red wine vinegar
2 teaspoons fresh lemon juice
3 tablespoons mayonnaise

1½ teaspoons SomerSweet
⅔ cup olive oil
¼ teaspoon salt
⅛ teaspoon black pepper

Combine vinegars, lemon juice, mayonnaise, and SomerSweet in a stainless-steel bowl. Drizzle in olive oil, whisking constantly, until mixture is creamy. Add salt and pepper.

For Level Two

For a Level Two dressing, omit the red wine vinegar and mayonnaise, and use 1 (5-ounce) container of fresh raspberries. Place all ingredients in a food processor or blender and pulse until smooth.

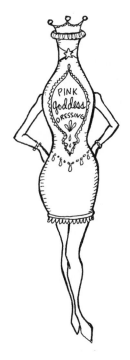

Crunchy Coleslaw

PRO/FATS AND VEGGIES—LEVEL ONE

SERVES 4

PREP TIME: 10 MINUTES

Fennel gives this coleslaw a new twist. For an extra-fast-and-easy coleslaw, look for preshredded cabbage in the produce section of your grocery store.

1 medium fennel bulb, trimmed and thinly
　　sliced
2 cups shredded green cabbage
2 cups shredded red cabbage
3 scallions, thinly sliced
½ cup mayonnaise
½ cup sour cream

2 teaspoons lemon juice
1 teaspoon SomerSweet
⅛ teaspoon Tabasco sauce
1 teaspoon apple cider vinegar
1 teaspoon celery seed (optional)
Salt and freshly ground black pepper

Place fennel, green cabbage, red cabbage, and scallions in a large mixing bowl. In a separate small bowl, stir together mayonnaise, sour cream, lemon juice, Somer-Sweet, Tabasco, and vinegar. Season with celery seed (optional), salt, and pepper. Toss dressing and vegetables together. Refrigerate until ready to serve.

Taco Salad

SERVES 4

Taco Salad is always satisfying for a Somersizer. Here's a fast version made with my Tex Mex Seasoning Blend. Of course, you can make it even faster with my packaged Somersize Taco Seasoning Mix.

PREP TIME: 8 MINUTES
COOKING TIME: 15 MINUTES

3 tablespoons vegetable oil
½ cup chopped onions
1 pound ground beef
1 tablespoon Tex Mex Seasoning Blend or
   a packet of your favorite seasoning mix
   (p. 275)
⅔ cup chopped tomato
½ cup sliced scallions

Salt and freshly ground black pepper
4 cups shredded iceberg lettuce (or your
   favorite salad greens)
1 cup shredded cheddar cheese
1½ cups sour cream
1 cup salsa
Cilantro sprigs, for garnish

Place a large skillet over medium-high heat. When hot, add oil and onions. Sauté for about 5 minutes. Add ground beef and sauté until browned, about 5 minutes. Drain off any excess fat. Add Tex Mex Seasoning Blend. Continue cooking for 3 more minutes. Remove from heat. Add tomatoes and scallions. Season with salt and pepper.

Divide the meat onto 4 plates. Top each with 1 cup of lettuce, cheddar cheese, sour cream, and salsa. Garnish with cilantro sprigs.

Vegetable Dishes

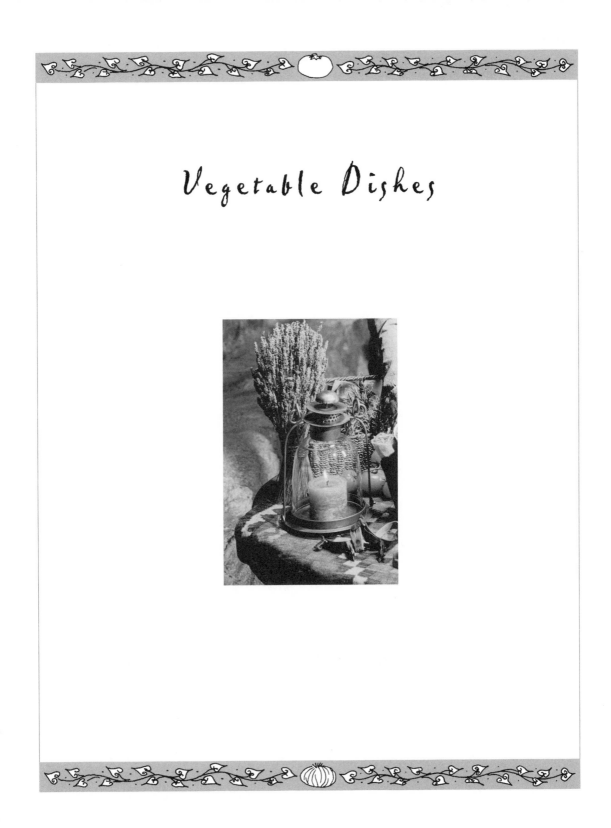

Somersize Fast and Easy Onion Rings

LEVEL ONE

SERVES 4

I make these on the weekend for a treat. They taste great with the Somersize Double Double Cheese-burger (p. 243), or just as a snack by themselves.

PREP TIME: 10 MINUTES
COOKING TIME: 15 MINUTES

5 eggs
4 large onions (14–16 ounces each)
Peanut or canola oil for deep frying
Salt

Somersize Ketchup (p. 245)

EQUIPMENT
Deep fryer

Place eggs in a large stainless-steel bowl. Peel onions. Cut into 1/2-inch-thick slices, horizontally. Separate slices into rings. Using paper towels, pat onion rings dry. This helps the egg to stick.

Heat oil to 375 degrees in a deep fryer or a large deep pot. Beat the eggs with a fork until blended. Dip onion rings in the egg mixture. Drop onion rings into hot oil.

Cook for about 2 minutes or until golden brown. Blot on paper towels. Sprinkle liberally with salt. Serve immediately with Somersize Ketchup.

Variation

For extra-crunchy onion rings, dip egg-coated onion rings in Somersize Bake and Fry Mix (page 235) before deep frying.

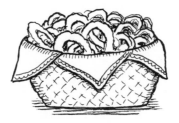

Cauliflower "Tater" Tots

PRO/FATS AND VEGGIES—LEVEL ONE

MAKES 50 TOTS

The Irish girl in me is always looking for ways to eat potatoes, or to at least trick my body into thinking it's eating potatoes. These "Tater" Tots are made with cauliflower, and they really do the trick. After you pipe them out, freeze them before you bake them. This helps to retain their beautiful shape. (If you don't have time for this step, the recipe works without it.) Get out your Somersize Ketchup (p. 245) and dig in! Your kids will love them!

PREP TIME: 10 MINUTES
COOKING TIME: 20 MINUTES

1 (1-pound) bag frozen cauliflower florets, or 1 pound fresh
2 tablespoons water
4 tablespoons (½ stick) butter, at room temperature

2 large egg yolks
1 cup grated Parmesan cheese
Salt and freshly ground black pepper

Preheat oven to 400 degrees. Place the cauliflower in a 2-quart microwave-safe casserole. Add the water to the cauliflower. Cover with plastic wrap and cook on high for 8 to 10 minutes, until very soft. Drain cauliflower and place in the work bowl of a food processor. Add butter, egg yolks, and Parmesan cheese. Process until mixture is smooth. Season with salt and pepper.

Place mixture in a piping bag fitted with a large plain tip, or put mixture in a large resealable bag and snip off a corner. Pipe cauliflower mixture in 1-inch lengths onto a greased baking sheet. Bake for 15 to 20 minutes, or until browned.

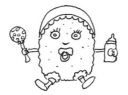

Garlic Sugar Snap Peas

PRO/FATS AND VEGGIES—LEVEL ONE

SERVES 4

Fresh sugar snap peas are a wonderful vegetable. Caroline served me these with her Ginger Scallion Grilled Mahi-Mahi (p. 283). The peas are loaded up with garlic and quickly stir-fried in olive oil. I have a daughter-in-law that I absolutely adore . . . and she's an awesome cook! I guess Bruce and I both lucked out.

PREP TIME: 3 MINUTES
COOKING TIME: 5 MINUTES

1 pound sugar snap peas
3 tablespoons olive oil
5 cloves garlic, minced

Juice of 1/2 lemon
Salt
White pepper

Wash and trim the snap peas. Place a sauté pan on medium-high heat. When hot, add the oil and the garlic and sauté for 1 minute. Add the snap peas and sauté until bright green and tender, about 3 minutes. Squeeze the lemon juice over the snap peas, then season with salt and white pepper to taste. Serve immediately.

Broiled Tomatoes

PRO/FATS AND VEGGIES—LEVEL ONE

SERVES 4

I am a tomato junkie. I eat them all the time—cooked, raw, baked, candied, grilled, and broiled. Speaking of broiled, here's a fast and easy broiled tomato that turns a simple chicken breast dinner into something special. You can use my Somersize Bake and Fry Mix (p. 235), or the following combination of Parmesan cheese and thyme.

2 tomatoes
2 tablespoons olive oil
Salt and freshly ground black pepper

¼ cup grated Parmesan cheese
1 teaspoon dried thyme

Slice the tomatoes in half crosswise. Place the tomatoes on a baking sheet, cut side up. Pour oil over the tomatoes. Sprinkle with salt, pepper, Parmesan cheese, and thyme. Broil for 5 minutes, or until the topping gets golden brown and bubbly. Serve immediately.

Cumin-Scented Zucchini

PRO/FATS AND VEGGIES—LEVEL ONE

SERVES 4

Toasting the cumin before adding the oil helps to release the heady aroma of the spice. Try this side dish with my In a Hurry Beef Curry (p. 270) or Moroccan Chicken (Eat Great, Lose Weight, p. 162).

6 medium zucchini (about 1 pound)
1 tablespoon cumin
3 tablespoons olive oil

3 cloves garlic, minced
Salt and freshly ground black pepper
Lemon wedges

Cut zucchini in half lengthwise. Cut each half into 2 pieces horizontally. Slice each strip into ½-inch pieces. Each piece will be triangular in shape.

Heat a 10-inch nonstick sauté pan over medium heat. Add cumin and stir for 10 seconds (to bring out the flavor). Add oil and heat for 30 seconds. Add garlic. Add zucchini. Turn heat to high and sauté for 2 minutes. Season with salt and pepper. Squeeze lemon juice over zucchini and serve.

Celery Root Purée

PRO/FATS AND VEGGIES—LEVEL ONE

SERVES 4

Adding chicken stock gives the celery root extra flavor. I have had a version of this in every book because it is a life-saving side dish for Somersizers. Try this with my Pot Roast . . . mmm, mmm.

PREP TIME: 2 MINUTES
COOKING TIME: 5 MINUTES

3 large celery roots
1 cup chicken stock
4 tablespoons (½ stick) unsalted butter, softened
¼ cup heavy cream, warmed

Salt and freshly ground black pepper

EQUIPMENT
Pressure cooker

Place steamer insert in the bottom of a 6-quart pressure cooker pan. Peel the celery root and cut into 1-inch pieces. Put celery roots on the steamer insert. Add chicken stock. Lock lid into place. Bring to pressure over high heat. Reduce heat and cook for 5 minutes. Use quick-steam-release method.

Drain celery root into a colander, then place in a food processor along with butter and cream. Purée until smooth. Season with salt and pepper before serving. Celery root can also be mashed with a potato masher.

Alternate Oven or Stovetop Method
You do not need the chicken stock for this method. Place about 5 cups of water in a large pot fitted with a steamer and a lid. Bring to a boil. Peel the celery root and cut into 1-inch pieces, then place on a steamer rack. Steam until very soft when poked with a fork, about 20 minutes. Transfer the celery root to a food processor. Add cream and butter and purée until smooth. Add additional cream or butter to achieve desired consistency. Season with salt and pepper.

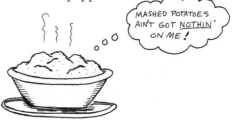

MASHED POTATOES AIN'T GOT NOTHIN' ON ME!

Zucchini Noodles Alfredo

PRO/FATS & VEGGIES—LEVEL ONE

MAKES 4 SERVINGS

Think your kids don't like zucchini? Think again. Zucchini noodles instead of pasta . . . what a revelation! In my last book, Eat, Cheat, and Melt the Fat Away, *I had a couple of recipes for zucchini noodles, one with pesto and one with meatballs and sauce. This creamy alfredo version is a real family favorite.*

PREP TIME: 5 MINUTES
COOKING TIME: 14 MINUTES

12 medium zucchini
2 tablespoons olive oil
6 cloves garlic, minced
2 cups heavy cream
2 tablespoons butter

1 cup grated Parmesan cheese
$\frac{1}{2}$ teaspoon salt
$\frac{1}{2}$ teaspoon freshly ground black pepper
2–3 tablespoons fresh chives, for garnish (optional)

With a sharp vegetable peeler, make long noodles by starting at the top of the zucchini and "peeling" ribbons down the length of the zucchini. Continue making ribbons as you turn the zucchini to get all the green part off first. Keep making ribbons until the center portion becomes too thin to peel. Set aside noodles.

Heat a medium saucepan. Add the olive oil and garlic and sauté for 1 to 2 minutes. Add the cream. Bring to a boil, then reduce heat and simmer until the mixture has a saucelike consistency, about 12 minutes.

Meanwhile, heat a large skillet on medium high and add the butter and zucchini noodles. Sauté noodles for 2 to 3 minutes.

Stir the Parmesan cheese into the sauce mixture until melted. Remove from heat. Season with the salt and pepper. Pour over zucchini noodles and toss to coat. Sprinkle with chives if desired.

Lemony Artichokes

SERVES 4

These make a great appetizer or first course and are perfect with my Artichoke and Onion Dip (p. 196). You may also use baby artichokes for this recipe. Serve four to five whole baby artichokes per person.

PREP TIME: 8 MINUTES
COOKING TIME: 3 MINUTES

4 medium artichokes, or 16 baby
   artichokes
2 lemons
2 tablespoons extra-virgin olive oil
2 cloves garlic, chopped
1 bay leaf
1 teaspoon whole black peppercorns

1 cup chicken or vegetable broth
1/2 cup white wine
1 teaspoon salt
5 sprigs parsley

EQUIPMENT
Pressure cooker

Using scissors, remove sharp tips from artichoke leaves. Cut each into quarters. Remove the choke. For baby artichokes, cut off tips only if your artichokes have sharp tips. Cut each artichoke in half. Place artichokes into a large bowl. Squeeze the juice from both lemons over artichokes and toss well. Reserve the lemon shells.

Heat oil in the pan of a pressure cooker (at least 6 quarts) over medium heat. Add garlic and sauté for 1 minute. Add artichokes, lemon shells, and remaining ingredients to pressure cooker. Lock lid in place. Bring to pressure over high heat. Reduce heat and cook for 3 minutes. Allow steam to release slowly.

Remove bay leaf and parsley. Place artichokes on a serving platter. Cool for 5 minutes before serving.

Alternate Stovetop Method
Prepare artichokes with lemon as descibed.

Heat oil in a large pot with tight-fitting lid over medium heat. Add garlic and sauté for 1 minute. Add artichokes, lemon shells, and remaining ingredients to pot. Bring liquid to a boil. Cover pot and reduce heat to low. Cook for 30–45 minutes, depending upon size (20 minutes for baby artichokes).

Remove bay leaf and parsley sprig. Place artichokes on a serving platter. Allow to cool for 5 minutes before serving.

Vegetable Fritters

PRO/FATS AND VEGGIES—LEVEL ONE

MAKES 4 FRITTERS

When you make a great side dish, your entrée can be simple as can be. Serve these vegetable fritters with a piece of London broil, a grilled chicken breast, or pan-fried lamb chops. They also go nicely with In a Hurry Beef Curry (p. 270).

PREP TIME: 4 MINUTES
COOKING TIME: 4 MINUTES

1/2 cup dehydrated onions
1 cup finely chopped vegetables
  (mushrooms, broccoli, zucchini, fennel,
  and bell peppers)

1 large egg white, beaten
Salt and freshly ground black pepper
Peanut or canola oil for frying

Place dehydrated onions in the bowl of a food processor and process for 1 minute.

Mix chopped vegetables with egg white. Season with salt and pepper. Stir in onions. Divide mixture into 4 portions and press to make patties.

Heat 1/4 inch oil in a skillet over medium heat. Fry fritters in hot oil until golden brown and crispy. Drain on paper towels. Serve hot.

Sweet Braised Leeks

PRO/FATS AND VEGGIES—LEVEL ONE

SERVES 4

I am a leek freak. These are sweet and buttery and oh so lovely! Serve with a piece of seared white fish on top for a fabulous dinner.

PREP TIME: 2 MINUTES
COOKING TIME: 14 MINUTES

1 teaspoon SomerSweet
1 cup chicken broth
4 large leeks, washed well and dark green tops discarded

2 tablespoons unsalted butter
1 tablespoon olive oil
1 cup red onions, halved and sliced thin
Salt and freshly ground black pepper

Dissolve SomerSweet in chicken broth and set aside. Cut leeks in half lengthwise, clean well, and set aside.

Heat butter and olive oil in a large skillet over medium heat. Add onions and sauté until soft and beginning to brown, about 5 minutes. Push onions to the sides of the skillet. Place leeks, cut side down, in a single layer in skillet. Let cook for 2 minutes. Pour chicken broth mixture over leeks. Bring to a boil, cover, and reduce heat. Cook for 6 minutes. Remove leeks and cover with foil to keep warm. Raise heat to high and cook sauce for 2 to 3 minutes, until thickened slightly. Spoon sauce over leeks before serving.

Alternate Microwave Method

In a glass baking dish, heat butter, oil, and onions on high for 2 minutes. Add leeks and chicken broth mixture. Cover with plastic wrap and heat on high for 3 minutes. Remove leeks and cover with foil to keep warm. Heat remaining sauce on high for 4 minutes to thicken slightly. Spoon sauce over leeks before serving. Season with salt and pepper.

Note on Cleaning Leeks

Remove the tough outer leaves and trim off most of the green part. Don't cut the root end yet. Cut leek in half lengthwise. Holding leek by the root end, place under cold running water and fan out the top part of the leek to rinse out any hidden dirt. Shake off excess water and cut off the roots.

Hometown Favorites

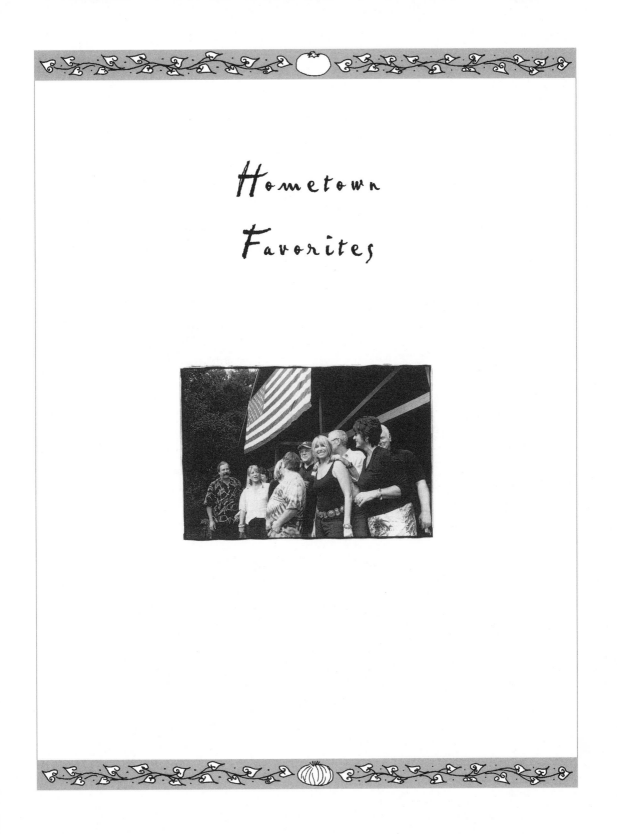

Somersize Shake It and Bake It Chicken

PRO/FATS AND VEGGIES—LEVEL ONE

SERVES 4

This is the heart of America—chicken that is coated, crispy, and baked to a golden brown. Nothing tastes more hometown than this. This recipe can be made with any part of the chicken, with or without skin, with or without bones. Great for picnics with my Crunchy Coleslaw (p. 220)!

PREP TIME: 5 MINUTES
COOKING TIME: 18 MINUTES

1 whole chicken fryer, cut up
2 cups Somersize Bake and Fry Mix
   (p. 235)

4 large eggs, beaten
Oil for misting

Heat oven to 375 degrees. Line a baking sheet with aluminum foil. Set aside.

Put Somersize Bake and Fry Mix in a large resealable bag. Dip one piece of chicken in beaten eggs, then place in resealable bag. Seal bag and shake to coat chicken. Place on paper towels. Repeat with the other chicken pieces.

Place chicken on prepared baking sheet. Lightly mist chicken with oil. Bake until golden brown, about 18 minutes. Serve hot or cold.

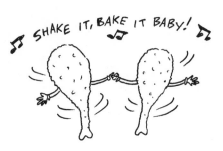

Somersize Bake and Fry Mix

PRO/FATS AND VEGGIES—LEVEL ONE

MAKES 1¼ CUPS

In every book I have a couple of recipes that are Somersize heroes. This is simply inspired, if I do say so myself! This incredible coating tricks you into thinking you are having bread crumbs. All you do is take your chicken, shrimp, fish, or pork chops and dip them in beaten egg, then shake them in a bag with Somersize Bake and Fry Mix. Then you just bake it or fry it! You'll love it!

PREP TIME: 2 MINUTES

2 cups dehydrated onion, about 5 ounces
2 teaspoons salt
½ teaspoon black pepper
½ teaspoon ground sage
1 teaspoon dried rosemary
1 teaspoon dried coriander

1 teaspoon dried thyme
½ teaspoon dried oregano
½ teaspoon paprika
¼ teaspoon red pepper flakes
2 bay leaves, crushed
1¼ cups grated Parmesan cheese

Put the dehydrated onion in the work bowl of a food processor. Process for 1 minute. Add the rest of the ingredients except the cheese and process for 30 seconds more. Add Parmesan and pulse to blend. Store refrigerated in an airtight container for 2 weeks.

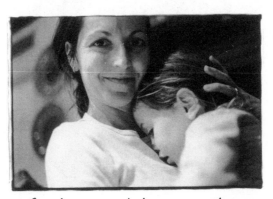

Caroline, one of the great mothers.

Somersize Chicken Nuggets

PRO/FATS AND VEGGIES—LEVEL ONE

SERVES 4

Kids love chicken nuggets dipped in ketchup or barbecue sauce. Now you can make them at home the Somersize way. Look for my line of condiments at SuzanneSomers.com.

4 boneless, skinless chicken breasts
Peanut oil for frying
4 large eggs, beaten
2 cups Somersize Bake and Fry Mix (p. 235)

EQUIPMENT
Deep Fryer

Cut chicken into 2 × 2-inch nuggets. Heat oil to 375 degrees in a deep fryer or deep pot. Dip the nuggets into the beaten egg, then roll in the Somersize Bake and Fry Mix. Fry in hot oil until deep, golden brown, about 5 minutes. Drain on paper towels. Serve immediately.

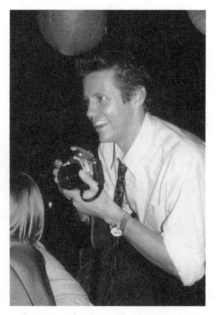

Bruce, the family historian.

Somersize Fish and Chips

PRO/FATS AND VEGGIES—LEVEL ONE

SERVES 4

Holy codfish! This is one of those "I can't believe I can eat this and still lose weight" recipes. Hot and crunchy, fresh and tasty. The "chips" are lovely zucchini fries. Serve with Somersize Tartar Sauce (p. 244) and Somersize Ketchup (p. 245).

PREP TIME: 2 MINUTES
COOKING TIME: 21 MINUTES

8 medium zucchini
2 pounds white fish (cod, orange roughy, mahi-mahi, red snapper, etc.)
6 eggs, beaten
4 cups Somersize Bake and Fry Mix (p. 235)

Peanut oil for deep frying

EQUIPMENT
Deep fryer

Preheat oven to 300 degrees. Heat oil to 375 degrees in a deep fryer or a large deep pot.

Cut zucchini into quarter-inch sticks. Set aside. Cut fish into 3 × 1-inch lengths. Set aside. Dip zucchini into beaten eggs, then roll in Somersize Bake and Fry Mix. Fry in hot oil until deep golden brown, about 3 minutes. Drain on paper towels. Place on a baking sheet and put in oven to keep warm.

Dip fish pieces in egg. Roll in Somersize Bake and Fry Mix. Fry, a few pieces at a time, in hot oil until deep golden brown, about 5 to 6 minutes. Drain on paper towels.

Serve with zucchini fries.

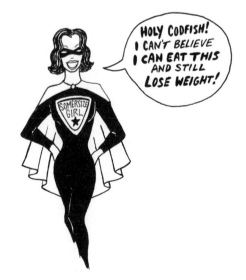

Chicken Pot Pie

PRO/FATS—LEVEL TWO

SERVES 4 TO 6

Chicken Pot Pie is one of those comfort foods that makes you feel like everything is going to be okay. My son, Bruce, always loved when I made him this delicious dinner. It's inherently un-Somersized because it's chicken and a crust, a combination of Pro/Fats and Carbos. That being said, I am known for my Chicken Pot Pie! When you feel like having a Level Two treat, try this recipe. It's a much better option than a pot pie with a crust made from white flour. It's great to make with leftover roasted chicken or reserved boiled chicken from making chicken stock. But it is also great with fresh boneless skinless chicken breasts. The end result looks intimidating, but it's really fast as can be. I swirl the thin, crispy layers into a beautiful rosette. It's almost too pretty to eat! You can prepare this the night before up to the point of putting the crust on top of the pie. Your family will love it, but it's pretty enough to serve to company. Enjoy!

PREP TIME: 10 MINUTES
COOKING TIME: 35 MINUTES

1 package whole-wheat phyllo dough, thawed
6 tablespoons olive oil
3 boneless, skinless chicken breasts cut into 1-inch fingers (or you can use 3 cups of boiled chicken or 3 cups of leftover roast chicken)
3 yellow onions, thinly sliced
1 clove garlic, chopped
2 sweet red peppers, thinly sliced, then cut in half

2 tablespoons butter
1 tablespoon whole-wheat flour
2 cups chicken broth
1/4 teaspoon red pepper flakes (or less to taste)
1/2 teaspoon salt (or more to taste)
Freshly ground black pepper
1 stick butter, melted (for phyllo crust)

Preheat oven to 350 degrees.

Heat a medium-size sauté pan (with straight sides) on high heat. Add olive oil.

If using raw chicken, sauté in olive oil until browned and cooked through, about 5 minutes. Remove with slotted spoon and reserve on plate.

Add sliced onions and fry them on medium heat for 15 minutes until golden brown. Add garlic and sauté for 2 minutes. Add sliced red peppers and sauté for 5 minutes more.

Add 2 tablespoons butter and stir it into the mixture. Add the whole-wheat flour and cook 2 minutes, stirring constantly. Then add the chicken broth, red pepper flakes, salt, and pepper. Reduce liquid for 5 minutes more. Add chicken meat and cook for another 2 to 5 minutes. Sauce should be thickened and brown in color. Place the hot filling in a baking dish.

This recipe can be made in advance up to this point. Reheat the filling before assembling the phyllo crust. When you are ready to assemble the pie, brush 5 sheets of whole-wheat phyllo with melted butter and arrange the phyllo atop the filling to resemble a flower (as pictured in photo demonstration).

Bake for 10 minutes (watch carefully). The crust should be lightly browned and crisp.

Serve immediately.

Mini-Pepperoni Pizzas

PRO/FATS AND VEGGIES—LEVEL ONE

MAKES 6 MINI-PIZZAS

My ladies on the website at SuzanneSomers.com inspired this pizza. I tried to contact the original creator of the cream cheese crust, but I never got a reply. Whoever you are, you are a super Somersizer! You've started a Somersize pizza revolution! Somersizers around the globe are now making "legal" pizza. Here's my version. Feel free to add whatever toppings you like. Since our ovens at home don't get as hot as pizza ovens, it adds a lot of flavor if you sauté your toppings first.

PREP TIME: 6 MINUTES
COOKING TIME: 25 MINUTES
COOLING TIME: 10 MINUTES

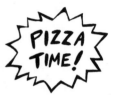

FOR THE CRUST
1 (8-ounce) package cream cheese, at room
   temperature
2 eggs
Salt and freshly ground black pepper
$1/4$ cup grated Parmesan cheese

FOR THE PIZZA
$1/3$ cup jarred Somersize Marinara Sauce
Pinch of cayenne pepper
$1/2$ teaspoon oregano
$1/2$ cup shredded mozzarella cheese
6 ounces pepperoni, sautéed

Preheat oven to 350 degrees. Butter a 9 × 13-inch baking dish. Set aside.

In a medium bowl, blend together cream cheese and eggs with a wooden spoon. Season with salt and pepper. Add Parmesan cheese and stir until combined. Pour into prepared baking dish. Bake for 17 minutes, or until golden brown. Let cream cheese crust cool for 10 minutes.

Meanwhile, mix together marinara sauce, cayenne pepper, and oregano. Set aside.

Raise heat to 400 degrees. Using a 4-inch round cookie cutter, and leaving the cream cheese crust in the baking dish, cut 6 rounds out of the crust. Discard the extra pieces of crust, leaving the 6 rounds in place. Top each crust with marinara sauce, cheese, and pepperoni. Bake for 8 minutes, or until cheese is bubbly.

SomerSails

SERVES 4

Your kids will love this! These darling zucchini boats are filled with your choice of ground beef, chicken, or turkey mixture that hark back to Sloppy Joes. Then they're topped with cheddar cheese sails. Dive in—they're delicious.

PREP TIME: 12 MINUTES
COOKING TIME: 12 MINUTES

4 medium zucchini
2 tablespoons olive oil
Salt and freshly ground black pepper
1 cup chopped onion
1 clove garlic, minced

1 pound ground turkey, chicken, or beef
1 packet Somersize Taco Seasoning, or
  your favorite packaged seasoning mix
1 cup jarred Somersize Marinara Sauce
4 slices cheddar cheese

Preheat oven to 350 degrees. Trim ends from zucchini. Using a vegetable peeler, remove a thin 2-inch section of peel from each zucchini to make a flat bottom. This will be the underside of the SomerSails. With a melon scoop or sharp paring knife, remove enough pulp from the other side to make a ½-inch-deep channel along the length of the zucchini. Take care not to cut all the way through.

Brush the inside of the zucchini with a tablespoon of the olive oil. Season with salt and pepper. Place the zucchini on a baking sheet. Bake for 10 minutes.

Meanwhile, heat the remaining table-spoon of oil in a sauté pan. Add onion and

sauté for 3 minutes. Add garlic and ground meat. Sauté for 5 minutes, or until meat has browned. Add Somersize Taco Seasoning Mix and Somersize Marinara Sauce. Bring to a boil. Reduce heat and simmer for 3 minutes.

To make sails, cut each slice of cheese in half diagonally twice, making 4 triangles. Using wooden skewers, pierce the cheese along a straight edge in two places to form a sail. Trim excess skewer with scissors.

Spoon meat mixture into each cooked zucchini boat. Place a sail into the base of each zucchini. Serve immediately before the cheese sail melts.

Somersize Macaroni and Cheese

PRO/FATS—LEVEL ONE

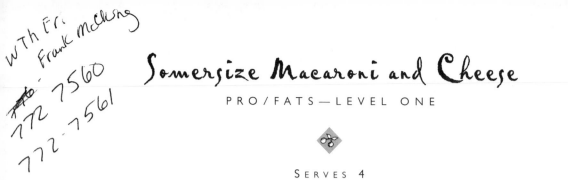

SERVES 4

Who says macaroni and cheese needs to come in a blue box! And who says it even needs macaroni? In this version I use Alan mother's awesome Egg Crêpes to make Somersize "noodles." Egg Crêpes take only a few minutes to make. I like to make a big batch and keep them in the freezer to thaw for dishes like this. Then a simple homemade cheese sauce tops it all off. This is a great dish to make ahead of time, but make sure to reheat this in the oven, not the microwave, or the cream will separate.

PREP TIME: 2 MINUTES
COOKING TIME: 32 MINUTES

Unsalted butter for greasing baking dish
4 cups heavy cream
2½ cups shredded cheddar cheese
Pinch of nutmeg

Pinch of ground cayenne pepper
8 Egg Crêpes (p. 188), sliced into ¼-inch strips
Salt and freshly ground black pepper

Preheat oven to 350 degrees. Butter an 8 × 8-inch glass baking dish. Set aside.

Place cream in a heavy medium saucepan. Bring to a boil, reduce heat slightly, and let boil gently for 10 minutes, or until reduced by half. Lower heat and add 1½ cups of cheddar cheese, nutmeg, and cayenne. Stir until the cheese melts and sauce is smooth.

Place sliced crêpes in prepared baking dish. Pour sauce over crêpes and stir to coat. Top with the remaining cheese. Bake for 20 minutes, or until cheese is bubbly and beginning to brown. Season with salt and pepper. Serve hot.

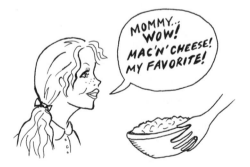

The Somersize Recipes

Somersize Double Double Cheeseburgers

PRO/FATS AND VEGGIES—LEVEL ONE

MAKES 4

There is a fast food restaurant in Los Angeles that serves this burger for all those who are trying to eliminate carbohydrates with their proteins. This burger is a Somersizer's dream. This is my "ode to the fast-food burger." Double burger, double cheese with fried onions, please . . . yes, we're Somersizing! Try these with my Secret Sauce and you'll never miss the bun and fries.

PREP TIME: 3 MINUTES
COOKING TIME: 7 MINUTES

1½ pounds ground sirloin
Salt and freshly ground black pepper
2 tablespoons olive oil
8 slices American cheese
1 head iceberg or limestone lettuce, leaves
    washed and separated

1 red onion, sliced
1 large tomato, sliced
8 dill pickle slices
8 tablespoons Somersize Secret Sauce
    (p. 244, or jarred)

Preheat broiler.

Form ground beef into 8 wide, thin patties. Season liberally with salt and pepper. Heat olive oil in a large skillet over medium-high heat. Add patties and cook for 3 minutes per side, or until meat is cooked through. Turn heat to very low.

Place the burgers on a baking sheet. Top each with a slice of cheese. Place under broiler until cheese melts. Remove from broiler.

Lay 4 large lettuce leaves on a work surface. Top each with 1 burger. Place a slice of onion and tomato and 2 slices of pickle on top of each. Generously spoon on the Somersize Secret Sauce. Stack the other 4 burgers on top to create 4 Double Doubles.

Top with more sauce, if desired. Add another lettuce leaf on top, then fold lettuce over the burgers. Wrap burgers in paper napkins and serve immediately.

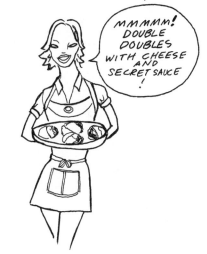

Hometown Favorites
243

Somersize Secret Sauce

LEVEL ONE

MAKES 1 CUP

Nothing makes a burger like Somersize Secret Sauce. Now you can have it without the sugar! You can buy my Somersize Secret Sauce ready-made, or use this easy recipe to make your own. Make sure to look for dill relish in your grocery store. Don't use sweet relish—it's loaded with sugar!

PREP TIME: 2 MINUTES

$^1/_2$ cup tomato paste
1 teaspoon SomerSweet
$^1/_2$ cup mayonnaise

1 tablespoon plus 1 teaspoon dill pickle
  relish
Salt and freshly ground black pepper

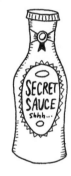

Place tomato paste, SomerSweet, mayonnaise, and relish in a mixing bowl. Stir thoroughly. Season lightly with salt and pepper. Store refrigerated in an airtight container. Keeps for about a week.

Somersize Tartar Sauce

PRO/FATS AND VEGGIES—LEVEL ONE

MAKES 1$^1/_2$ CUPS

Again, here's a condiment that is hard to find without sugar. Somersize Tartar Sauce is made with SomerSweet and it tastes great with Somersize Fish and Chips (p. 237). Buy mine at Suzanne Somers.com or make it yourself.

1 cup mayonnaise
1/3 cup dill pickle relish
1/4 teaspoon Worcestershire sauce
1 tablespoon finely chopped onion

2 teaspoons chopped fresh dill (optional)
2 tablespoons lemon juice
Salt and freshly ground black pepper
   to taste

Place all ingredients in a mixing bowl. Stir until well blended. Store in refrigerator in an airtight container. It will keep for 5 or 6 days.

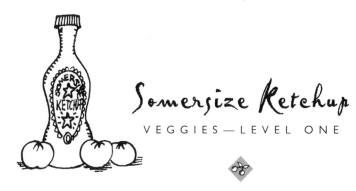

Somersize Ketchup
VEGGIES—LEVEL ONE

MAKES 1 1/2 QUARTS

Regular ketchup is made up of more than 25 percent sugar! My Somersize Ketchup is made with SomerSweet. You can buy it on my website, or make your own.

2 cups apple cider vinegar
1 cinnamon stick
1 teaspoon whole black peppercorns
1/4 teaspoon whole allspice
1 (28-ounce) can tomato sauce
1 (12-ounce) can tomato paste

3 tablespoons SomerSweet
1/4 teaspoon Worcestershire sauce
1 teaspoon lemon juice
Salt and freshly ground black pepper
   to taste

Combine vinegar, cinnamon, peppercorns, and allspice in a small saucepan. Bring ingredients to a boil over medium heat. Boil for 2 minutes. Remove from heat. Cover pan and allow mixture to steep for 1 hour.

Pour mixture through a fine sieve into a large stainless-steel mixing bowl. Discard the cinnamon, allspice, and peppercorns. Add tomato sauce, tomato paste, Somer-Sweet, Worcestershire sauce, and lemon juice to seasoned mixture. Stir until smooth. Season with salt and pepper. Store covered in the refrigerator.

Turkey Chili Cheese Fries

PRO/FATS AND VEGGIES—LEVEL ONE

SERVES 6 TO 8

American Graffiti . . . Richard Dreyfuss . . . and a whisper from the blonde in the Thunderbird, "I love you." Do you think I was talking about Richard or the chili fries from Mel's Drive-In? This dish will tantalize your taste buds and send you on a trip down memory lane where we used to meet at the diner to share a heaping mound of french fries covered with chili and cheese. Those were the days. When I'm feeling nostalgic, I make these awesome zucchini fries and cover them with my Twenty-Minute Chili (p. 265), made with ground turkey, and cheese. Doo-wop, doo-wop, doo-wop.

PREP TIME: 4 MINUTES
COOKING TIME: 15 MINUTES

8 to 10 medium zucchini
Peanut oil for frying
4 eggs, beaten
2 cups grated Parmesan cheese, or 2 cups
  Somersize Bake and Fry Mix (p. 235)
1 recipe Twenty-Minute Chili
  made with ground turkey

2 cups shredded cheddar cheese

EQUIPMENT
Deep fryer

Trim ends from zucchini. Cut each zucchini in half lengthwise. Cut each half into 3 strips to form fries.

Heat oil to 375 degrees in a deep fryer or large deep pot. Dip fries into beaten egg. Coat fries with Parmesan cheese or Somersize Bake and Fry Mix. Cook in hot oil until golden brown. Place fries on individual plates or in shallow bowls. Spoon turkey chili over fries and sprinkle with cheddar cheese. Allow cheese to melt slightly before serving.

Turkey Taco Wraps

PRO/FATS AND VEGGIES—LEVEL ONE

MAKES 4

Tacos are such crowd pleasers. These are made with ground turkey, then wrapped in a lettuce leaf. For Level Two you may wrap them in whole-wheat tortillas. Kids love them! Make them with my Somersize Tex Mex Blend, or my packaged Somersize Taco Seasoning.

PREP TIME: 6 MINUTES
COOKING TIME: 10 MINUTES

1 tablespoon olive oil
1/3 cup diced red onion
1 pound ground turkey
2 teaspoons Somersize Tex Mex Seasoning
   Blend (p. 275), or 1 packet Somersize
   Taco Seasoning
1/2 teaspoon salt
1/2 cup diced tomato

1/3 cup sliced scallions
1/4 cup chopped cilantro
1 jalapeño, seeded and finely chopped
   (optional)
1 head of iceberg or butter lettuce
1 cup shredded cheddar cheese
Sour cream and salsa, for garnish

Place a large skillet over medium-high heat. Add oil and onions. Sauté for 3 to 4 minutes, until onions become translucent. Add turkey and sauté until brown, about 5 minutes. Add Tex Mex Seasoning Blend and salt. Cook for 1 minute more. Remove from heat and stir in tomato, scallions, cilantro, and jalapeño.

Lay 2 lettuce leaves on a clean work sur-face. Spoon 1/4 cup cheese, 2/3 cup ground turkey mixture, salsa, and sour cream onto the lettuce. Roll up lettuce leaves in cone shapes.

For Level Two:
Instead of lettuce leaves, place ingredients down the center of a whole-wheat tortilla.

Vegetable Calzones

MAKES 4

With a whole-wheat crust and a nonfat ricotta cheese and spinach filling, you can make a Level One calzone—and it's yummy! For Level Two we add the full-fat cheeses, like mozzarella and Parmesan, for a more traditional gooey calzone. You'll need a bread maker to make the crust.

PREP TIME: 5 MINUTES
BREAD MAKER/PROOFING TIME: 1 1/2 HOURS
BAKING TIME: 25 MINUTES

FOR THE DOUGH
3 cups whole-wheat flour, plus more for
   dusting
3/4 teaspoon salt
1 cup nonfat milk
1/4 cup nonfat yogurt

2 1/4 teaspoons bread machine yeast, or
   1 packet active dry yeast
1 recipe Spinach Ricotta Filling (p. 249)

EQUIPMENT
Bread maker

Mix together whole-wheat flour and salt. Set aside.

Place nonfat milk and nonfat yogurt in a small saucepan. Heat on low until mixture reaches a temperature of 120 degrees on a thermometer. Pour mixture into bread maker. Add dry ingredients. Make a 1-inch well in the center of the dry mixture. Sprinkle in yeast. Set machine to dough cycle and start.

When cycle is complete, preheat oven to 375 degrees. Remove dough and place on a lightly floured surface. Cut into 4 equal portions. Form each piece of dough into a flat disk. Roll each disk into a circle about 10 inches in diameter. Place a quarter of the Spinach Ricotta Filling on one side of the dough, leaving 3/4-inch border. Brush border with water. Fold dough over filling to make a half circle. Seal the edges together. Bake for 10 minutes. Remove from oven, cover with foil, and bake for an additional 15 minutes.

For a glossy sheen brush calzone with beaten egg white before baking.

Spinach Ricotta Filling

PRO/FATS AND VEGGIES—LEVEL ONE

FILLS 4 CALZONES

This classic mixture is traditionally used to stuff raviolis, to layer lasagna, or to fill calzones. It's Level One on its own, but when you add it to carbohydrates, it becomes Level Two. If you'd like to make an Almost Level One calzone, use this filling but omit the mozzarella and Parmesan cheeses and use egg white only.

PREP TIME: 2 MINUTES

2 (10-ounce) packages frozen chopped spinach, thawed and drained
3 cups ricotta cheese
3 cups shredded mozzarella cheese
1 cup grated Parmesan cheese
2 cup chopped onions

5 cloves garlic, minced
$\frac{1}{4}$ teaspoon nutmeg
2 teaspoons salt
$\frac{1}{2}$ teaspoon black pepper
3 large eggs, beaten

Mix all ingredients together in a large mixing bowl. Store refrigerated in an airtight container until use.

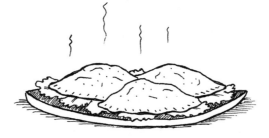

Chicken Fried Steak with Creamy Mushroom Sauce

PRO/FATS AND VEGGIES—LEVEL ONE

SERVES 4

Nothing says Middle America like chicken fried steak. But you won't find any white flour or thick goopy sauces in this one, just a delicious creamy mushroom sauce over a crispy fried steak.

PREP TIME: 5 MINUTES
COOKING TIME: 6 MINUTES

1 pound beef tip steak
2 large eggs, beaten
2 cups Somersize Bake and Fry Mix (p. 235) or 2 cups grated Parmesan cheese

Oil for frying
1 recipe Creamy Mushroom Sauce (p. 251)

Cut steak into 4 even portions. Place steak between 2 sheets of plastic wrap. Using a meat tenderizer or a small heavy frying pan, pound meat until 1/2 inch thick. Dry meat with paper towels.

Place eggs in a mixing bowl. Place Somersize Bake and Fry Mix in a second mixing bowl. Dip steaks in egg and then coat in Somersize Bake and Fry Mix. Repeat with remaining steaks.

Heat 1/2 inch of oil in a large skillet. Add steaks and cook until coating is golden brown, about 2 to 3 minutes on each side.

Serve with hot Creamy Mushroom Sauce.

Creamy Mushroom Sauce

PRO/FATS AND VEGGIES—LEVEL ONE

SERVES 6

This versatile sauce will dress up any grilled chicken breast or meat. Try it on my Chicken Fried Steak (p. 250). For a spicier variation, try adding cracked peppercorns, or for fish add a handful of capers.

PREP TIME: 2 MINUTES
COOKING TIME: 19 MINUTES

3 tablespoons olive oil
6 ounces sliced mushrooms
3 cloves garlic, minced

1 cup chicken broth
1½ cups heavy cream
Salt and freshly ground black pepper

Place a large skillet over medium heat. When hot, add oil, then mushrooms. Sauté mushrooms for about 8 minutes, until they are browned and crusty. Add garlic. Sauté for an additional 2 minutes. Add chicken broth and bring to a boil, scraping any bits off the bottom of the pan. Reduce heat and simmer for 6 minutes, or until almost dry. Add cream. Bring to a boil. Let boil for 3 minutes. Remove from heat. Season with salt and pepper.

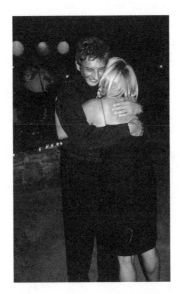

My pal Barry Manilow.

Soft Whole-Wheat Pretzels

CARBOS—ALMOST LEVEL ONE

MAKES 12

There's nothing like a soft pretzel with coarse salt and French's Yellow Mustard. Too bad they don't sell these at the ball park . . . we could Somersize and watch baseball! These are an Almost Level One treat because we combine egg whites with the Carbos.

PREP TIME: 20 MINUTES
BREAD MAKER/PROOFING TIME: 1 1/2 HOURS
RESTING TIME: 15 MINUTES
COOKING TIME: 22 MINUTES

4 cups whole-wheat flour
2 teaspoons SomerSweet
1½ teaspoons salt
1½ cups nonfat milk
3 tablespoons nonfat yogurt
1 packet (1½ ounces) active dry yeast

2 egg whites, beaten
Coarse salt

EQUIPMENT
Bread maker

Mix together flour, SomerSweet, and salt. Set aside.

Place milk and yogurt in a small saucepan. Heat on low until mixture reaches a temperature of 120 degrees on a thermometer. Place mixture in bread maker. Add flour mixture.

Make a well in the flour mixture about 1 inch deep. Pour in yeast. Set bread maker to dough cycle. Start bread maker. When cycle is completed, remove dough.

Preheat oven to 350 degrees. Cut dough into quarters. Cut each quarter into 3 pieces to make a total of 12 pieces of

dough. Roll each piece of dough into a rope 18 to 20 inches long. Allow dough to rest for 15 minutes. Bring ends together to form a circle. Pinch ends to seal. Pick up dough at seam, twist, and bring seam to lower edge of circle to form a pretzel shape. Pinch dough to secure in place. Brush pretzels with egg white. Place on a baking sheet and bake for 15 minutes. Remove from oven. Brush again with egg white and sprinkle with coarse salt. Bake for 7 minutes longer. The pretzels should be golden brown.

Poultry

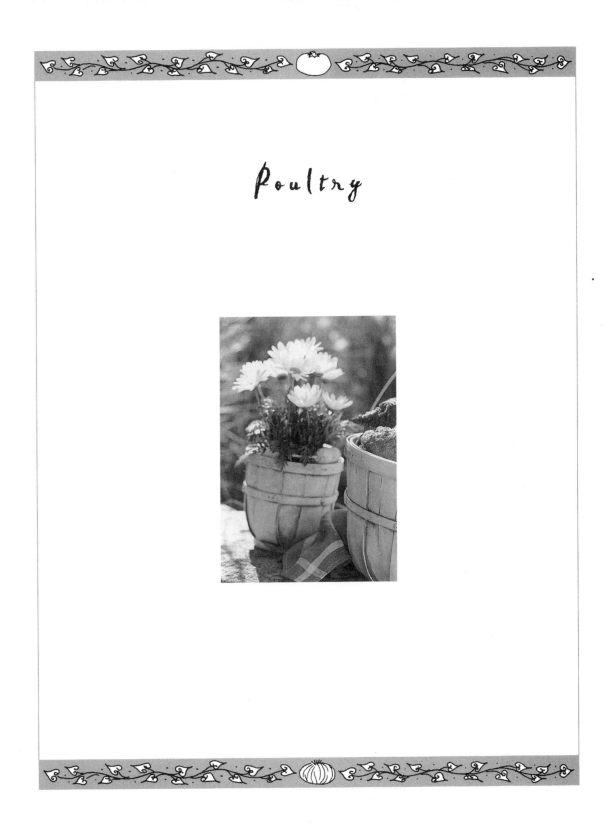

Creamy Chicken and Leek Stew

PRO/FATS AND VEGGIES—LEVEL ONE

SERVES 4

My husband, Alan, loves leeks. This is one of his favorite meals. If you're in a real time crunch, buy a roasted chicken and shred the meat.

PREP TIME: 10 MINUTES
COOKING TIME: 20 MINUTES

4 tablespoons unsalted butter
6 ounces mushrooms, sliced
4 stalks celery, chopped
3 medium leeks, thinly sliced
   (white part only)
½ cup dry white wine
1 cup heavy cream
1 (14.5-ounce) can chicken broth

4 boneless, skinless chicken breasts, cut
   into 1-inch pieces
2 tablespoons chopped fresh tarragon, or
   2 teaspoons dried
1 (8-ounce) package cream cheese, at room
   temperature
Salt and freshly ground black pepper

Heat butter in a large saucepan over high heat. Add mushrooms, celery, and leeks. Sauté, stirring constantly, for 3 minutes. Add wine, cream, and chicken broth. Bring mixture to a boil. Cook for 7 minutes. Reduce heat, add chicken and tarragon, and simmer for 10 minutes. Stir in cream cheese until blended. Season with salt and pepper.

Note on Cleaning Leeks
To clean leeks, remove the tough outer leaves and trim off most of the green part. Don't cut the root end yet. Cut leek in half lengthwise. Holding leek by the root end, place under cold running water and fan out the top part of the leek to rinse out any hidden dirt. Shake off excess water and cut off the roots.

Chicken Kiev

SERVES 4

This classic Russian dish is perfect for Somersize entertaining; a boneless chicken breast is wrapped around chilled herbed butter. Roll them a day in advance for an easy dinner party.

PREP TIME: 10 MINUTES
COOKING TIME: 19 MINUTES

4 boneless, skinless chicken breasts
Salt and freshly ground black pepper
4 tablespoons (1/2 stick) unsalted butter, chilled
2 tablespoons fresh chives or chopped whole scallions

3 large eggs, beaten
1/2 cup grated Parmesan cheese
Olive oil for frying

Preheat oven to 350 degrees. Place chicken breasts between 2 sheets of plastic wrap. Using a meat tenderizer or a small heavy saucepan, pound chicken until it is a quarter inch thick. Season chicken with salt and pepper.

Place 1 tablespoon of chilled butter in the center of each chicken breast. Sprinkle with chives or scallions. Fold the two shorter edges over the butter. Fold one of the long ends over, then the other end, forming a package. Dip in beaten egg, then dredge in cheese. (Up to this point, dish can be made a day in advance and chilled.)

Heat about 1/2 inch of oil in a large sauté pan. Place chicken breasts, seam side down, into the hot oil and cook for 2 minutes. Turn the chicken and cook on the other side for an additional 2 minutes.

Place the chicken on a baking sheet and bake for about 15 minutes. Serve immediately.

Chicken in a Balsamic Dijon Sauce

PRO/FATS AND VEGGIES—LEVEL ONE

SERVES 4

This dish is not only fast and easy, but it's also an impressive meal for your family and friends. The creamy sauce has balsamic vinegar and a hint of Dijon for a truly gourmet flavor.

PREP TIME: 2 MINUTES
COOKING TIME: 25 MINUTES

2 tablespoons unsalted butter
4 boneless, skinless chicken breasts
1/2 cup chopped onions
1 cup heavy cream

2 tablespoons balsamic vinegar
1/2 tablespoon Dijon mustard
2 tablespoons chopped fresh parsley
Salt and freshly ground black pepper

Place a large skillet over medium-high heat. When pan is hot, add butter and melt. Add chicken breasts and cook for 6 minutes. Turn chicken over and cook for another 6 minutes. Remove chicken from skillet and transfer to a plate. Cover with aluminum foil to keep warm.

Add onions to skillet and cook for 5 to 7 minutes, scraping any bits off the bottom of the pan. Add cream and vinegar. Bring mixture to a boil, reduce heat, and simmer for 4 minutes. Stir in mustard and parsley. Season with salt and pepper. Spoon sauce over chicken and serve.

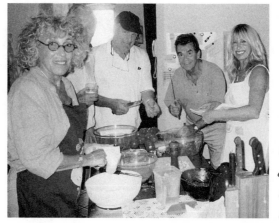

As friends, we all cook together. Susie, Alan, Guido, Dick Clark, and me.

Stuffed Bells

PRO/FATS AND VEGGIES—LEVEL ONE

SERVES 4

I love one-pot meals. These stuffed bell peppers take only 10 minutes to prepare, then they slow cook in your slow cooker, and voilà—dinner! If you have the time and would like some extra flavor, first sauté the onions and mushrooms in olive oil until they are caramelized (about 10 to 15 minutes), then add the rest of the ingredients and stuff the peppers. You may use whatever color pepper you like. I prefer red, yellow, or orange, but if you're a fan of the green, go for it. For variation, you may add a packet of my Somersize Onion Dip Mix or my Roasted Pepper Dip Mix.

PREP TIME: 10 MINUTES
SLOW COOKING TIME: 3 1/2 HOURS ON HIGH,
OR 7 HOURS ON LOW

1 pound ground turkey, chicken, or beef
1/4 cup (1/2 stick) unsalted butter, at room temperature
1/2 teaspoon salt
Pinch of cayenne pepper or 2 shakes Tabasco sauce
1/4 teaspoon black pepper
1/2 teaspoon dried oregano
1/4 teaspoon ground cumin
1 (8-ounce) can crushed tomatoes

1 medium chopped onion
6 ounces mushrooms, sliced
1 (4-ounce) can diced green chilies
4 red bell peppers, tops sliced off, membranes and seeds removed
1 cup shredded jack, mozzarella, or cheddar cheese

EQUIPMENT
Slow cooker

In a medium bowl, combine ground meat, butter, salt, cayenne and black pepper, oregano, cumin, tomatoes, onions, mushrooms, and chilies. Stuff the bell peppers with the meat mixture. Place upright in a slow cooker on high for 3 1/2 hours, or low for 7 hours. Thirty minutes before peppers are finished cooking, sprinkle each one with cheese.

Alternate Oven Method
You can also bake these in a glass baking dish for 1 hour at 350 degrees.

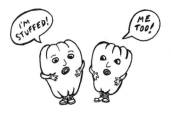

Coq au Vin

PRO/FATS AND VEGGIES—LEVEL ONE

SERVES 4

Alan and I have spent many, many summers vacationing in France. This classic dish is a French housewife's staple. It usually takes hours of braising in the red wine, herbs, and mushrooms to create the tender, falling-off-the-bone chicken. In this version I make it in my Fast and Easy Cooker, and it's quicker than running out to buy fast food. Serve with buttered green beans and watch them rave! I have also included an oven method if you do not have a pressure cooker.

PREP TIME: 5 MINUTES
COOKING TIME: 45 TO 50 MINUTES

4 slices bacon
1 to 2 tablespoons olive oil
1 whole chicken (3½ to 4 pounds), cut into 8 pieces
1 cup chopped onions
2 stalks celery, chopped
6 ounces mushrooms, sliced
4 cloves garlic, finely chopped
1½ cups dry red wine

½ cup chicken broth
1 bay leaf
6 fresh thyme sprigs, or 1 tablespoon ground
¼ cup finely minced fresh parsley
Salt and freshly ground black pepper

EQUIPMENT
Pressure cooker

In a large sauté pan, fry bacon until crisp over high heat. Remove bacon from the pan and set aside. Add olive oil to the pan. Brown chicken pieces in hot oil. Remove chicken and set aside.

Add onions to pan. Sauté for 5 to 7 minutes, until browned. Add celery and mushrooms and sauté for 7 minutes more. Add garlic and sauté for 1 minute. Pour wine and chicken broth into pan. Raise heat to

high and scrape any bits off the bottom of the pan. Remove pan from heat.

Place reserved chicken pieces in pressure cooker pot. Pour wine-vegetable mixture over chicken. Add bay leaf and thyme. Crumble reserved bacon into cooker. Lock lid into place. Bring to pressure over high heat. Reduce heat and cook for 10 minutes. Release pressure slowly.

Remove chicken and place on a serving

platter. Discard bay leaf. Add parsley to sauce. Raise heat and bring to a boil. Reduce heat and simmer until sauce is reduced by half, about 10 minutes. Season sauce with salt and pepper. Pour sauce over chicken pieces.

Alternate Oven Method

Preheat oven to 350 degrees.

Place reserved chicken pieces in a glass or ovenproof casserole dish. Pour wine-vegetable mixture over chicken. Add bay leaf and thyme. Crumble reserved bacon over chicken. Season the casserole with salt and pepper. Place casserole, uncovered, in the oven. Bake for $1\frac{1}{2}$ to 2 hours. (Chicken is cooked when a leg or thigh is cut into and the juices run clear.)

Remove chicken to a platter, keeping it warm. Remove bay leaf. Transfer sauce to a saucepan and place over high heat. Bring sauce to a boil and reduce by half, about 10 minutes. Add parsley. Season sauce with salt and pepper. Pour sauce over chicken.

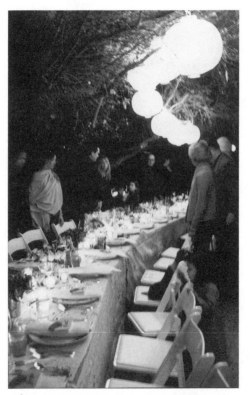

Everyone preparing to sit down for Thanksgiving dinner in the garden at our home in the desert.

Saltimbocca in a Tarragon Butter Sauce

PRO/FATS AND VEGGIES—LEVEL ONE

SERVES 4

The literal Italian translation of Saltimbocca is "jump mouth." The original Roman recipe calls for veal topped with prosciutto. In this Somersize version, I use thinly sliced chicken breasts topped with prosciutto or Black Forest ham.

PREP TIME: 10 MINUTES
COOKING TIME: 12 MINUTES

4 boneless, skinless chicken breasts
Salt and freshly ground black pepper
2 tablespoons whole fresh tarragon leaves
   plus 2 teaspoons chopped leaves
8 thin slices of prosciutto or Black Forest
   ham

½ cup (1 stick) unsalted butter
1 cup chicken broth
8 toothpicks

Cut chicken breasts horizontally to make them half as thick. Cover the 8 halves with plastic wrap. Using a meat tenderizer or a small heavy saucepan, pound chicken breasts until they are about ⅛ inch thick. Remove plastic wrap and season chicken with salt and pepper. Sprinkle whole tarragon leaves on top of chicken. Lay one slice of prosciutto on top of tarragon. Roll chicken breasts up with prosciutto on the inside. Secure with toothpicks. Season outside with salt and pepper.

Heat a large sauté pan on medium-high heat. When hot, add ½ of the stick of butter, then the chicken. Sauté chicken for 2 minutes. Turn and cook for an additional 2 minutes. Remove chicken and cover with foil to keep warm.

Add broth and 2 teaspoons chopped tarragon leaves to sauté pan, scraping any bits off the bottom of the pan. Bring to a boil. Let boil for 3 to 4 minutes. Reduce heat, add the remaining butter, and stir until butter has melted. Remove toothpicks from chicken. Return chicken to sauté pan. Simmer on low for 4 minutes, turning chicken halfway through cooking. Serve with sauce spooned over top of chicken.

Chicken Parmigiana

SERVES 4

Quick, easy dinners like this make buying a pressure cooker a must for weeknight cooking.

PREP TIME: 2 MINUTES
COOKING TIME: 5 MINUTES

2 tablespoons unsalted butter, softened
4 boneless, skinless chicken breasts
1 (32-ounce) jar Somersize Marinara
   Sauce, about 3 cups
6 ounces mushrooms, sliced
1 tablespoon Italian seasoning

Salt and freshly ground black pepper
1½ cups grated mozzarella cheese

EQUIPMENT
Pressure cooker

Grease the bottom of the pressure cooker pot with the butter. Lay the chicken breasts in a single layer on the bottom of the cooker. Pour the marinara sauce over the chicken breasts. Scatter the sliced mushrooms over the chicken breasts. Sprinkle with the Italian seasoning. Season with salt and pepper.

Divide the grated cheese into quarters and place on top of each chicken breast. Lock lid into place. Bring to pressure over high heat. Reduce heat and cook for 5 minutes. Use quick-steam-release method.

Remove lid. Serve immediately.

Alternate Oven Method
Preheat oven to 350 degrees.

Grease the bottom of a glass or oven-proof baking dish with the butter. Lay the chicken breasts in a single layer on the bottom of the dish. Pour the marinara sauce over the chicken breast. Scatter the sliced mushrooms over the chicken breasts. Sprinkle with Italian seasoning. Season with salt and pepper.

Divide the grated cheese into quarters and place on top of each chicken breast. Cover the baking dish with a lid or aluminum foil and bake for 30 to 40 minutes in the oven.

Uncover dish, and brown the tops of the chicken breasts for 5 to 10 minutes. Serve immediately.

Garlic Chicken

PRO/FATS AND VEGGIES—LEVEL ONE

SERVES 6

If you want a change of pace from regular roasted chicken, try this tasty alternative. Use my Lemon Olive Oil (p. 279) for extra flavor.

PREP TIME: 5 MINUTES

COOKING TIME: 7 MINUTES

SLOW COOKING TIME: 3 1/2 HOURS ON HIGH,
7 HOURS ON LOW

2½ to 3 pounds chicken thighs and legs
Salt and freshly ground black pepper
⅓ cup plus 2 tablespoons olive oil
1 large red onion, cut into 8 wedges
12 cloves garlic, crushed
   (about 3 tablespoons)
1 jalapeño, peeled and sliced

6 sprigs fresh rosemary
1 cup lemon juice
1 (14-ounce) can chicken broth
Lemon wedges

EQUIPMENT
Slow cooker

Rinse chicken and pat dry with paper towels. Season liberally with salt and pepper. Place a large heavy skillet over medium-high heat. When hot, add ⅓ cup olive oil. Place chicken in skillet, skin side down, and cook until skin is golden brown, about 7 minutes. Season with salt and pepper.

Put onion wedges in the bottom of slow cooker. Place chicken on top of onion wedges. (Reserve pan with chicken drip-

pings.) Sprinkle crushed garlic and jalapeño slices over chicken. Top with rosemary.

In the sauté pan containing the chicken drippings, mix together lemon juice and chicken broth. Cook for 5 to 6 minutes, scraping bits off the bottom of the pan. Pour over chicken. Drizzle with 2 table-spoons olive oil. Cover and cook on high for 3½ hours, or on low for 7 hours. Garnish with lemon wedges.

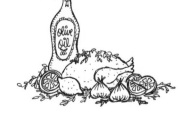

Beef

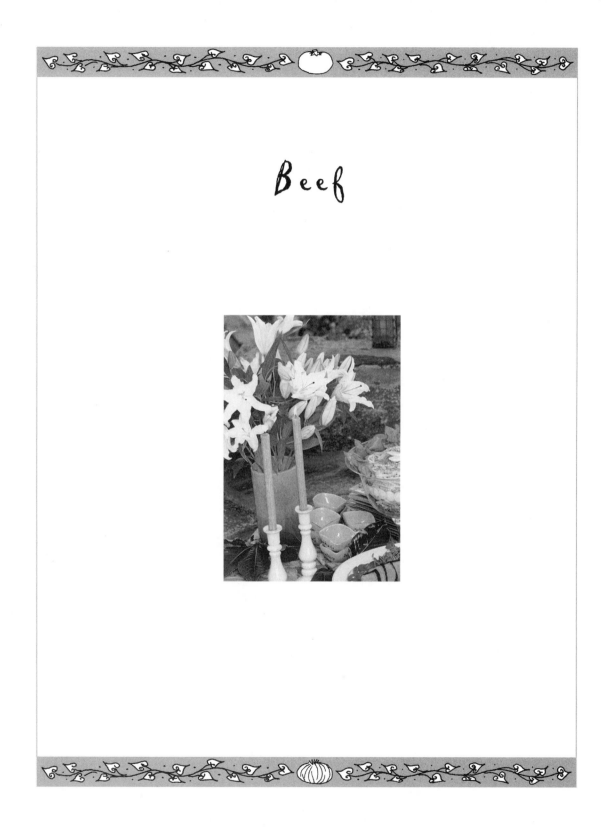

Mini-Mini Meatloaves

PRO/FATS AND VEGGIES—LEVEL ONE

MAKES 6 SERVINGS

Mini-Mini Meatloaves are fun to eat, and they take much less time to cook than they do in a standard loaf pan.

PREP TIME: 8 MINUTES
COOKING TIME: 20 MINUTES

Butter for greasing pan
1½ pounds lean ground beef or turkey
1½ cups finely chopped onions
3 stalks celery, finely chopped
3 eggs
3 tablespoons Somersize Ketchup (p. 245)

4 cloves garlic, finely chopped
2¼ teaspoons salt
½ teaspoon pepper
1½ teaspoons dried thyme
1 (32-ounce) jar Somersize Marinara
    Sauce, about 3 cups

Preheat oven to 350 degrees. Butter a 12-cup muffin tin.

In a large bowl, mix together ground beef, onions, celery, eggs, ketchup, garlic, salt, pepper, and thyme. Spoon mixture into prepared pan. Bake for 20 minutes, or until meatloaves are cooked through.

Heat marinara sauce in a small saucepan until hot. Set aside.

Remove meatloaves from oven. Place an inverted baking sheet (baking sheet should have an edge of at least ½ inch to keep grease from dripping everywhere) over the top of the muffin tin. Carefully invert muffin tin and baking sheet together. Unmold meatloaves onto baking sheet.

Serve each meatloaf with ½ cup marinara sauce.

Variation

If baking in a standard loaf pan, increase the cooking time to 45 to 60 minutes.

Twenty-Minute Chili

PRO/FATS—LEVEL ONE

SERVES 4 TO 6

Chili is one of those very personal recipes . . . everyone thinks his or her own is the best! I guess I'm no exception to the rule. Top this with lots of shredded cheddar cheese and sour cream. Or try my Somersize Chili Seasoning.

PREP TIME 5 MINUTES
COOKING TIME 25 MINUTES

3 tablespoons olive oil

2 large red onions, finely chopped

6 cloves garlic, finely minced

2 pounds fresh ground beef or ground turkey

1 (28-ounce) can plum tomatoes (in juice), coarsely chopped in Cuisinart, or squeezed by hand

$\frac{2}{3}$ cup good red wine

1 (14-ounce) can chicken broth

$\frac{1}{4}$ cup chopped Italian parsley

$1\frac{1}{2}$ teaspoons salt (or to taste)

$\frac{1}{4}$ teaspoon ground pepper (or to taste)

1 teaspoon SomerSweet

4 teaspoons ground cumin

$1\frac{1}{2}$ tablespoons ground chili powder

$1\frac{1}{2}$ teaspoons ground oregano

$\frac{1}{2}$ cup shredded cheddar cheese (optional)

1 small carton sour cream (optional)

1 bunch cilantro (optional)

Heat a skillet over medium high. Add olive oil and chopped onions and cook until soft and slightly browned, about 5 minutes.

Add garlic and cook 1 minute more.

Add ground turkey and cook with the onion mixture until browned and almost cooked through, about 6 minutes.

Add tomatoes and cook for 3 minutes.

Add wine to the boiling mixture and cook 2 minutes or until the alcohol is cooked away.

Add chicken broth, parsley, salt, pepper, SomerSweet, and spices. Cook 5 minutes more.

Serve in bowls with shredded cheddar cheese, sour cream, and cilantro.

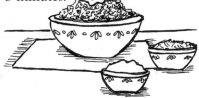

Beef Fajitas

PRO/FATS AND VEGGIES—LEVEL ONE

SERVES 8 TO 10

Instead of tortillas, I wrap these fajitas in Alan's mother's Egg Crêpes. These fajitas are also great in a lettuce cup for extra crunch.

PREP TIME: 6 MINUTES
COOKING TIME: 8 MINUTES

1 pound sirloin steak, cut into 1½-inch strips
2 tablespoons Tex Mex Seasoning Blend (p. 275), or 2 tablespoons fajita seasoning
2 tablespoons fresh lime juice
3 tablespoons olive oil
1 large onion, sliced
2 red bell peppers, sliced into ¼-inch strips

3 cloves garlic, crushed
8 to 10 Egg Crêpes (p. 188)

GARNISH
Sour cream
Salsa
Shredded cheese
Chopped cilantro
Lime wedges

Toss together steak, Tex Mex Seasoning Blend, and lime juice in a bowl. Set aside.

Heat oil in a large sauté pan over medium heat. Add onion and cook for 3 minutes. Add peppers and garlic and cook for 2 more minutes. Raise heat to high and add steak. Cook for 2 minutes.

Heat crêpes in a warm oven for 5 minutes, or microwave for 1 minute. Place fajita mixture on crêpes and serve with garnishes of your choice.

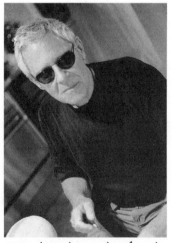

My handsome husband.

Somersize Lasagna

SERVES 4

What's great about lasagna are the layers of sauce and bubbling cheese. You'll never miss the pasta in this fabulous version! And the Egg Crêpes cut the baking time in half compared to lasagna made with pasta.

PREP TIME: 4 MINUTES
COOKING TIME: 40 MINUTES

Butter for greasing the baking dish
1 cup chopped onions
2 tablespoons olive oil
1 pound ground beef
1 (32-ounce) jar Somersize Marinara
    Sauce, about 3 cups
1 clove garlic, crushed
$1/4$ cup grated Parmesan cheese

$1^1/2$ cups full-fat ricotta cheese
1 (10-ounce) package frozen chopped
    spinach, thawed and drained
$1/4$ teaspoon nutmeg
Salt and freshly ground black pepper
$2^1/2$ cups shredded mozzarella cheese
4 Egg Crêpes (p. 188)

Preheat oven to 350 degrees. Butter an 8 × 8-inch glass baking dish. Set aside.

In a large heavy sauté pan over medium-high heat, sauté onions in olive oil for 2 minutes. Add ground beef and sauté for 3 minutes. Add marinara sauce and garlic. Simmer for 5 minutes.

In a medium bowl, combine Parmesan and ricotta cheese, spinach, and nutmeg. Season with salt and pepper.

Place $1^1/4$ cups ground beef mixture in the bottom of the prepared pan. Top with $1/2$ cup mozzarella. Lay one egg crêpe over mozzarella. Spread 1 cup of the spinach mixture on top of the egg crêpe. Top spinach mixture with another egg crêpe. Repeat layers, finishing with the remaining mozzarella cheese. Bake for 30 minutes, until cheese is melted and beginning to brown. Serve hot.

TRATTORIA
della
SOMERSIZIO
ITALIANO
buon appetito!

Cheeseburger Pie

SERVES 6

Here is a fast and deliciously easy midweek dinner that is perfect when you're pressed for time. You can make hundreds of variations of this recipe: add a packet of Somersize Dip Mix, or some green Ortega chilies, or broccoli florets, or a different type of cheese—use your imagination!

PREP TIME: 8 MINUTES
COOKING TIME: 15 MINUTES

Butter for greasing baking dish
1 pound ground beef or turkey
1 small onion, chopped
1 cup heavy cream

3 eggs, beaten
4 cups shredded cheddar cheese
Salt and freshly ground black pepper

Preheat oven to 350 degrees. Butter a 13 × 9-inch glass baking dish. Set aside.

Brown ground beef in a large skillet over medium heat. Add onions and cook for an additional 3 minutes, stirring constantly. Remove pan from heat. Add cream, eggs, and 3 cups of the cheese. Stir well. Season with salt and pepper. Pour mixture into prepared baking dish. Sprinkle with remaining cheese. Bake for 15 to 20 minutes, or until cheese begins to brown.

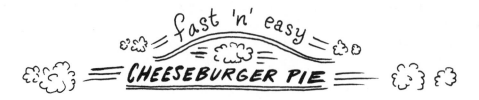

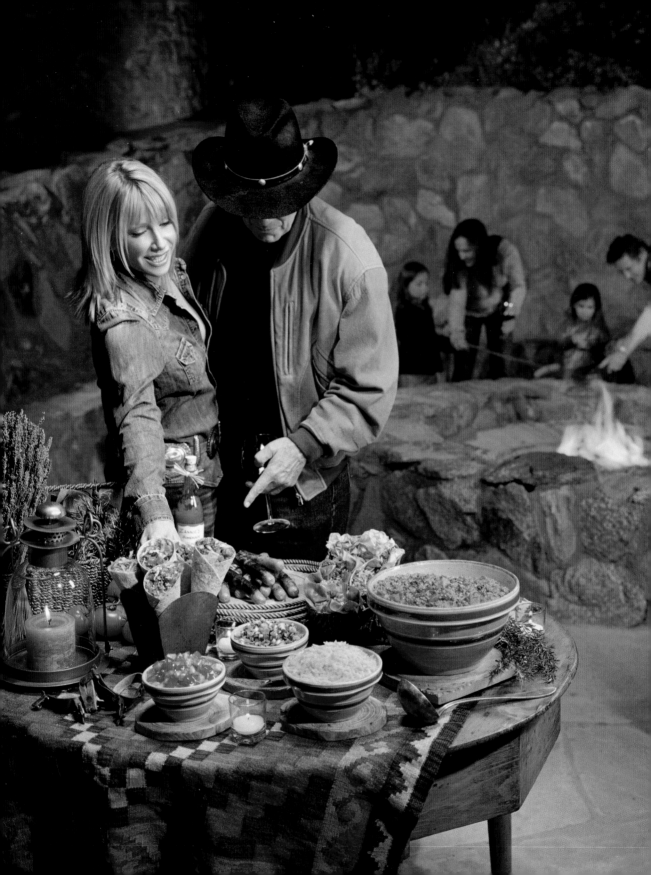

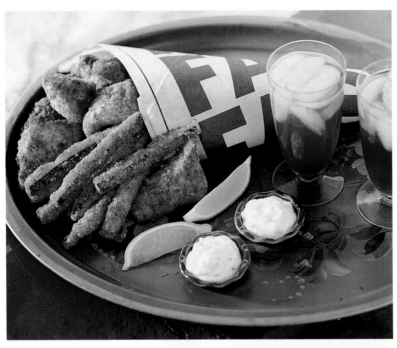

Somersize Fish
and Chips with
Somersize
Tartar Sauce

Previous page:
Family barbecue fun.
Here we have Turkey
Taco Wraps and Twenty
Minute Chili with
salsa, cheddar, and sour
cream.

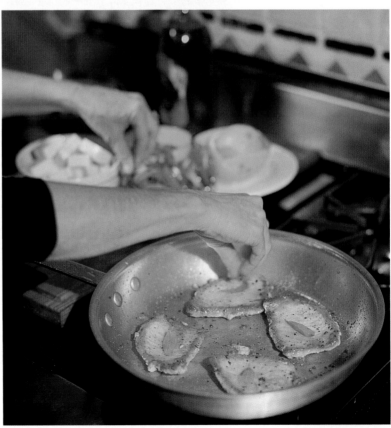

Quickly sauté
medallions in butter
and olive oil and . . .

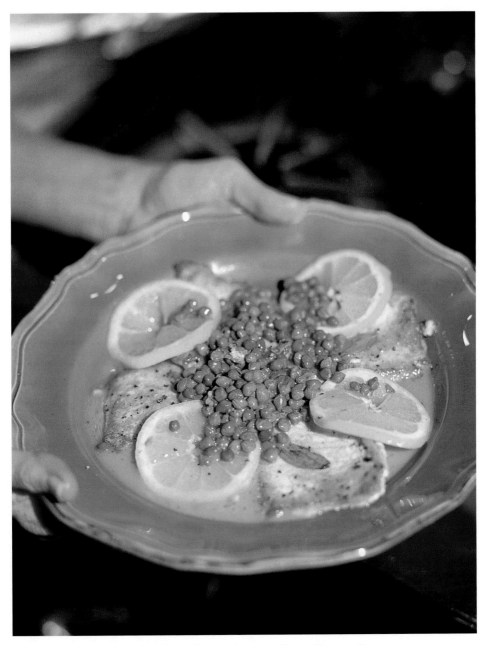

. . . Voilà! Pork Paillards with Caper Butter Sauce.

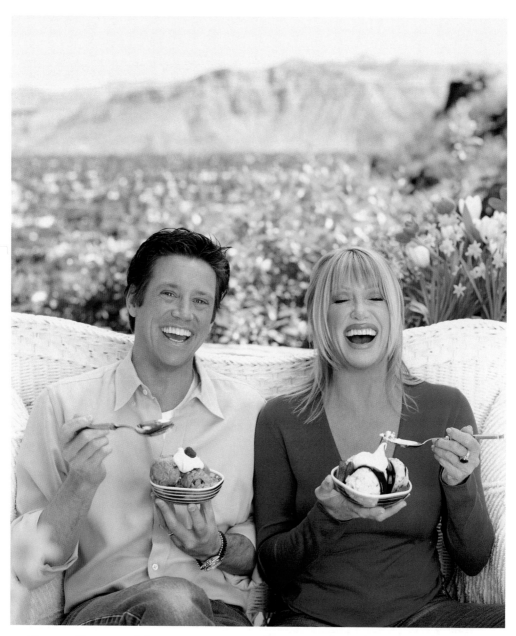

My son, Bruce, and I enjoying guilt-free Somersize Coffee Toffee Ice Cream and Strawberry Ice Cream with Somersize Dipping and Coating Fudge Sauce.

Opposite: A backyard birthday party for my granddaughter with Chocolate Cupcakes with Whipped Cream Filling and Jiggly Fruit Gels.

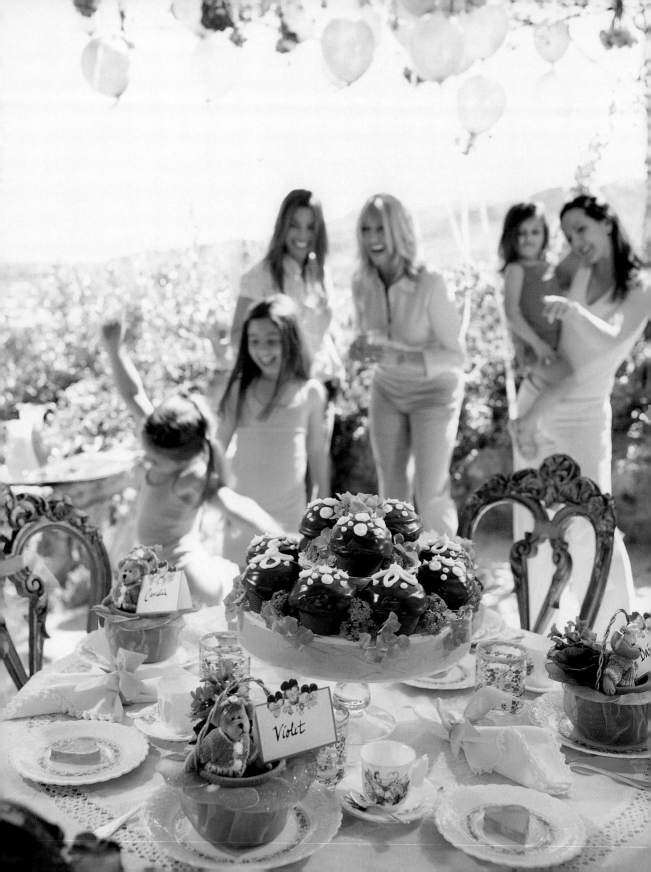

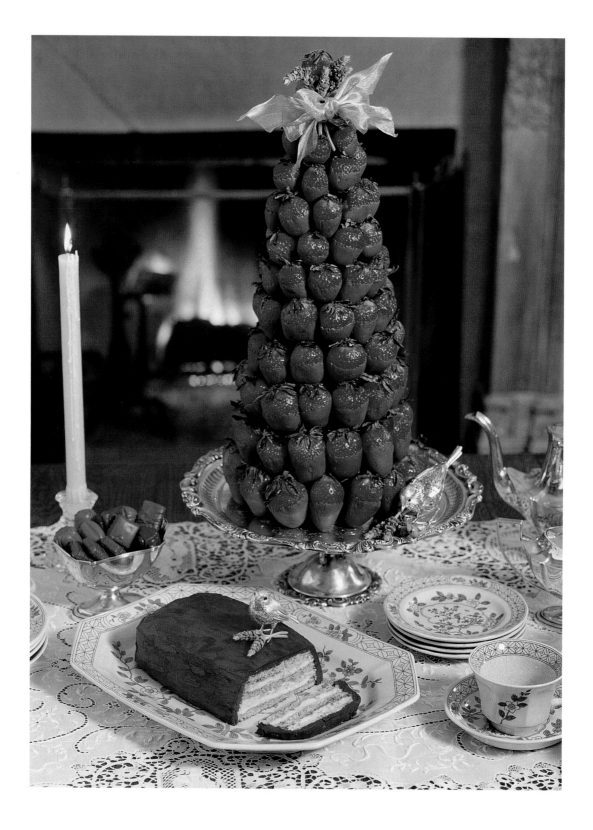

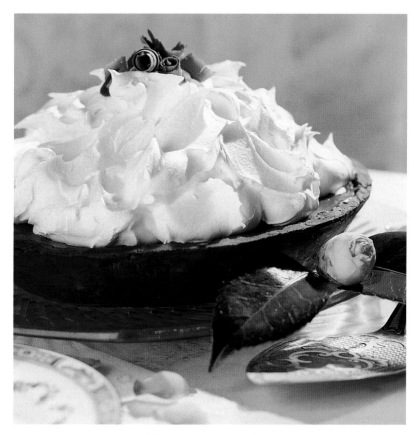

Chocolate Cream Pie

Opposite: This is a beautiful way to enjoy the holidays.
Croquembouche made from Chocolate-Dipped Strawberries and
Boston Cream Pie Cake.

Following page: My granddaughter and I love Somersicles!

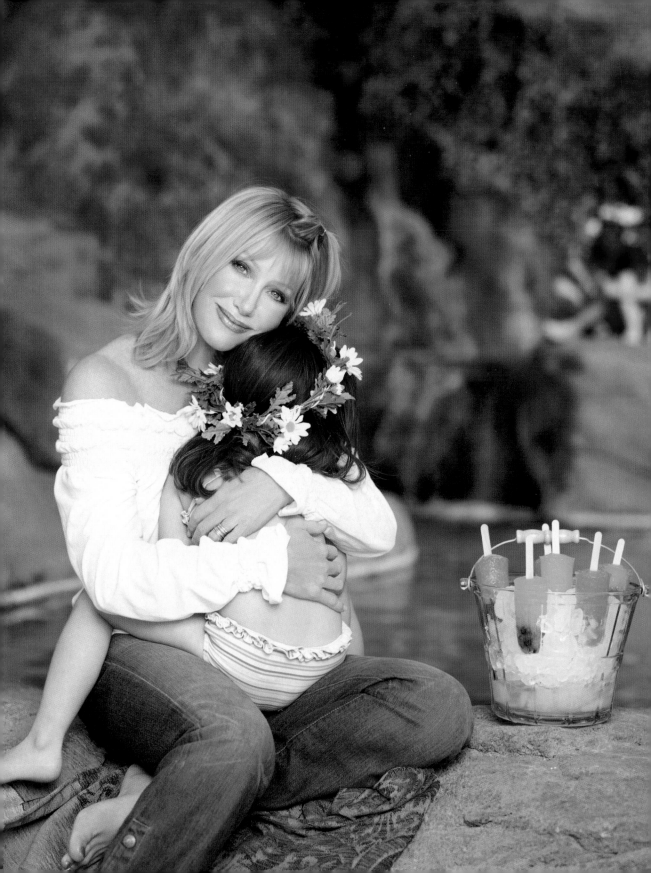

Old-Fashioned Beef Stew

PRO / FATS AND VEGGIES—LEVEL ONE

SERVES 6

The great thing about a slow cooker is that you set it and forget it. It takes five minutes to make this in the morning. You'll thank yourself at the end of the day. Or, you can use a pressure cooker and be done in about 20 minutes. Easy!

PREP TIME: 5 MINUTES
COOKING TIME: 4 TO 8 HOURS

1 tablespoon olive oil
2 pounds beef stewing meat
Salt and freshly ground black pepper
2 cloves garlic, minced
1 (14.5-ounce) can diced tomatoes
1 (8-ounce) can tomato sauce
1 (14.5-ounce) can beef broth
2 teaspoons Worcestershire sauce

2 teaspoons dried thyme
1 bay leaf
8 ounces mushrooms, sliced
4 stalks celery, chopped
8 ounces pearl onions, peeled

EQUIPMENT
Slow cooker or pressure cooker

Heat olive oil in a large skillet over medium-high heat. Season beef with salt and pepper. Brown in olive oil in small batches. When beef is browned, put into slow cooker. Add the rest of the ingredients. Stir to combine. Cook on high for 4 hours, or on low for 8 hours. Discard bay leaf before serving.

Alternate Pressure Cooker Method
Season beef with salt and pepper. Place the pan of a pressure cooker (at least 6-quarts) on medium-high heat. Add the olive oil and one fourth of the beef. Brown the beef, then remove from pan and set aside while you brown the other batches of beef. Once all the beef is browned, place all of it back into the pan. Add the remaining ingredients and stir to combine. Lock pressure lid into place. Bring to pressure over high heat. Lower heat and cook for 20 minutes. Release pressure slowly. Discard bay leaf. Season with salt and pepper before serving.

In a Hurry Beef Curry

PRO/FATS AND VEGGIES—LEVEL ONE

SERVES 6

This is one of my favorite recipes in this book. Serve it over my Cumin-Scented Zucchini (p. 227) with a dollop of my Cucumber Dill Dip (p.197) to cool the spice. Fabulous! For a really fast prep time, look for precut meat in your supermarket. It is often labeled "stir-fry." Curry paste is a blend of curry powder, chilies, vinegar, and other spices. This dish can also be made with cubed chicken, veal, lamb, or even with peeled shrimp.

PREP TIME: 3 MINUTES
COOKING TIME: 22 MINUTES

2 tablespoons olive oil
1 pound top round or sirloin steak, sliced
   into ¼-inch-thick pieces
1 medium onion, chopped
1 bell pepper, chopped

1 (14-ounce) can diced tomatoes
⅔ cup sugar-free mild curry paste, or
   ½ cup sugar-free hot curry paste
¾ teaspoon SomerSweet
½ cup heavy cream

Place a large sauté pan over medium-high heat. When hot, add olive oil and beef. Sauté for 2 to 3 minutes until browned. Remove steak from pan and set aside. Add onions to pan and cook for 2 minutes. Add peppers and cook for another 2 minutes. Stir in tomatoes, curry paste, SomerSweet, and heavy cream. Bring to a boil, reduce heat, and simmer for 10 minutes. Return steak to pan and simmer for 5 minutes. Serve hot.

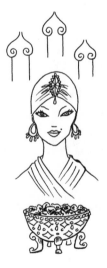

Sixty-Minute Pot Roast

PRO/FATS AND VEGGIES—LEVEL ONE

SERVES 6

Pot roast usually takes hours to cook. This hearty version can be prepared and cooked in a pressure cooker in just an hour! I have always loved my mother's recipe—this is like coming home. Serve it with my Celery Root Purée (p. 228).

PREP TIME: 5 MINUTES
COOKING TIME: 60 MINUTES

3 tablespoons vegetable or peanut oil

5 pounds rump roast

1 cup chopped onions

1 leek, cleaned and sliced (green and white parts)

3 cloves garlic, chopped

2 cups red wine

1 (14-ounce) can beef broth, plus more if necessary

1 (6-ounce) can tomato paste

2 bay leaves

1 tablespoon dried oregano or Italian seasoning

Salt and freshly ground black pepper

EQUIPMENT
Pressure cooker

Heat oil in the large pan of a pressure cooker (at least 6 quarts) over medium heat. Add roast and brown on all sides, about 2 minutes per side. Remove roast from pan using large tongs. Set aside.

Add onions and leeks to pan. Sauté for 2 minutes, adding more oil if necessary. Add garlic and sauté for an additional minute. Pour wine and beef broth into pan. Add tomato paste, bay leaves, and oregano. Stir until mixture is smooth.

Return meat to pan. Lock pressure lid into place. Bring to pressure over high heat. Reduce heat and cook for 55 minutes. Allow steam to release slowly. Place roast on a serving platter. Season juices with salt and pepper. Spoon juices over pot roast before serving.

Alternate Oven Braising Method
Preheat oven to 350 degrees.

In a large sauté pan, brown roast and vegetables following directions above.

Place roast and vegetables in an oven-proof pan with liquid ingredients and seasonings.

Cover and let cook for 3 to 4 hours or until roast is tender, checking occasionally to see if additional beef broth is necessary.

Pork

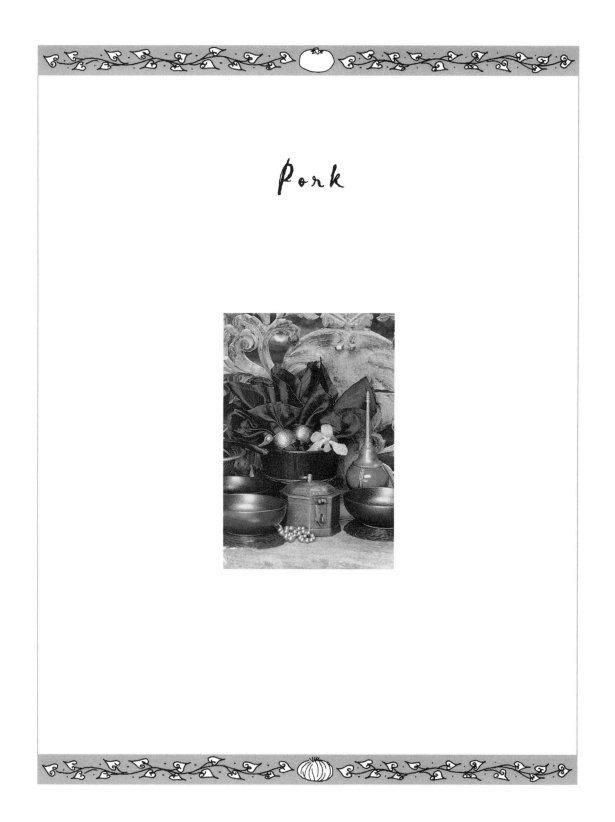

Creamy Tex Mex Pork Chops

PRO/FATS AND VEGGIES—LEVEL ONE

SERVES 4

A squeeze of fresh lime juice at the very end really kicks up the flavor of these delicious pork chops.

PREP TIME: 4 MINUTES
COOKING TIME: 10 MINUTES

4 boneless pork chops
Salt and freshly ground black pepper
2 teaspoons Tex Mex Seasoning Blend
   (p. 275), or fajita seasoning
4 tablespoons (½ stick) unsalted butter

1 cup heavy cream
1 package Somersize Salsa Dip Mix, or
   1 cup salsa, drained
Lime wedges

Place pork chops on a plastic-covered work surface. Cover with plastic wrap. Using a meat tenderizer, pound pork chops until they are ½ inch thick. Season each pork chop with salt, pepper, and ¼ teaspoon Tex Mex Seasoning Blend. Turn chops over and season again.

Heat butter in a large skillet over medium heat. Add pork chops to pan. Sauté for 2½ minutes. Turn pork chops over and cook for an additional 2 minutes. Remove from pan and transfer onto a serving platter. Cover with foil to keep warm.

Add cream and contents of dip mix (or drained salsa) to sauté pan. Bring to a boil. Reduce heat to low and simmer for 2 minutes, stirring constantly. Season with salt and pepper. Spoon sauce over pork chops. Squeeze lime juice over chops and serve.

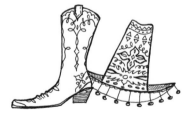

Tex Mex Seasoning Blend

VEGGIES—LEVEL ONE

MAKES ABOUT ¹/₂ CUP

I love the flavor of fajita seasoning, but most are made with sugar. Here's my version. I keep this in my pantry to season fajitas, pork chops, or chicken, or to add a quick kick to eggs!

PREP TIME: 5 MINUTES

1 tablespoon plus 1 teaspoon cayenne
    pepper
2 tablespoons plus 2 teaspoons dried
    oregano
2 tablespoons plus 2 teaspoons ground
    cumin

1 tablespoon plus 1 teaspoon ground
    coriander
2 teaspoons black pepper
2 teaspoons sea salt

Combine all ingredients in a jar or resealable plastic bag. Shake until blended. Store in an airtight container for up to 6 months.

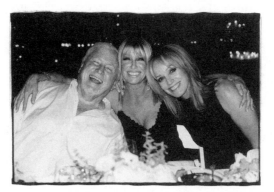

*Merv Griffin, me, and Susan Anton
having a ball at my birthday party.*

Baby-Back Barbecue Ribs

PRO/FATS AND VEGGIES—LEVEL ONE

SERVES 2

Alan loves ribs. It could be his all-time favorite food. These are incredibly tender when made in a pressure cooker, and they only take 15 minutes! You can also make them in the oven. I have Somersize Barbecue Sauce available, or you can make your own (p.277).

PREP TIME: 2 MINUTES
COOKING TIME: 15 MINUTES

1 rack (about 2 pounds) baby-back pork
   ribs
1³⁄₄ cups Somersize Barbecue Sauce
2¹⁄₂ cups water
¹⁄₃ cup peanut oil

4 scallions, chopped
   (white and green parts)

EQUIPMENT
Pressure cooker

Cut ribs into 4 sections. Coat both sides of ribs with Somersize Barbecue Sauce. Pour water and peanut oil into pan of pressure cooker (at least a 6-quart pan). Stir to combine. Layer ribs in pressure cooker. Sprinkle with scallions. Lock lid into place. Bring to pressure over high heat. Reduce heat and cook for 15 minutes. Use the quick-steam-release method. Allow ribs to cool slightly before handling.

Alternate Oven Method
Preheat oven to 350 degrees. Combine barbecue sauce, water, and peanut oil in a medium bowl. Cut ribs into 4 sections. Coat both sides of ribs with sauce. Place ribs in a shallow baking pan and cook for about 1 hour, or until meat comes easily off the bone, basting every 15 minutes with remaining sauce. Garnish with scallions before serving.

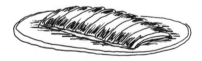

Somersize Barbecue Sauce

VEGGIES—LEVEL ONE

MAKES 1 3/4 CUPS

Make it or buy it—your choice. My Somersize Barbecue Sauce is available at SuzanneSomers.com, along with all my Somersize food, or you can make your own. This recipe is for an old-fashioned chunky barbecue sauce. For a smooth texture, purée the sauce in a blender or food processor. This sauce keeps for a week—double the recipe so you always have some on hand.

PREP TIME: 3 MINUTES
COOKING TIME: 15 MINUTES

1/4 cup hot water
1 teaspoon instant coffee granules, or 1/4 cup strong-brewed coffee
1 cup jarred Somersize Marinara Sauce, or 1 cup tomato sauce
1/2 cup chopped onions
2 tablespoons tomato paste
3 tablespoons red wine or apple cider vinegar

2 tablespoons Worcestershire sauce
3 tablespoons Dijon mustard
1 teaspoon Liquid Smoke
1/4 teaspoon cayenne pepper
Tabasco sauce (optional)
2 tablespoons SomerSweet
Salt and freshly ground black pepper

Mix water and coffee granules together. Pour into a 2 1/2-quart saucepan. Add all ingredients except the SomerSweet, salt, and pepper. Bring to a boil over medium heat. Reduce heat and simmer for 15 minutes. Stir in SomerSweet. Season with salt and pepper. Let cool, cover, and refrigerate.

Pork Paillards with Caper Butter Sauce

PRO/FATS AND VEGGIES—LEVEL ONE

SERVES 4

My favorite hot and fast recipes include the winning combination of lemon, capers, and butter. I love it on chicken breasts, veal, pounded turkey, and petrale sole. Now you can try it with thinly pounded pork. This really delivers.

PREP TIME: 5 MINUTES
COOKING TIME: 17 MINUTES

4 (4–6 ounces each) boneless pork chops
8 tablespoons unsalted butter, softened
2 tablespoons Lemon Olive Oil (p. 279) or
    regular olive oil
½ cup finely chopped onions
½ cup chicken broth
2 tablespoons lemon juice
2 tablespoons capers
Salt and freshly ground black pepper
Lemon slices, for garnish

Place pork chops on a plastic-covered work surface and cover with another piece of plastic wrap. Using a meat tenderizer or a small heavy saucepan, pound pork chops to half-inch thickness.

Place a large sauté pan over medium-high heat. Add 4 tablespoons butter and swirl until melted. Add the pork chops and sauté for 3 minutes. Turn and sauté an additional 3 minutes. Remove from pan and transfer onto serving plates. Add olive oil and onions to pan. Sauté for 5 minutes, scraping any bits off the bottom of the pan. Add chicken broth to pan and continue scraping the bits from the pan to release the flavor. Let reduce until thick and syrupy, about 5 minutes. Reduce heat to low. Add remaining butter and stir until melted. Add lemon juice and capers. Season with salt and pepper. Spoon sauce over pork chops. Garnish with lemon slices.

Lemon Olive Oil

PRO/FATS—LEVEL ONE

MAKES 1 1/2 CUPS

I love shopping in fancy food stores. There's nothing more beautiful than those long thin bottles filled with expensive flavored oils. But they're also pricey! Here's an easy way to make your own flavored oil. This is delightful on salads, or anywhere you want a hint of lemon with your oil. The peel creates an amazing flavor.

PREP TIME: 2 MINUTES
STANDING TIME: 2 1/2 HOURS

1 1/2 cups extra-virgin olive oil
4 whole lemons, each cut into 8 wedges,
　with peel on

Place olive oil and lemons in the bowl of a food processor. Process for 30 seconds until mixture is the consistency of chunky salsa. Pour into a stainless-steel bowl. Cover and allow mixture to stand for 2 hours. Place a sieve over another stainless-steel bowl. Pour mixture into sieve. Allow oil to drain through sieve for 1/2 hour.

Gently press down pulp to extract as much liquid as possible. Pour lemon olive oil into a bottle. Keep in a cool, dry place for up to a month.

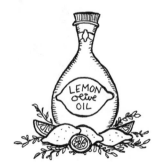

Peppered Pork Tenderloin

PRO/FATS AND VEGGIES—ALMOST LEVEL ONE

SERVES 4

This is my kind of dinner—cook it hot and fast, then deglaze the pan with brandy, butter, and cream. It's Somersize cooking at its best. The small amount of brandy makes this Almost Level One. If you are doing well, you should not have a problem.

PREP TIME: 3 MINUTES
COOKING TIME: 7 MINUTES

1 tablespoon coarsely ground black pepper
1½ to 2 pounds pork tenderloin
½ cup (1 stick) unsalted butter
3 cloves garlic, chopped

3 tablespoons brandy
¼ cup heavy cream
Salt and freshly ground black pepper

Sprinkle pepper on all sides of tenderloin. Gently press pepper into pork. Slice pork into ¼-inch-thick slices.

Place a large skillet over medium-high heat. Add ½ stick butter and stir until melted. Add pork to butter and sauté for 2 minutes. Turn pork over and sauté for an additional 2 minutes. Add garlic to pan and sauté for 30 seconds. Reduce heat to low. Add brandy and cook for 2 minutes. Add remaining butter to pan and stir until melted. Add cream and heat until warm. Season with salt and pepper. Serve sauce over pork slices.

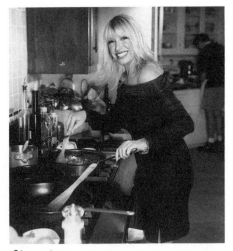

I'm always cooking.

Seafood

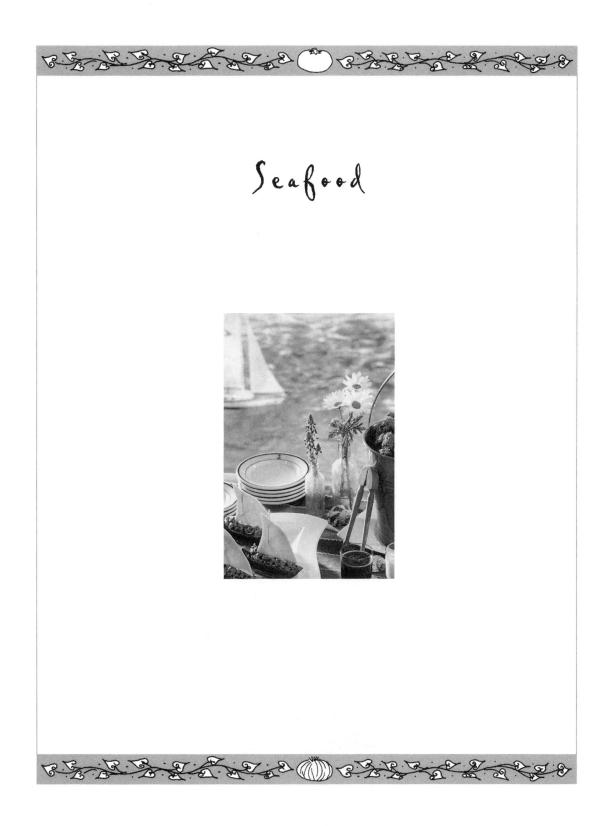

Salmon Baked in Parchment

PRO/FATS AND VEGGIES—LEVEL ONE

SERVES 4

This is such an easy way to cook fish, and it keeps it really moist. For thinner or thicker cuts of fish, simply adjust the cooking time. Look for parchment paper in the baking section of your grocery store, or use a paper sandwich bag instead.

PREP TIME: 5 MINUTES
COOKING TIME: 18 MINUTES

1 lemon, cut into 8 slices
4 tablespoons unsalted butter
4 sprigs fresh herbs, such as basil, tarragon, dill, thyme, or rosemary

4 salmon fillets (4–5 ounces each)
Salt and freshly ground black pepper
1 cup chopped onions

Preheat oven to 400 degrees. Lay one piece of parchment, about 10 inches square, on a work surface. Place two lemon slices side by side in center of parchment. Dot the lemon slices with a quarter of the butter. Lay one herb sprig on top. Sprinkle a salmon fillet with salt and pepper, then place, skin side up, on top of the herbs. Sprinkle skin side with salt and pepper. Mound a quarter of the chopped onions on top of the salmon.

Fold two opposite sides of the parchment up and over the salmon. Take the open ends and fold over salmon to seal. Place parchment, seam side down, on a greased baking sheet. Repeat with the other salmon fillets. Bake for 18 to 20 minutes.

To serve, place parchment packet on a dinner plate, then cut an X into the top of parchment with a sharp knife and pull open slightly.

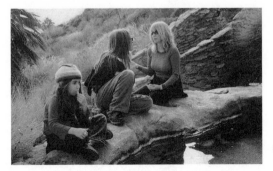

I love sharing a private moment with my girls.

The Somersize Recipes

Ginger Scallion Grilled Mahi-Mahi

PRO/FATS AND VEGGIES—LEVEL ONE

SERVES 2

I love to go to dinner at Bruce and Caroline's house. The girls are darling and the food is always spectacular. Last time we were there, Bruce grilled mahi-mahi steaks with Caroline's delicious Gingered Soy Sauce. Serve this with Garlic Sugar Snap Peas (p. 226) for a fresh, clean dinner.

PREP TIME: 2 MINUTES
MARINATING TIME: 10 MINUTES
COOKING TIME: 6 MINUTES

2 mahi-mahi steaks or your favorite fish
1 cup Gingered Soy Sauce (p. 201)
Juice of 1 lime
6 scallions, whole

Place the mahi-mahi, Gingered Soy Sauce, and lime juice in a resealable plastic bag. Marinate for at least 10 minutes, or up to several hours.

Preheat grill to medium high. Remove fish from bag, reserving marinade. Place fish and scallions on grill. Grill for 3 minutes per side. Brush scallions with marinade, turning as necessary.

Serve immediately.

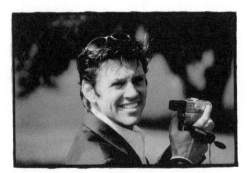

My son Bruce—just because I thought you might enjoy looking at him as much as I do.

Scallop Kabobs

MAKES 5 KABOBS

Recently Alan and I went to Catalina Island for a taste of charming seaside living. We also had a taste of delicious seafood, including a scallop kabob. Now I make them at home. I don't like my scallops too thick. Slice them about ½ inch thick for best results.

PREP TIME: 15 MINUTES
MARINATING TIME: 1 HOUR
COOK TIME: 12 MINUTES

2 tablespoons lemon juice (about 1 lemon)
⅓ cup lime juice (about 5 limes)
3 cloves garlic, chopped
½ cup olive oil
½ teaspoon salt
¼ teaspoon black pepper
1 pound large scallops

1 large red bell pepper, cut into 1-inch pieces
1 large onion, quartered and cut into 1-inch pieces
½ pound medium-size whole button mushrooms (about 15)
Chopped chives, for garnish

To make the marinade, mix together the lemon juice, lime juice, garlic, olive oil, salt, and pepper in a medium bowl. Whisk until smooth and slightly thickened. Add scallops and toss to coat with the marinade. Cover and refrigerate for 1 hour.

To make the kabobs, alternate red bell peppers, onions, mushrooms, and scallops on 12-inch wooden or metal skewers. Lay skewers in a shallow pan. Pour marinade over kabobs.

Preheat grill. Grill for 5 to 6 minutes per side, or until cooked through. Sprinkle with chopped chives before serving.

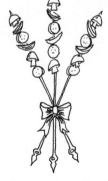

The Somersize Recipes

Chilantro Lime Grilled Tuna

PRO/FATS—LEVEL ONE

MAKES 4 SERVINGS

Tuna steaks are easy to prepare and they taste great fresh off the grill. These are marinated in olive oil, cilantro, and lime juice.

PREP TIME: 2 MINUTES
MARINATING TIME: 1 HOUR
COOK TIME: 6 TO 10 MINUTES

⅓ cup lime juice (about 5 limes)
⅔ cup olive oil
¼ cup chopped cilantro
5 cloves garlic, chopped

¼ teaspoon salt
¼ teaspoon black pepper
4 (½-inch-thick) tuna steaks
(4–5 ounces each)

To make the marinade, place the lime juice, olive oil, cilantro, garlic, salt, and pepper in a bowl. Whisk until mixture emulsifies and becomes thick. Place tuna steaks in a large resealable plastic bag. Pour marinade into bag. Seal and refrigerate for 1 hour.

Preheat grill. Remove tuna from marinade. Grill for 2 to 3 minutes per side, or until tuna is cooked to preferred doneness.

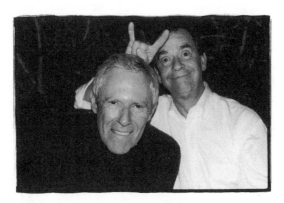

*Dick Clark and Alan—
friends for years.*

Desserts

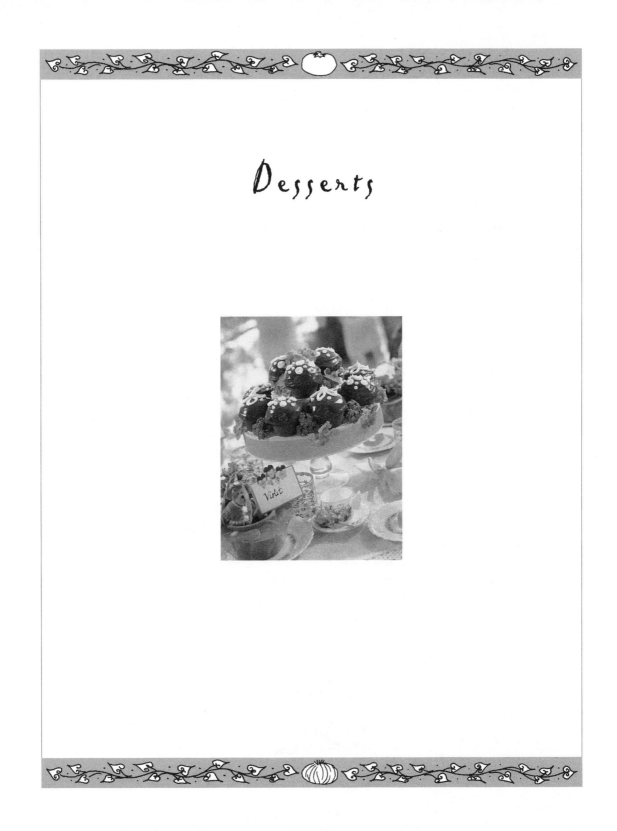

Lemon Crème Fraîche Ice Cream

PRO/FATS—LEVEL ONE

MAKES 1 QUART

This light, lemony ice cream will knock your socks off. My husband, Alan, likes to put this ice cream into ramekins straight out of the ice cream maker, refreeze for several hours, and then sprinkle the tops with SomerSweet. Right before serving, I use our kitchen torch to caramelize the SomerSweet for a brûlée topping. It's ice cream and crème brûlée rolled into one. If you can't find crème fraîche in your supermarket, you can use my recipe in Get Skinny on Fabulous Food *(p. 152) or you can use sour cream.*

PREP TIME: 10 MINUTES
CHILLING TIME: 30 MINUTES

4 large egg yolks, beaten
3 cups crème fraîche (or sour cream, at
    room temperature)
3 tablespoons plus 2 teaspoons SomerSweet

¾ teaspoon pure lemon extract

EQUIPMENT
Ice cream maker

Pour egg yolks into a stainless-steel bowl. Add 1 cup of crème fraîche to eggs, whisking constantly. Set aside. Place remaining crème fraîche in a medium saucepan over low heat. Heat, stirring constantly, until warm. Do not let crème fraîche boil. Slowly pour crème fraîche into egg mixture. Add SomerSweet and lemon extract.

Whisk well. Place bowl on top of a saucepan of simmering water. Whisk until mixture thickens and reads 170 degrees on an instant-read thermometer. Allow mixture to cool to room temperature, about 30 minutes. Refrigerate for at least 2 hours, or overnight. Freeze in ice cream maker according to manufacturer's directions.

Pink Kiddie Ice Cream

PRO/FATS—ALMOST LEVEL ONE

MAKES 1 QUART

This is the easiest ice cream you will ever make! All you need is heavy cream, half-and-half, Somer-Sweet, and a packet of my Somersize Peach-Mango Drink Mix. My grandchildren call it Zannie's Kool-Aid Ice Cream.

PREP TIME: 2 MINUTES
CHILLING TIME: 20 MINUTES
ICE CREAM MAKER TIME: 10 TO 15 MINUTES

2½ cups heavy whipping cream
1 cup half and half
1 package Somersize Peach-Mango Drink
   Mix

1 tablespoon SomerSweet

EQUIPMENT
Ice cream maker

Pour cream and half-and-half into a large mixing bowl. Sprinkle contents of drink mix over cream. Whisk until drink mix is completely dissolved. Add SomerSweet.

Whisk until SomerSweet is dissolved, about 1 minute. Chill for at least 20 minutes. Pour mixture into ice cream maker. Freeze according to manufacturer's directions.

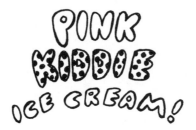

Somersize Dipping and Coating Fudge Sauce

PRO/FATS—ALMOST LEVEL ONE

MAKES 2 CUPS

The secret to this velvety sauce is to keep the cream from boiling. Keep this fudgy delight on hand in the refrigerator for dipping fruit or truffles, for covering cakes, or just for eating by the spoonful! I find Hershey's unsweetened baking chocolate works the best with SomerSweet. Of course, you can also buy my Somersize Triple Hot Fudge Sauce already made.

PREP TIME: 10 MINUTES

6 ounces unsweetened chocolate,
   broken up
1¼ cups heavy cream
2 tablespoons unsalted butter, softened

3 tablespoons plus 2 teaspoons SomerSweet
½ teaspoon vanilla extract
½ cup sour cream
Pinch of baking soda

Place chocolate in a small heavy-bottomed saucepan. Heat on low until chocolate has melted. Add heavy cream to pan. Cook on medium heat, stirring constantly, until small bubbles appear around the edges or an instant-read thermometer inserted in the liquid reads between 90 and 100 degrees. Remove pan from heat.

Stir until the chocolate is dissolved and the mixture is smooth. The mixture will be thick. Add butter and stir until smooth. Add the remaining ingredients and stir well. Use fudge sauce while still warm, or refrigerate in an airtight container.

Chocolate-Dipped Strawberries

ALMOST LEVEL ONE

MAKES 16 TO 20 DIPPED STRAWBERRIES
PREP TIME: 10 MINUTES

Don't be intimidated by the photograph of the chocolate strawberry Croquembouche in the photo insert. It's really easy to make. Look for a cone-shaped Styrofoam "tree" from your local art supply store and cover it in aluminum foil. Then insert toothpicks into the tree and secure the dipped strawberries to the cone by attaching them to the toothpicks. You will need about four pounds of strawberries and four cups of Somersize Dipping and Coating Fudge Sauce to decorate a two-foot tree.

TO DIP STRAWBERRIES
1 pound of strawberries, stems attached
1 cup Somersize Dipping and Coating
    Fudge Sauce (p. 290) or 1 jar Somersize
    Triple Hot Fudge Sauce

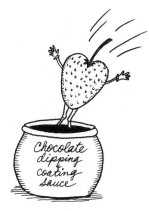

Line a baking sheet with parchment or waxed paper. Wipe strawberries with a damp cloth and dry with a soft cloth. Hold strawberries by stems and dip three-quarters of each berry into the Somersize Dipping and Coating Fudge Sauce. Place on prepared baking sheet.

Refrigerate for 1 hour until firm.

Cherry Chocolate Trifle

ALMOST LEVEL ONE

SERVES 8

This easy-to-make trifle combines four of my favorite flavors: cherries, chocolate, custard, and whipped cream. I use frozen cherries so you can enjoy it all year round. Use a pretty glass bowl for a lovely presentation.

PREP TIME: 20 MINUTES
COOKING TIME: 10 MINUTES

FOR THE CHOCOLATE
TRIFLE CAKE

Butter for greasing the pan
3 ounces unsweetened baking chocolate
5 tablespoons unsalted butter
3 large eggs, separated, at room
   temperature

Preheat oven to 400 degrees.

Butter the sides and bottom of a jelly roll pan. (A jelly roll pan is a sheet pan with low sides.)

Line the pan with parchment paper. Butter the parchment paper. Set pan aside. Place chocolate and butter in a small heavy-bottomed saucepan. Over low heat, stir until chocolate and unsalted butter have melted.

Place egg yolks in a medium mixing bowl. Beat on high speed until light and

¼ cup plus 1 tablespoon SomerSweet
2 teaspoons vanilla extract
⅛ teaspoon baking soda

FOR THE TRIFLE

1 cooled Chocolate Trifle Cake
1 (16-ounce) package frozen cherries,
   thawed and juices reserved
1 prepared Somersize Crème Brûlèe Mix
   or 1 recipe Vanilla Custard (p. 293)
1 recipe Perfectly Whipped Cream (p. 305)

pale in color, about 8 minutes. Add ¼ cup SomerSweet, vanilla, and baking soda. Beat for 1 more minute. Fold egg-yolk mixture into chocolate mixture.

Place egg whites in a clean medium stainless-steel bowl. Beat on high speed until frothy. Add remaining tablespoon of SomerSweet. Continue to beat until egg whites form stiff peaks. Stir one third of the white mixture into chocolate mixture. Carefully fold remaining egg whites into chocolate mixture until combined.

Spoon batter into prepared pan. Bake for 8 to 10 minutes until firm.

Cool completely.

To assemble the trifle, cut up cooled chocolate trifle cake into 1-inch pieces and place into the bottom of a 2½-quart glass bowl. Pour thawed cherries and cherry juice over cake. Spoon prepared crème brûlée or Vanilla Custard over cherries. Top with Perfectly Whipped Cream.

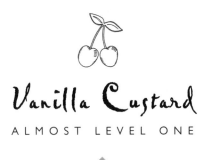

Vanilla Custard

ALMOST LEVEL ONE

MAKES ABOUT 2 CUPS

Nothing is more comforting than a dish of custard. As a child, Bruce's favorite dessert was custard. I use this in several recipes as a filling. Or you can serve it in a dish with a dollop of whipped cream. Yum. The cornstarch makes it Almost Level One.

PREP TIME: 10 MINUTES
COOLING TIME: 1 HOUR
CHILLING TIME: 2 HOURS

8 large egg yolks, beaten
2 tablespoons cornstarch
1½ cups heavy cream

1 tablespoon plus 1 teaspoon SomerSweet
½ teaspoon vanilla

Combine egg yolks and cornstarch in a medium stainless-steel bowl. Pour cream into a heavy-bottomed saucepan.

Heat cream on low until small bubbles appear around the outside edge or until an instant-read thermometer inserted reads 120 degrees. Slowly pour cream over eggs, stirring constantly. Place bowl over a saucepan of simmering water.

Cook for 4 to 5 minutes, stirring constantly until mixture thickens, or until an instant-read thermometer inserted in the custard reads 160 degrees.

Add SomerSweet and vanilla. Stir until SomerSweet dissolves.

Cover surface with plastic wrap. Allow custard to cool to room temperature, about 1 hour. Refrigerate for at least 2 hours or until set.

Frozen Chocolate Coffee Bombe

PRO/FATS AND VEGGIES—ALMOST LEVEL ONE

SERVES 6

A bombe is a dome-shaped frozen dessert, often filled with layers of ice cream, meringue, or cake. This Somersize version is very simple . . . coffee ice cream with a chocolate dome. It's made in a bowl, then inverted and sliced like a cake. Try it for your next birthday celebration or party at home. It's a French sensation!

PREP TIME: 10 MINUTES
CHILLING TIME: 3 HOURS

1 recipe Somersize Dipping and Coating
   Fudge Sauce, at room temperature
   (p. 290), or 1 jar Somersize Triple Hot
   Fudge

1 recipe Somersize Coffee Toffee Ice
   Cream, softened (p. 302)

Pour Somersize Dipping and Coating Fudge Sauce into a clean 1 1/2-quart stainless-steel or glass bowl. The bowl is your mold. Tilt the bowl to coat the sides with sauce. Take a pastry brush and brush the chocolate all the way to the edge. (You may have to paint in stages, letting the chocolate set up between strokes.) Place in refrigerator until completely set, about 1 hour.

Fill chocolate-lined bowl with softened Somersize Coffee Toffee Ice Cream all the way to the top. Place in freezer for at least 2 hours.

To unmold, place bombe bowl in a larger bowl of hot water for 30 seconds. Place a serving platter on top of bombe bowl and invert. Remove bowl. If bombe will not unmold, place a warm damp tea towel on outside of bowl for 30 seconds. Once you have unmolded the bombe, return to freezer until ready to use. Slice with a knife that has been run under warm water.

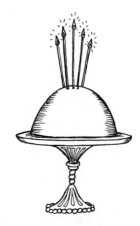

Bittersweet Chocolate "Bread" Pudding with Brandy Cream Sauce

ALMOST LEVEL ONE

❧

SERVES 4 TO 6

Bread pudding is traditionally made with chunks of bread that are then dipped in an egg mixture. In this version I use my Chocolate Trifle Cake to replace the bread. The finished product looks like an earthquake. Count on it shaking up your family and friends!

PREP TIME: 20 MINUTES
COOKING TIME: 30 MINUTES

FOR THE BREAD PUDDING
Butter for greasing baking dish
1 recipe Chocolate Trifle Cake (p. 292)
2 cups heavy cream
$^{1}/_{4}$ cup brandy
4 large eggs, beaten
3 tablespoons SomerSweet
1 teaspoon vanilla extract

FOR THE BRANDY SAUCE
$1^{1}/_{2}$ cups heavy cream
$^{1}/_{4}$ cup brandy
1 tablespoon SomerSweet

Preheat oven to 350 degrees. Butter an 8 × 8-inch glass baking dish. Set aside.

Cut chocolate trifle cake into 1-inch square pieces. Place into the prepared pan. Bring cream and brandy to boil in a small saucepan. Reduce heat and simmer for 5 minutes.

Place beaten eggs in a large stainless-steel bowl. Add 1 cup brandy–cream mixture to eggs. Whisk for 30 seconds. Add remaining brandy–cream, SomerSweet, and vanilla. Stir until SomerSweet is dissolved.

Pour custard over cake. Allow mixture to stand for 10 minutes so that the cake absorbs the liquid. Bake for 30 minutes.

For the Brandy Sauce
While waiting for cake to bake, mix together heavy cream and brandy in a small saucepan. Bring to a boil. Reduce heat, simmer, and cook for 20 minutes over low heat until reduced. Stir in SomerSweet. Serve over warm bread pudding.

Boston Cream Pie Cake

LEVEL TWO

SERVES 8

I absolutely love Boston Cream Pie. In this recipe I took the flavors of a traditional Boston Cream Pie and turned it into an easy and elegant cake! Great for an afternoon snack or to serve at your next party. It's Level Two because of the combination of whole-wheat flour and the Pro/Fats.

PREP TIME: 20 MINUTES
COOKING TIME: 10 MINUTES
CHILLING TIME: 60 MINUTES

FOR THE EASY GÉNOISE CAKE
Butter for greasing pan
$\frac{1}{2}$ cup whole-wheat flour
$\frac{1}{8}$ teaspoon salt
3 eggs, at room temperature
2 egg yolks, at room temperature
$\frac{1}{4}$ cup SomerSweet
1 teaspoon vanilla extract
1 tablespoon butter, melted and slightly
   cooled

FOR THE FILLING
1 prepared package Somersize Crème
   Brûlée Mix made with 1$\frac{1}{2}$ cups heavy
   cream or 1 recipe Vanilla Custard
   (p. 293)

TOPPING
1 recipe Somersize Dipping and Coating
   Fudge Sauce (p. 290) or 1 jar Somersize
   Triple Hot Fudge Sauce

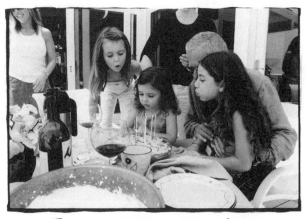

The grandchildren all love Alan.

Preheat oven to 400 degrees. Lightly butter a jelly roll pan and set aside. Mix whole-wheat flour and salt together in a small bowl. Set aside.

Place eggs, yolks, and SomerSweet into another medium mixing bowl. Beat on high until eggs are light and pale. Eggs have been sufficiently beaten when beaters are lifted out of bowl and eggs drip back into bowl in a ribbon that rests visibly on the surface. If egg ribbons sink into mixture, beat for a few more minutes. Add vanilla and beat for 30 seconds. Sprinkle half the flour over the egg mixture. Using a large spatula, carefully fold in remaining flour. Pour melted butter down the edge of bowl into the batter. Carefully fold butter into mixture. Spoon into prepared pan. Smooth evenly with a spatula.

Bake for 10 minutes, until cake is lightly golden brown. Remove from oven and cool for 20 minutes.

While cake is cooling, line a 1½-quart loaf pan with a double thickness of plastic wrap, allowing 2 inches to hang over each end.

Cut cooled cake into 3 pieces, each about 7 × 4 inches. Place 1 slice of cake in bottom of prepared loaf pan. Spoon half of the crème brûlée or Vanilla Custard over cake layer. Place another layer on top. Spoon remaining custard on top of second layer. Place remaining layer on top of custard. Refrigerate assembled cake for at least 1 hour.

Remove cake from refrigerator. Place a cooling rack on top of pan. Invert pan and cooling rack together. Remove plastic wrap. Place a cookie sheet under the cooling rack to catch any extra "frosting." The Somersize Fudge Dipping and Coating Sauce should be slightly warm, but thickened so that it sticks to the cake. Pour over cake and lightly smooth with a spatula. Serve immediately or refrigerate until frosting is firm.

Mixed Berry Steamed Pudding

LEVEL TWO

SERVES 6

Serve this delicious pudding with my Spiced Whipped Cream (p. 299).

PREP TIME: 6 MINUTES
COOKING TIME: 25 MINUTES

Unsalted butter for greasing mold or bowl
2/3 cup whole-wheat flour
4 tablespoons unsalted butter, melted
1/4 cup SomerSweet
1 cup heavy cream
1 teaspoon cinnamon
4 eggs, beaten

1 teaspoon vanilla extract
2 pounds frozen mixed berries, thawed and drained
1 recipe Spiced Whipped Cream

EQUIPMENT
Pressure cooker

Butter a 1-quart pudding mold or bowl. Place all ingredients except the berries in a large mixing bowl. Stir ingredients together until a thick batter forms. Carefully fold in berries, being careful to keep fruit whole. Pour berry mixture into prepared mold. Place lid onto mold. (If using a bowl, see note at end of recipe for directions.)

Place mold on a trivet set inside pressure cooker. Add 3 cups water to pressure cooker. Lock lid into place. Bring to pressure over high heat. Reduce heat and cook for 25 minutes. Allow pressure to release slowly.

Using oven mitts or hot pads, remove mold from cooker. Remove lid from mold. Invert pudding onto serving plate. Unmold

pudding. Serve warm with Spiced Whipped Cream.

Alternate Stovetop Method
Prepare batter and pour into mold or bowl as directed.

Place mold on a rack in a large stock pot filled with enough water to come halfway up the sides of the mold. Cover and simmer on low heat for 1 hour and 15 minutes.

Remove the pudding mold from the pot and let cool for 10 minutes. To unmold, remove the lid and gently shake until the pudding pulls away from the sides. Carefully invert onto a serving plate. If it sticks, gently tap the mold with a wooden spoon.

Note

Use a stainless-steel kitchen bowl 8 inches in diameter and at least 3 inches deep. For a lid, cut four 12-inch foil squares and layer them over the top. Take a string and tie it around the foil to secure the flaps so no water gets in. Cook as directed.

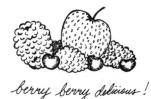

berry berry delicious!

Spiced Whipped Cream
PRO/FATS—LEVEL ONE

SERVES 6

This spiced whipped cream is a wonderful twist on regular whipped cream. Use this wherever you would use regular whipped cream—it's great with my Mixed Berry Steamed Pudding (p. 298), with chocolate cake, or as a layer in my Cherry Chocolate Trifle (p. 292).

PREP TIME: 4 MINUTES

1 cup heavy cream, chilled
2 teaspoons SomerSweet
1/2 teaspoon vanilla extract

1/2 teaspoon cinnamon
1/2 teaspoon nutmeg
Pinch of allspice

Pour heavy cream into a large stainless-steel bowl. Beat with an electric mixer at high speed until frothy. Add remaining ingredients and continue to beat until soft peaks form. Cover and chill until you are ready to use.

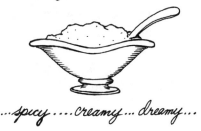

...spicy....creamy...dreamy...

Chocolate Cream Pie

ALMOST LEVEL ONE

SERVES 8

Now you don't have to pass on the pie! This pie has a delicious all-chocolate crust with no flour, which makes it Almost Level One. To make the chocolate custard you can use my Somersize Chocolate Mousse Mix, or follow the recipe below to make it from scratch.

PREP TIME: 20 MINUTES
CHILLING TIME: 2 HOURS

FOR THE CRUST
¾ cup heavy cream
4 ounces unsweetened chocolate, broken
  up
1 tablespoon SomerSweet
1 teaspoon vanilla extract
¼ teaspoon baking soda

FOR THE FILLING
1 prepared package Somersize Chocolate
  Mousse Mix or 1 recipe Chocolate
  Custard (p. 301)

FOR THE TOPPING
2 cups heavy cream
1 tablespoon SomerSweet
1 teaspoon vanilla extract
1 tablespoon cocoa powder

For the Crust

Heat cream in a small heavy-bottomed saucepan over medium heat. When bubbles appear around the edge of the pan, remove from heat. Do not let cream boil. Add chocolate and stir until smooth. Add remaining ingredients and stir well. Pour chocolate mixture into the bottom of a 9-inch glass pie pan. Smooth along the edge of the pie pan to create the crust. Refrigerate until set, about 1 hour.

Pour cooled chocolate mousse into chocolate crust.

For the Topping

Place cream into a mixing bowl. Beat on high speed until frothy. Add remaining ingredients and continue beating until cream forms stiff peaks. Mound cream on top of pie. Chill until ready to serve.

Chocolate Custard

MAKES: 8 SERVINGS

Chocolate custard! Am I dreaming? No, Somersizing!

PREP TIME: 20 MINUTES
CHILLING TIME: 2 TO 3 HOURS

6 egg yolks, beaten
2 ounces unsweetened chocolate
  (preferably Hershey's)

2 cups heavy cream
1 tablespoon plus 2 teaspoons SomerSweet
½ teaspoon vanilla extract

Place egg yolks into a stainless-steel bowl. In a small heavy-bottomed saucepan, melt chocolate over low heat. Add cream, SomerSweet, and vanilla.

Heat mixture, stirring occasionally, until small bubbles appear around the edges or until an instant-read thermometer inserted into the mixture reads 120 degrees.

Pour cream mixture over egg yolks, stirring constantly. Place bowl over a saucepan of simmering water and cook until mixture thickens slightly or until an instant-read thermometer inserted in the custard reads 160 degrees. Remove bowl from saucepan.

Cover the surface of the custard with a layer of plastic wrap. Cool to room temperature, about 1 hour. Refrigerate for at least 2 hours until set.

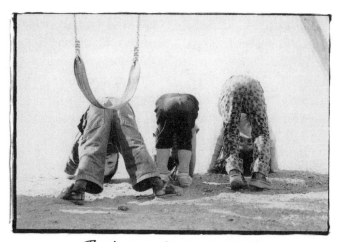

They're cute from any angle.

Somersize Coffee Toffee Ice Cream

PRO/FATS—ALMOST LEVEL ONE

MAKES 1 QUART

I have a Somersize Coffee Ice Cream Mix if you want to make this in a snap. Or simply follow the easy instructions below for a delicious combination of Coffee Ice Cream with chunks of my Somer-Sweet English Style Butter Toffee. This is great with my Somersize Hot Caramel on top.

PREP TIME: 60 MINUTES

CHILLING TIME: 30 TO 45 MINUTES

5 large egg yolks, beaten
2½ cups heavy whipping cream
3 tablespoons instant decaffeinated coffee granules
3 tablespoons plus 2 teaspoons SomerSweet
1 teaspoon vanilla extract

1 cup half-and-half
SomerSweet English Style Butter Toffee, cut into ¼-inch chunks

EQUIPMENT
Ice cream maker

Place egg yolks in a stainless-steel bowl. Set aside. Heat 1½ cups of cream in a small saucepan over low heat until small bubbles appear on the outer edge. If you use an instant-read thermometer, the temperature of the cream should read about 120 degrees.

Pour half of the hot cream over the egg yolks, stirring constantly. Place bowl over a simmering pan of water.

Cook, whisking slowly, until mixture thickens slightly, about 4 minutes, or until a thermometer inserted into the mixture reads 160 degrees. Add decaf coffee granules, SomerSweet, and vanilla. Whisk until coffee has dissolved.

Stir in remaining 1 cup of cream and the half-and-half. Refrigerate for 2 hours, or overnight. Freeze in an ice cream maker following the manufacturer's instructions. During the last 5 minutes, sprinkle in the toffee chunks.

Strawberry Ice Cream

ALMOST LEVEL ONE

MAKES 1 QUART

I love to make strawberry ice cream in the middle of the summer when the berries are bursting with ripeness. Of course, frozen berries make this recipe a snap all year long. Plus, the frozen berries cool the mixture so you don't have to wait for it to chill before pouring it into your ice cream maker.

PREP TIME: 12 MINUTES

4 large egg yolks
½ cup half-and-half
2 cups heavy whipping cream

1 (16-ounce) package frozen strawberries
    or 2 cups fresh
2 tablespoons plus 1 teaspoon SomerSweet

Place egg yolks in a medium stainless-steel bowl and whisk for 2 to 3 minutes, until pale yellow. Set aside. Heat half-and-half and cream in a small heavy-bottomed saucepan over medium heat until bubbles appear around the edge. Remove from heat. Pour half of the hot cream mixture over egg yolks, stirring constantly for 2 to 3 minutes. Add remaining cream mixture and continue whisking for another minute.

Place the stainless-steel bowl over a saucepan of simmering water. Stir egg–cream mixture for 3 minutes until slightly thickened.

Place fresh or frozen strawberries into the bowl of a food processor or blender. Pour thickened egg–cream mixture over fruit and allow mixture to sit for 5 minutes. Add SomerSweet. Pulse mixture until fruit is chopped but still chunky. If using frozen berries there is no need to chill the mixture. Simply follow the ice cream maker instructions as directed. If using fresh berries, chill the ice cream mixture for at least 2 hours, or overnight, then follow the ice cream maker instructions as directed.

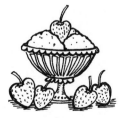

Raspberry Meringue Cake

ALMOST LEVEL ONE

MAKES 6 TO 8 SERVINGS

I could write a whole dessert book around this fabulous meringue cake. It came from my pal Merv Griffin, who loves SomerSweet. His personal chef, David Mantessi, created this fabulous soft, airy meringue cake, and it's a real winner. The addition of the raspberries makes this Almost Level One, but it's only a minor imbalance. You can make this cake even faster by purchasing just the egg whites available in the refrigerator section of your grocery store. Serve the extra raspberry purée over ice cream.

PREP TIME: 12 MINUTES
COOKING TIME: 1 HOUR

9 egg whites (about 1 cup), at room temperature
1/3 cup SomerSweet
1/2 teaspoon water

Pinch of salt
1/4 cup Raspberry Purée (p. 305)
1 recipe Perfectly Whipped Cream (p. 305)

Preheat oven to 250 degrees. Line a non-stick 8- or 9-inch round springform pan with wax paper or parchment paper.

Place egg whites in a clean stainless-steel bowl of an electric mixer. Beat on medium speed until frothy. Add SomerSweet, water, and salt. Increase speed to high and beat until egg whites form stiff peaks, about 6 minutes. Do not let egg whites get too dry.

Spoon meringue into prepared pan. Distribute meringue evenly over bottom of springform pan, taking care not to deflate the batter. Bake in the center of oven for 1 hour. Remove cake from oven and allow to cool for 5 minutes. Carefully run a thin-bladed knife or metal spatula around the edge of the cake to loosen it. Remove out-side edge of springform pan. Run a spatula underneath the cake to loosen it from the wax paper underneath. Transfer cake onto a serving platter.

For Raspberry Whipped Cream

Fold Raspberry Purée into Perfectly Whipped Cream recipe. Using a spatula, smooth over top and sides of cake. Serve immediately or refrigerate.

Note

If you want extra Raspberry Purée, double the recipe and use half to make the Raspberry Whipped Cream and half to spoon onto each plate. Garnish with whole raspberries or a mint leaf.

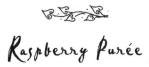

Raspberry Purée

MAKES 1 CUP

PREP TIME: 5 MINUTES

1 (12-ounce) package frozen raspberries,
  thawed
1 tablespoon SomerSweet
1 teaspoon vanilla extract

Place all ingredients in the bowl of a food processor or blender. Blend until smooth. Taste and add more SomerSweet if needed.

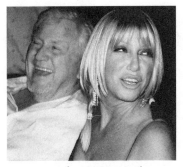

My pal Merv and me.
We've been friends for years.

Perfectly Whipped Cream

PRO/FATS AND VEGGIES—LEVEL ONE

MAKES ABOUT 3 CUPS

Fat is your friend . . . fat is your friend . . . fat is your friend. I guess whipped cream is your best friend!

PREP TIME: 3 MINUTES

2 cups heavy whipping cream
1 teaspoon vanilla extract

2 teaspoons SomerSweet

With an electric mixer, whip the cream until it starts to thicken. Add the vanilla and the SomerSweet. Continue whipping until soft peaks form.

Chocolate Cupcakes with Whipped Cream Filling

LEVEL TWO

MAKES 12

Kids love Hostess cupcakes from the grocery store (and so do I!). Here's my Somersize version. No one will ever notice the missing sugar. You'll notice the missing sugar "meltdown." I made these into a "birthday cake" for my granddaughter's birthday. They were a big hit.

PREP TIME: 20 MINUTES
COOKING TIME: 10 MINUTES
COOLING TIME: 30 MINUTES

FOR THE CUPCAKES
Unsalted butter for greasing muffin tins
1 1/3 cups whole-wheat flour
1/2 cup SomerSweet
2/3 cup unsweetened cocoa powder
1 teaspoon baking powder
1 teaspoon baking soda
1 1/2 teaspoons salt
3 egg whites
2/3 cup mayonnaise
2 teaspoons vanilla extract
1/3 cup heavy cream

1 cup water
2 tablespoons instant decaf coffee granules

FOR THE FILLING
2/3 cup heavy cream
1/2 teaspoon vanilla extract
1 teaspoon SomerSweet

FOR THE FROSTING
1 recipe Somersize Dipping and Coating
   Fudge Sauce (p. 290) or 1 jar Somersize
   Triple Hot Fudge Sauce

Preheat oven to 350 degrees. Grease a 12-cup muffin tin and set aside. Take 2 tablespoons of the flour and coat the muffin tin. Tap out excess flour.

Mix together the remaining flour, SomerSweet, cocoa powder, baking powder, baking soda, and salt in a medium-size bowl.

In a separate bowl, beat the egg whites until frothy. Add mayonnaise, vanilla, cream, water, and coffee. Whisk until well blended.

Pour the wet mixture into the dry ingredients and stir thoroughly until the batter is smooth. Divide batter among the muffin tins. Bake for 10 minutes, or until a toothpick inserted into center comes out clean.

Cool on a wire rack for 10 minutes. Remove cupcakes from muffin tins and cool completely before filling, about 20 minutes.

When muffins are cool, use a melon baller to scoop a hole from the bottom of each cupcake. Reserve the piece of cake to use as a plug. Using the melon baller, enlarge the hole in the center of the cupcake. Set cupcakes aside.

With an electric mixer, whip the cream until it starts to thicken. Add the vanilla and SomerSweet. Continue whipping until soft peaks form.

Using a small spoon or butter knife, fill cupcake holes with the whipped cream. Use reserved cupcake bottoms to plug the holes. Place right side up on a piece of wax paper.

Carefully reheat the Somersize Dipping and Coating Fudge Sauce in a microwave on high for 30 seconds. Stir well. Repeat heating and stirring until mixture is smooth. Do not overheat or sauce will separate. Spoon sauce carefully over tops of cupcakes.

Variation
Mix $1/4$ cup cocoa powder into the filling for a chocolate-filled cupcake. You can also put any extra filling in a pastry bag and use it to decorate the tops of the cupcakes.

Lemon-Lime Jiggly Fruit Gels

FRUIT—LEVEL ONE

MAKES 4 SERVINGS

When I was a kid, my mother made Jell-O for me and I loved it. I had no idea how much sugar was in it, though. Now I've made my own Jiggly Fruit Gels with no sugar! What a treat. It's not clear, but it's jiggly and wiggly, and the kids love it. You can make it in a glass baking dish and then slice it into cubes and serve it in pretty glasses.

PREP TIME: 8 MINUTES
CHILLING TIME: 2 HOURS

3 cups water
3 (1/4-ounce) packets unflavored gelatin
1/4 cup plus 2 tablespoons fresh lemon juice
  (about 4 lemons)
1/4 cup fresh lime juice (6–8 limes)

1/2 teaspoon pure lemon extract
Green food coloring (optional)
3 tablespoons SomerSweet
Perfectly Whipped Cream, for garnish
  (p. 305)

Place water in a small saucepan. Sprinkle gelatin over water. Allow gelatin to soften for 5 minutes. Heat gelatin on low, stirring constantly until it has dissolved. Stir in lemon juice, lime juice, lemon extract, food coloring, and SomerSweet. Stir until SomerSweet has dissolved. Pour mixture into an 8 × 8-inch baking dish. Refrigerate for at least 2 hours. Cut into cubes and serve with Perfectly Whipped Cream.

Variation

To make ice pops, follow recipe for fruit gels as directed, increasing SomerSweet to 4 tablespoons. Pour into ice pop molds.

Allow to cool to room temperature. Freeze for at least 4 hours. To unmold pops, dip mold into hot water for 10 to 20 seconds. As an alternative to the molds, use disposable fluted plastic champagne glasses. Freeze for about 1 hour, then insert sticks and continue to freeze until solid, about 3 hours more.

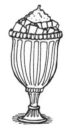

Orange Jiggly Fruit Gels

FRUIT—LEVEL ONE

MAKES 4 SERVINGS

Something between a gelatin and a pudding, but better than both. My fruit gels have a fresh, fruity taste that everyone will enjoy. Add chopped chunks of mango or berries for even more fruity fun.

PREP TIME: 8 MINUTES
CHILLING TIME: 2 HOURS

2 cups orange juice
1 cup water
3 (1/4-ounce) packets unflavored gelatin
3/4 teaspoon orange extract

1 tablespoon SomerSweet
Chunks of fruit (optional)
Perfectly Whipped Cream for Almost
    Level One garnish (p. 305)

Place orange juice in a mixing bowl. Set aside.

Place water in a small saucepan. Sprinkle gelatin over water. Allow gelatin to soften for 5 minutes. Heat gelatin on low, stirring constantly until gelatin has dissolved. Pour gelatin mixture into orange juice. Stir well. Add orange extract and SomerSweet. Stir until SomerSweet has dissolved. Pour into an 8 × 8-inch baking dish. Add optional chunks of fruit. Refrigerate for at least 2 hours. Cut into cubes and serve with Perfectly Whipped Cream.

Variation
To make ice pops, follow recipe for fruit gels as directed, increasing SomerSweet to 2 tablespoons. Pour into molds. Allow to cool to room temperature. Freeze for at least 4 hours. To unmold ice pops, dip mold into hot water for 10 to 20 seconds. As an alternative to the molds, use disposable fluted plastic champagne glasses. Freeze for about 1 hour, then insert sticks and continue to freeze until solid, about 3 hours more.

Blueberry Jiggly Fruit Gels

FRUIT—LEVEL ONE

MAKES 4 SERVINGS

More jiggly fun!

PREP TIME: 8 MINUTES
CHILLING TIME: 2 HOURS

1 pound frozen blueberries, thawed
1 cup water
3 ($^1/_4$-ounce) packets unflavored gelatin

1 tablespoon SomerSweet
Perfectly Whipped Cream for Almost
 Level One garnish (p. 305)

Place thawed blueberries with juice in the bowl of a food processor. Add $^1/_2$ cup of the water. Process until smooth. Place blueberry purée in a sieve set over a bowl. Allow mixture to drain, gently pressing on the blueberries to extract all juices.

Place remaining $^1/_2$ cup water in a small saucepan. Sprinkle gelatin over water. Allow gelatin to soften for 5 minutes. Heat gelatin on low, stirring constantly until gelatin has dissolved. Add SomerSweet and stir until dissolved. Pour gelatin mixture into blueberry juice. Pour mixture into an 8 × 8-inch baking dish. Refrigerate for at least 2 hours. Cut into cubes and serve with Perfectly Whipped Cream.

Variation
To make ice pops, follow recipe for fruit gels as directed, increasing SomerSweet to 2 tablespoons. Pour into molds. Allow to cool to room temperature. Freeze for at least 4 hours. To unmold pops, dip mold into hot water for 10 to 20 seconds. As an alternative to molds, use disposable fluted plastic champagne glasses. Freeze for about 1 hour, then insert sticks and continue to freeze until solid, about 3 hours more.

Raspberry Jiggly Fruit Gels

FRUIT—LEVEL ONE

MAKES 4 SERVINGS

This is great with chunks of mango and raspberries.

PREP TIME: 8 MINUTES
CHILLING TIME: 2 HOURS

1 pound frozen raspberries, thawed
1 cup orange juice
1 cup water
3 (¼-ounce) packets unflavored gelatin

1 tablespoon plus 1 teaspoon SomerSweet
Chunks of assorted fruit (optional)
Perfectly Whipped Cream, for garnish
  (p. 305)

Place thawed raspberries in the bowl of a food processor or blender. Add orange juice. Process until smooth. Place raspberry purée in a sieve set over a bowl. Allow mixture to drain, gently pressing to extract all the juices.

Place water in a small saucepan. Sprinkle gelatin over water. Allow gelatin to soften for 5 minutes. Heat gelatin on low, stirring constantly until gelatin has dissolved. Add SomerSweet and stir until dissolved. Pour gelatin mixture into orange–raspberry juice. Pour mixture into an 8 × 8-inch baking dish. Add optional chunks of fruit. Refrigerate for at least 2 hours. Cut into cubes and serve with Perfectly Whipped Cream.

Variation

To make ice pops, follow recipe for fruit gels as directed, increasing SomerSweet to 2 tablespoons. Pour into ice pop molds. Allow to cool to room temperature. Freeze for at least 4 hours. To unmold pops, dip mold into hot water for 10 to 20 seconds. As an alternative to the molds, use disposable fluted plastic champagne glasses. Freeze for about 1 hour, then insert sticks and continue to freeze until solid, about 3 hours more.

Somersicles

SERVES 8 TO 10

Kids love frozen desserts on a stick. Now you can make homemade ice pops without any sugar. Use unsweetened fruit juice or my Somersize Drink Mixes.

2 cups diced fruit or berries
1 packet Peach-Mango or Lemon-Lime
    Somersize Drink Mix
1 cup cold water, or fruit juice

2 envelopes unflavored gelatin
3 cups water, heated to boiling

EQUIPMENT
Ice pop molds

Divide the fruit into the bottom of ice pop molds. Stir contents of drink mix package with 1 cup cold water. Sprinkle gelatin over cold water mixture. Let mixture soften for 2 minutes. Add hot water and stir until gelatin has dissolved, about 4 minutes. Pour into molds.

Allow to cool to room temperature.

Freeze for at least 4 hours. To unmold pops, dip mold into hot water for 10 to 20 seconds.

As an alternative to the molds, use disposable fluted plastic champagne glasses. Freeze for about 1 hour, then insert sticks and continue to freeze until solid, about 3 hours more.

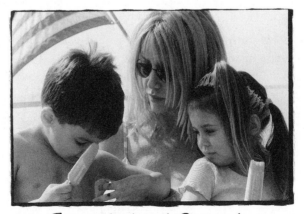

*The grandkids with Somersicles.
They're both such a treat.*

Appendix

When I first discovered this remarkable way of eating I was determined to find medical research to make sure my program was not only effective, but safe. If raised insulin levels are responsible for weight, increased cholesterol, hypertension, heart disease, and certain types of cancer, why aren't doctors telling us to worry about our sugar intake?

Surprisingly, finding the medical backup was not difficult at all. The effects of high insulin levels (resulting from overeating sugar/carbohydrates/caffeine or from stress) and their relationship to weight gain, abnormal cholesterol levels, coronary heart disease, and Type II diabetes have been documented in numerous medical studies that span more than thirty years! This is hardly new information.

Specifically, I want to share three articles linking high insulin levels to these diseases. The first is from *The New England Journal of Medicine.* "Risk Factors for Coronary Artery Disease in Healthy Persons with Hyperinsulinemia and Normal Glucose Tolerance" (Vol. 320, March 16, 1989) concluded that healthy persons with hyperinsulinemia and normal glucose levels are at higher risk for coronary artery disease, as compared with a well-matched group of healthy subjects with normal insulin levels.

The second article is from *Diabetes Care,* "Insulin Resistance: A Multifaceted Syndrome Responsible for NIDDM, Obesity, Hypertension, Dyslipidemia, and Atherosclerotic Cardiovascular Disease" (Vol. 14, no. 3, March 1991). I'll share with you a passage from the summary:

Much evidence has begun to accumulate that chronic day-long hyperinsulinemia is associated with the development of hypertension [high blood pressure], hyperlipidemia [high cholesterol and triglycerides], and atherosclerosis [clogged arteries]. In a sense, insulin resistance can be viewed as a large iceberg submerged just below the surface of the water. The physician recognizes only the tip of the iceberg—diabetes, obesity, hypertension, hypertriglyceridemia, diminished HDL-chol, and atherosclerosis—which extrude above the surface, and complete insulin resistance may be missed.

The third article, also from *Diabetes Care,* "Insulin and Atheroma: A 20-Year Perspective" (Vol. 13, no. 6, June 1990), outlines the research on the subject of insulin for the last twenty years. This comprehensive study concludes:

> The fact that hyperinsulinemia has been shown to have an independent predictive correlation with cardiovascular disease and that insulin has biological actions on arterial tissue, lipid metabolism, and renal sodium handling suggest that the primary abnormality may be hyperinsulinemia due to insulin resistance.

Check out these articles for yourself.

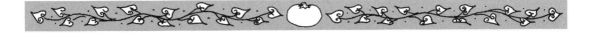

Reference Guide

Here is a complete list of all the foods available in each of the categories:

PRO/FATS

CHEESE
American
asiago
Babybel
bel paese
blue
Bonbel
Brie
buffalo mozzarella
Camembert
cheddar
Colby
cream cheese
farmer
feta
fontina
goat
gouda

Gruyère
Havarti
hoop
Jarlsberg
Limburger
mascarpone
Monterey jack
mozzarella
Muenster
Parmesan
pecorino
provolone
queso blanco
ricotta
Romano
Roquefort
string
Swiss

OTHER DAIRY PRODUCTS
butter
cream
eggs
margarine
mayonnaise
sour cream
whey protein

FISH
anchovy
bass
bluefish
bonito
burbot
carp
catfish

cod
eel
flatfish
flounder
gefilte fish
grouper
haddock
halibut
herring
mackerel
mahi-mahi
monkfish
ocean perch
orange roughy
pollack
pompano
red snapper
sablefish

salmon
sardine
sea bass
shark
smelt
snapper
sole
sturgeon
swordfish
tripe
trout
tuna
turbot
whitefish
wolf fish
yellowtail

MEAT
bacon
Canadian bacon
beef
bologna
bratwurst
capocollo
cold cuts
frog's legs
ham
hot dogs
lamb
pastrami
pepperoni
pork
prosciutto
rabbit
salami

sausage
veal
venison

OILS
canola oil
chili oil
olive oil
peanut oil
safflower oil
sesame oil
vegetable oil

POULTRY
capon
chicken
Cornish game hen
duck
goose

guinea hen
pheasant
quail
squab
turkey

SEAFOOD
abalone
caviar
clams
crab
crayfish
lobster
mussels
octopus
oysters
scallops
shrimp
squid

CARBOS

BEANS
adzuki beans
anasazi beans
black beans
black-eyed peas
cannellini beans
fava beans
garbanzo beans
great northern beans
green peas
kidney beans
lentils
lima beans
mung beans
navy beans
pinto beans
red beans
split peas
white beans

BREADS, BAGELS, CRACKERS, HOT CEREALS, COLD CEREALS, OR PASTA MADE FROM WHOLE GRAINS
amaranth
barley
bran
brown rice
buckwheat
kamut
millet
oat
pumpernickel
rye
spelt
wheat

NONFAT DAIRY PRODUCTS
nonfat cottage cheese
nonfat milk
nonfat rice milk
nonfat ricotta cheese
nonfat sour cream
nonfat soy milk
nonfat yogurt

RICE
brown rice
brown rice cakes
wild rice

VEGGIES

alfalfa sprouts
artichoke
arugula
asparagus
bamboo shoots
basil
bean sprouts
beet greens
bok choy
broccoli
brussels sprouts
cabbage
cauliflower
celery
chervil
chicory greens
chives
cilantro
clover sprouts
collard greens
crookneck squash

cucumber
daikon
dandelion greens
dill weed
eggplant
endive
escarole
fennel
garlic
ginger
green beans
horseradish
jícama
kale
kohlrabi
leeks
lettuce
   Boston or bibb
   frisée
   iceberg
   limestone

red oak
romaine
mushrooms
mustard greens
okra
onion
parsley
peppers
   bell peppers
   cherry peppers
   chili peppers
   pepperoncini
   piccalilli
pickles (except sweet)
purslane
radicchio
radish
rhubarb
rosemary
sage
salsify

sauerkraut
scallions
shallots
snow peas
spinach
sugar snap peas
Swiss chard
tarragon
thyme
tomatillo
tomato
tomato (green)
turnip
turnip greens
water chestnut
watercress
wax beans
yard-long beans
yellow beans
zucchini

FRUIT

apples
apricots
Asian pear
berries
   blackberry
   blueberry
   boysenberry
   cranberry
   currant
   elderberry
   gooseberry
   mulberry
   ollalaberry
   raspberry

strawberry
cherimoya
cherry
crabapple
fig
grapefruit
grapes
guava
kiwi
kumquat
lemon
lime
loquat
lychee

mandarin oranges
mangoes
melons
   cantaloupe
   casaba
   Crenshaw
   honeydew
   orange flesh
   sharlyn
   watermelon
nectarines
oranges
papaya
passion fruit

peaches
pears
persimmon
pineapple
plums
pomegranate
prickly pear
pommelo
quince
star fruit
tamarind
tangerine

YOUR ONE-PAGE REFERENCE GUIDE

For the first few days or weeks on the program, you might want to make a copy of this page and slip it into your purse or wallet. Somersizing will soon become second nature to you, but this summary will help remind you of the plan until you no longer need it for reference.

1. Eliminate all Funky Foods.
2. Eat Fruits alone, on an empty stomach.
3. Eat Proteins/Fats with Veggies.
4. Eat Carbos with Veggies and no fat.
5. Keep Proteins/Fats separate from Carbos.
6. Wait three hours between meals if switching from a Proteins/Fats meal to a Carbos meal, or vice versa.
7. Do not skip meals. Eat three meals a day, and eat until you feel satisfied and comfortably full.

PROTEINS AND FATS

Butter	Mayonnaise
Cheese	Meat
Cream	Oil
Eggs	Poultry
Fish	Sour cream

VEGGIES

Asparagus	Green beans
Broccoli	Lettuce
Cauliflower	Mushrooms
Celery	Spinach
Cucumber	Tomato
Eggplant	Zucchini

CARBOS

Beans	Whole-grain
Nonfat milk	breads, cereals,
products	pastas
Nonfat soy milk	

FRUITS

Apples	Oranges
Berries	Papaya
Grapes	Peaches
Mangoes	Pears
Melons	Plums
Nectarines	

Eliminate Funky Foods

SUGAR

Beets	Maple syrup
Carrots	Molasses
Corn syrup	Sugar
Honey	

STARCHES

Bananas	Potatoes
Corn	Sweet potatoes
Pasta made from	White flour
semolina or	White rice
white flour	Winter squashes
Popcorn	(acorn, butternut)

COMBO PROTEINS/FATS AND CARBOS

Avocados	Nuts
Buttermilk	Olives
Coconuts	Tofu
Liver	
Low-fat or	
whole milk	

CAFFEINE AND ALCOHOL

Alcoholic beverages
Caffeinated coffees, teas, and sodas
Cocoa (including unsweetened cocoa)

Bibliography

Anderson, K. M., W. P. Castelli, and D. Levy. "Cholesterol and Mortality: 30 Years of Follow-up from the Framingham Study," *JAMA* 257 (1987): 2176–80.

Anderson-Parrado, Patricia. "Type II Diabetes and Obesity: An All-Too-Common Combination." *Better Nutrition*. April 1998. FINDarticles.com. 2 Jan. 2002. <http://www.findarticles.com/cf_0/m0FKA /n4_v60/20471628/print.jhtml>

Applegate, Liz. "Fats as Fuel? A Little More Fat in Your Diet May Help You on Your Next Run," *Runner's World* 29, no. 6 (June 1994): 24.

Atkins, Robert C. "Artificial Sugar: A Sweet and Dangerous Lure," *Dr. Atkins' Health Revelations* (April 1994): 1.

Barlow, Sarah E., M.D., MPH, and William H. Dietz, M.D. Ph.D. "Obesity Evaluation and Treatment: Expert Committee Recommendations." *Pediatrics*. 3 Sept. 1998. Pediatrics .org. 11 Dec. 2001 <http://www.pediatrics.org/cgi/content /full/102/3/e29>

Brown, David. "Linkage of Breast Cancer, Dietary Fat Is Discounted," *The Washington Post* 119, no. 65 (February 8, 1996): A5, col. 1.

"Brown University Child and Adolescent Behavior Letter: Childhood Obesity." *American Diabetes Association*. June 2000. FINDarticles.com. 19 Dec. 2001. <http://www.findarticles.com/cf_0/m0537 /6_16/62801487/print.jhtml>

Carlson, L. A., L. E. Bottiger, and P. E. Anfeldt. "Risk Factors for Myocardial Infarction in the Stockholm Prospective Study: A 14-year Follow-up Focusing on the Role of Plasma Triglycerides and Cholesterol," *Acta Med Scand* 206 (1979): 351–60.

Clark, Nancy. "Fat and Fiction: Dispelling the Myths About Fat in a Healthy Diet," *American Fitness* 15, no. 3 (May–June 1997): 59.

Critser, Greg. "Let Them Eat Fat." (brief article) *Harper's Magazine*. March 2000. FINDarticles.com. 11 Dec. 2001.

<http://www.findarticles.com/cf_dls /m1111/1798_300/60102141/print.jhtml>

DeFronzo, R. A. "Insulin Secretion, Insulin Resistance, and Obesity." *Int J Obes* 6 (Suppl. 1) (1982): 72–82.

DeFronzo, R. A., and E. Ferrannini. "Insulin Resistance: A Multifaceted Syndrome Responsible for NIDDM, Obesity, Hypertension, Dyslipemia, and Atherosclerotic Cardiovascular Disease," *Diabetes Care* 14, no. 3 (March 1991): 173.

"Evidence Proves Sugar-Sweetened Beverages Contributing to Obesity in Children." (brief article) *Nutrition Research Newsletter.* Mar. 2001. FINDarticles.com. 11 Dec. 2001. <http://www.findarticles.com/cf_0/m0887 /3_20/72606626/print.jhtml>

Fackelmann, K. "Hidden Hazards: Do High Blood Insulin Levels Foretell Heart Disease?" *Science News* 136 (September 16, 1989): 184.

"Fatter Parents, Fatter Kids: Childhood Obesity Is a Hefty Problem." *CNN In-Depth Health.* 8 Sept. 1998. CNN interactive. 11 Dec. 2001. <http://www.cnn.com/HEALTH/9809/08 /child.obesity/>

Fontbonne, A. "Why Can High Insulin Levels Indicate a Risk Factor for Coronary Heart Disease?" *Diabetologia* 37 (1994): 953–55.

Foster, G. D., H. R. Wyatt, J.O. Hill, et al. "Evaluation of the Atkins Diet: A Randomized Controlled Trial. *Obes Res.* 2001; 9 (suppl 3): 0132.

Garn, Stanley, Ph.D. "Obesity." *Gale Encyclopedia of Childhood and Adolescence.* FINDarticles .com. 11 Dec. 2001. <http://www.findarticles.com/cf_dls/g2602 /0004/2602000409/pl/article.jhtml>

Grundy, Scott M. "Cholesterol and Coronary Disease," *JAMA* 256 (1986): 2849–58.

———. "Fats and Oil Consumption to Combat Metabolic Complications and Obesity," *American Journal of Clinical Nutrition* 67, no. 3

(March 1998): 5275.

Howe, Maggy. "Good Fats, Bad Fats," *Country Living* 21, no. 1 (January 1998): 50.

Hughes, Zondra. "What to Do If Your Child Is Too Fat." *Ebony.* July 2000. FINDarticles .com. 11 Dec. 2001. <http://www.findarticles.com/cf_dls/m1077 /9_55/63165394/print.jhtml>

Jenkins, J. A., et al. "Starchy Foods and Glycemic Index," *Diabetes Care* 11, no. 2 (February 1998): 149.

Ludwig, David S., Karen E. Peterson, and Steven L. Gortmaker. "Relation Between Consumption of Sugar-Sweetened Drinks and Childhood Obesity: A Prospective, Observational Analysis." *The Lancet.* 17 Feb. 2001: Vol. 357.

Modann, M., H. Halkin, S. Almog, et al. "Hyperinsulinemia: A Link Between Hypertension, Obesity, and Glucose Intolerance," *J Clin Invest* 75 (1985): 809–17.

"New Study Links Over-Consumption of Soft and Fruit Drinks to Childhood Obesity." *Business Wire.* 16 Feb. 2001. FINDarticles .com. 11 Dec. 2001. <http://www.findarticles.com/cf_0/m0EIN /2001_Feb_16/70505490/print.jhtml>

"Obesity Overview." *Spotlight Health.* 11 Dec. 2001. <http://www.spotlighthealth.com/morbid _obesity/obesity_overview/index.html>

"What is Morbid Obesity?" *Spotlight Health.* 11 Dec. 2001. <http://www.spotlighthealth.com /morbid_obesity/obesity_overview/what _is_morbid_obesity?html>

"What is Morbid Obesity? Related Health Problems." *Spotlight Health.* 11 Dec. 2001. <http://www.spotlighthealth.com /morbid_obesity/obesity_overview /related_problems.html>

"How Is Obesity Diagnosed?" *Spotlight Health*. 11 Dec. 2001. <http://www.spotlighthealth.com/morbid_obesity/obesity_overview/identify_morbid_obesity.html>

"Understanding the Body Mass Index (BMI)?" *Spotlight Health*. 11 Dec. 2001. <http://www.spotlighthealth.com/morbid_obesity/obesity_overview/bmi.html>

"Obesity: Statistics." *Spotlight Health*. 11 Dec. 2001. <http://www.spotlighthealth.com/morbid_obesity/obesity_overview/oo_obesity_statistics.html>

Page, Douglas. "Give Fat a Break," *Muscle and Fitness* 58, no. 5 (May 1997): 58.

Pollare, T., H. Lithell, and C. Berne. "Insulin Resistance Is a Characteristic Feature of Primary Hypertension Independent of Obesity," *Metabolism* 39 (1990): 167–74.

Raloff, Janet. "High Fat Diets Help Athletes Perform," *Science News* 149, no. 18 (May 4, 1996): 287.

Reaven, G. M. "Banting Lecture: Role of Insulin Resistance in Human Disease," *Diabetes* 37 (1988): 1595–1607.

Reaven, G. M., C. B. Hollenbeck, and Y-DI Chen. "Relationship between Glucose Tolerance, Insulin Secretion, and Insulin Action in Non-Obese Individuals with Varying Degrees of Glucose Tolerance," *Diabetologia* 32 (1989): 52–55.

Reppert, Bertha, and Sharon Mikkelson. "Stevia (Stevia rebaudiana 'honeyleaf ')," *American Health and Herbs* (1998): 1–7.

Schechter, Steven. "Fat Intake Can Boost Weight Loss, If We Are Selective About Our Choices," *Better Nutrition* 59, no. 6 (June 1997): 26.

Schwarzbein, Diana, and Nancy Deville. *The Schwarzbein Principle*. Calif.: Health Communications, Inc., 1999.

Shapiro, Laura. "In Sugar We Trust," *Newsweek* (July 13, 1998): 72.

Sowers, J. R., M. Nyby, N. Stern, F. Beck, S. Baron, R. Catania, and N. Vlachis. "Blood Pressure and Hormone Changes Associated with Weight Reduction in the Obese," *Hypertension* 4 (1982): 686–91.

Stout, Robert W. "Insulin and Atheroma Twenty Year Perspective." *Diabetes Care* 13, no. 6 (June 1990): 631.

Taubes, Gary. "What If It's All Been a Big Fat Lie?" *NY Times*. 7 July 2002. NYTimes.com. 8 July 2002 <http://www.nytimes.com/2002/07/07/magazine/07FAT.html?ex=1027151477&ei=1&en=bb41d22c6b88108>

"Type 2 Diabetes in Children and Adolescents." *American Diabetes Association*. 19 Dec. 2001 <http://www.diabetes.org/ada/consensus/pg381.htm>

Wingard, D. L., E. L. Barrett-Connor, and A. Ferrara. "Is Insulin Really a Heart Disease Risk Factor?" *Diabetes Care* 18 (1995): 1299–1304.

Yancy, W. S., J. R. Guyton, R. P. Bakst, et al. "A Randomized Controlled Trial of a Very-Low-Carbohydrate Diet with Nutritional Supplements Versus a Low-Fat/Low-Calorie Diet. *Obes Res*. 2001; 9 (suppl 3): 17.

Zavaroni, I., et al. "Risk Factors for Coronary Artery Disease in Healthy Persons with Hyperinsulinemia and Normal Glucose Tolerance," *NEJM* 320 (March 16, 1989): 702.

Index

dinner
    best choices for, 11–12, 14, 94
    Level One, 91–93
    scheduling time for, 53–54
Dip, Artichoke and Onion, 196
Dip, Cucumber Dill, 197
disease, causes of, 37, 56
dressing. *See* Salad Dressing
drinks
    diet drinks, 38
    juices, 146
    questions about, 134–37
    soft drinks, 38, 43–44, 118
    water, 118, 135
    Watermelon Icy, 192

*E*ating disorders, 63, 64
edamame, 167
Egg Beaters, 137
Egg(s)
    -in-a-Pan Casserole, South-
        western, 183
    Crêpes, 188
    Florentine, Easy, 184
    and Ham Sandwiches, Green,
        181
    nutrients in, 36–37, 137, 138
    and Sausage Breakfast Enchi-
        ladas, 186
    Spinach "Bread," 182
emotional swings, 19
Enchiladas, Sausage and Egg
    Breakfast, 186
energy, 3, 12–13, 22–23, 59–60,
    83
estrogen, 37
exercise
    for children, 43, 50–51
    effect on bone strength, 64
    effect on insulin, 71, 120
    importance of, 57–59, 120
    recommendations for, 153
    statistics on, 41

*F*ajitas, Beef, 266
family meals, 48–49, 53–54,
    151–52
farina, 126

fast-food, 113–15
fat-free foods, 12, 163
fat-free movement, 23, 25, 26
fat-free sprays, 137
fat reserves, 3, 13, 22–23, 26, 30,
    70
fats, dietary. *See also* Pro/Fats
    group
    controversy over, 29–32, 34,
        35–36
    importance of, 33, 37, 82–83
    insulin and, 30
    metabolizing of, 30
    types of, 33
fatty acids, 36, 83
Fennel, Red Onion, and Hearts
    of Palm Salad, 218
Feta Vinaigrette, Tomato and
    Cucumber Salad with, 215
fiber
    in All-Bran cereal, 128–29
    in berries, 105, 144
    in brown rice, 24
    in complex carbohydrates, 83
    for digestion, 155
    in fruits, 84–85
    insulin and, 24, 128–29
    in low-glycemic foods, 86
    psyllium fiber, 172
    in vegetables, 83–84, 171
fish. *See* Seafood
flavored extracts, 168
flax meal, 128
flaxseed, 165
flaxseed oil, 174
flours, 79, 124, 126–27, 143–44
Free Foods, 85
free radicals, 38
Fritters, Vegetable, 231
fructose, 77
Fruit. *See also specific fruits*
    for breakfast, 88–90
    in Fruits group, 10, 317
    Gels, Jiggly, Blueberry, 310
    Gels, Jiggly, Lemon Lime, 308
    Gels, Jiggly, Orange, 309
    Gels, Jiggly, Raspberry, 311
    guidelines for eating, 84–85,
        105–6
    juices, about, 85, 146

questions about, 144–46
Somersicles, 312
Fruits group, 10, 84–85, 88–90,
    317
frying foods, 33
Fudge Sauce, Somersize Dipping
    and Coating, 290
Funky Foods
    bad combo foods, 80–81
    caffeine and alcohol, 81
    dairy products, 87
    insulin-raising effect of, 9
    in Level Two, 106
    starches, 79–80
    sugars, 77, 79
    vegetables, 86

*G*arlic Chicken, 262
Garlic Sugar Snap Peas, 226
ginger, benefits of, 61
Ginger Chicken Wontons, 199
Ginger Scallion Grilled Mahi
    Mahi, 283
Gingered Soy Sauce, 201
glucose, 83
glycemic index, 85–86
glycogen, 18
Gorgonzola Cheese and Shrimp
    Scampi Salad, 212
grains. *See* whole grains
Grape-Nuts cereal, 128
gravies, 166–67
grocery shopping, 49–50, 164
gum, 129

*H*alf-and-half, 138–39
Ham
    Easy Eggs Florentine, 184
    and Eggs Sandwiches, Green,
        181
    Saltimbocca in a Tarragon But-
        ter Sauce, 260
HDL cholesterol, 34, 36, 140
health-related questions, 148–51
heart disease, 24, 31, 70
herbal supplements, 59–61
high blood pressure, 37, 71
hominy, 157

hormonal imbalances. *See also* cravings
  health problems from, 23, 37
  from raised insulin levels, 23, 37
  therapy for, 98
  weight gain from, 173
hormones. *See also* insulin; serotonin
  female, 37–38, 148, 173–74
  male, 64
HRT (hormone replacement therapy), 173–74
hyperglycemia, 86
hyperinsulinemia, 25–26
hyperinsulinism, 42
hypoglycemia, 65–66
hypothyroidism, 150

Ice Cream
  Lemon Crème Fraîche, 288
  Pink Kiddie, 289
  questions about, 141, 142
  Somersize Coffee Toffee, 302
  Strawberry, 303
iced tea, 134
ideal body composition, 69–70
indigestion, 61
insulin
  blood pressure and, 71
  caffeine and, 44, 81, 82, 136–37
  carbohydrates and, 24–27
  cholesterol and, 23, 31, 32, 35
  dietary fats and, 30
  exercise and, 71, 120
  fat reserves and, 3, 22–23, 26, 30
  fiber and, 24, 128–29
  function of, 22–23
  heart disease and, 24, 31, 70
  hormonal imbalances from, 23, 37
  kidneys and, 71
  protein and, 30
  raised levels of, 23, 32, 35, 37, 71
  resistance, 22–24, 26, 31, 37–38, 70, 81
  sugar and, 24–27

Irish Oatmeal Pancakes with Raspberry Sauce, 188–89

Jams, 128
Jell-O, 162
juices, 146
junk food, 44–46, 49

Kabobs, Scallop, 284
kasha, 124–25
ketchup, 163
Ketchup, Somersize, 245
kidneys, 71

Lactose intolerance, 140
Lasagna, Somersize, 267
LDL cholesterol, 34, 36, 140
Leek and Chicken Stew, Creamy, 254
Leeks, Sweet Braised, 232
Lemon Crème Fraîche Ice Cream, 288
Lemon Lime Jiggly Fruit Gels, 308
Lemon Olive Oil, 279
Lemony Artichokes, 230
Lentil, Red, Cumin Soup, 204
Level One
  breakfasts, 88–91
  cheating in, 51–53, 96–97
  lunches and dinners, 91–93
  sample week on, 98–100
  transitioning from, 153
Level Two
  Bad Combo foods in, 106
  cheating in, 102–4
  desserts in, 106–7
  Funky Foods in, 106
  meal plans for, 108–10
  mixing food groups in, 104–6
  moderation needed for, 103–4, 107–8
  sugar in, 106
  transitioning to, 153
  wine and chocolate in, 108
liver, 150

lunch
  best choices for, 11–12, 14, 94, 165
  brown-bag, 115–17, 155, 165
  Level One, 91–93

Macaroni and Cheese, Somersize, 242
Mahi Mahi, Ginger Scallion Grilled, 283
Malt-O-Meal cereal, 126
malted barley extract, 169–70
margarine, 33, 140
mayonnaise, 163
meals. *See also* breakfast; dinner; lunch
  family meals, 48–49, 53–54, 151–52
  finding rhythm for, 93–94, 157
  Level One, 88–93
  Level Two, 108–10
  scheduling times for, 53–54
  skipping, 11, 118–19
Meatloaves, Mini-Mini, 264
meats. *See also* Beef; Pork
  in Pro/Fats group, 316
  questions about, 146–48
The Melt, 24, 50, 149–50
menopause, 37–38, 62, 150–51, 173–74
menstruation, 150
metabolic aging, 37–38
metabolism
  decreasing, 23, 51
  herbal supplements for, 59–60
  increasing, 51, 66
midsection, 23, 26, 70, 81, 149
milk, 87, 132, 138, 139
minerals, 172
Minestrone, Fast and Easy, 210
moderation, 94–95, 103–4, 107–8
Molly McButter, 138
monounsaturated fats, 33
motivation, 69–73
muscles, lean, 120
Mushroom Sauce, Creamy, 251
mustard, 164
Mustard Dipping Sauce, Chinese-Style Hot, 200

Taco Salad, 221
Taco Wraps, Turkey, 247
tamoxifen, 173
taro root, 166
Tartar Sauce, Somersize, 244–45
tea, 134, 136, 140–41
teenagers, 43, 152
television, 50
testosterone, 37, 64
Tex Mex Black Bean Soup, 208
Tex Mex Pork Chops, Creamy, 274
Tex Mex Seasoning Blend, 275
toast, spreads for, 128, 130
Toffee Coffee Ice Cream, Somersize, 302
tofu, 170
tofu cheese, 131
Tomato(es), 171
    Broiled, 226–27
    Cherry, and Buffalo Mozzarella Salad, 214
    and Cucumber Salad with Feta Vinaigrette, 215
    Somersize Barbecue Sauce, 277
    Somersize Ketchup, 245
    Soup, Eight-Minute Creamy, 207
tortillas, 125
trans fats, 33–34, 138
Trifle, Cherry Chocolate, 292–93
Tuna, Cilantro Lime Grilled, 285
Turkey
    Cheeseburger Pie, 268
    Chili Cheese Fries, 246
    Mini-Mini Meatloaves, 264
    Somersails, 241
    Stuffed Bells, 257
    Taco Wraps, 247
    Twenty-Minute Chili, 265
Type II diabetes, 26, 37, 42, 72

Unsaturated fats, 33, 83

Vanilla Custard, 293
Vegetable(s). *See also* Veggies group; *specific vegetables*
    Calzones, 248
    Fast and Easy Minestrone, 210
    fiber in, 83–84, 171
    Fritters, 231
    high-starch, 86, 171–72
    low-starch, 83–84, 86, 171–72, 317
    Pinwheels, 202
    recipes for, 224–32
vegetarians, 80, 131, 154
veggie burgers, 171
Veggies group
    at breakfast, 90–91
    at dinner, 91–92, 92–93
    at lunch, 91–92, 92–93, 116–17
    mixing with Carbos, 13
    mixing with Pro/Fats, 13
    vegetables in, 9, 83–84, 86, 171–72, 317
Vinaigrette, Citrus-Serrano, 217
Vitamin A, 38, 83
Vitamin C, 38
Vitamin D, 63, 64, 83
Vitamin E, 38, 83
Vitamin K, 83
vitamins, 172

Water chestnut starch, 126
water intake, 118, 135
water weight, 18
Watermelon Icy, 192
weight-loss, temporary, 18–19
weight-loss products, 172–73
wheat allergies, 125
wheat germ, 158
Whipped Cream, Perfectly, 305
Whipped Cream, Spiced, 299
White Bean Rosemary Spread, 198
white flour, 79, 80
white rice, 79, 80
whole grains, 24–25, 125–29, 316
wild rice, 80, 160
wine, 81, 108, 122–23
Wontons, Ginger Chicken, 199

Yams, 79, 161
yeast, 125
yogurt, 87, 132, 137–38, 139, 140
yucca root, 172

Zucchini
    Cumin-Scented, 227
    Noodles Alfredo, 229
    Somersails, 241
    Somersize Fish and Chips, 237
    Turkey Chili Cheese Fries, 246

About the Author

SUZANNE SOMERS is the author of ten books, including the *New York Times* bestsellers *Keeping Secrets; Eat Great, Lose Weight; Get Skinny on Fabulous Food*; and *Eat, Cheat, and Melt the Fat Away*. The former star of the hit television programs *Three's Company* and *Step by Step*, Suzanne is one of the most respected and trusted brand names in the world, representing cosmetics and skincare products, apparel, jewelry, a computerized facial fitness system, fitness products, and a dessert line called SomerSweet.

CONVERSION CHART
EQUIVALENT IMPERIAL AND METRIC MEASUREMENTS

American cooks use standard containers, the 8-ounce cup and a tablespoon that takes exactly 16 level fillings to fill that cup level. Measuring by cup makes it very difficult to give weight equivalents, as a cup of densely packed butter will weigh considerably more than a cup of flour. The easiest way therefore to deal with cup measurements in recipes is to take the amount by volume rather than by weight. Thus the equation reads:

1 cup = 240 ml = 8 fl. oz.   1/2 cup = 120 ml = 4 fl. oz.

It is possible to buy a set of American cup measures in major stores around the world.

In the States, butter is often measured in sticks. One stick is the equivalent of 8 tablespoons. One tablespoon of butter is therefore the equivalent to ½ ounce/15 grams.

SOLID MEASURES

U.S. and Imperial Measures		Metric Measures	
Ounces	Pounds	Grams	Kilos
1		28	
2		56	
3½		100	
4	¼	112	
5		140	
6		168	
8	½	225	
9		250	¼
12	¾	340	
16	1	450	
18		500	½
20	1¼	560	
24	1½	675	
27		750	¾
28	1¾	780	
32	2	900	
36	2¼	1000	1
40	2½	1100	
48	3	1350	
54		1500	1½
64	4	1800	
72	4½	2000	2
80	5	2250	2¼
90		2500	2½
100	6	2800	2¾

LIQUID MEASURES

Fluid Ounces	U.S.	Imperial	Milliliters
	1 teaspoon	1 teaspoon	5
¼	2 teaspoons	1 dessertspoon	10
½	1 tablespoon	1 tablespoon	14
1	2 tablespoons	2 tablespoons	28
2	¼ cup	4 tablespoons	56
4	½ cup		110
5		¼ pint or 1 gill	140
6	¾ cup		170
8	1 cup		225
9			250
10	1¼ cups	½ pint	280
12	1½ cups		340
15		¾ pint	420
16	2 cups		450
18	2¼ cups		500
20	2½ cups	1 pint	560
24	3 cups		675
25		1¼ pints	700
27	3½ cups		750
30	3¾ cups	1½ pints	840
32	4 cups or 1 quart		900
35		1¾ pints	980
36	4½ cups		1000
40	5 cups	2 pints or 1 quart	1120
48	6 cups		1350
50		2½ pints	1400
60	7½ cups	3 pints	1680
64	8 cups or 2 quarts		1800
72	9 cups		2000

OVEN TEMPERATURE EQUIVALENTS

Fahrenheit	Celsius	Gas Mark	Description
225	110	¼	Cool
250	130	½	
275	140	1	Very Slow
300	150	2	
325	170	3	Slow
350	180	4	Moderate
375	190	5	
400	200	6	Moderately Hot
425	220	7	Fairly Hot
450	230	8	Hot
475	240	9	Very Hot
500	250	10	Extremely Hot

EQUIVALENTS FOR INGREDIENTS

all-purpose flour—plain flour
arugula—rocket
confectioners' sugar—icing sugar
cornstarch—cornflour
eggplant—aubergine
granulated sugar—castor sugar
half and half—12% fat milk
lima beans—broad beans
scallion—spring onion
shortening—white fat
squash—courgettes or marrow
unbleached flour—strong, white flour
vanilla bean—vanilla pod
zest—rind
zucchini—courgettes